Food and Beverage Consumption and Health Series

FRUIT JUICES: PROPERTIES, CONSUMPTION AND NUTRITION

Food and Beverage Consumption and Health Series

Handbook of Green Tea and Health Research
Helen McKinley and Mark Jamieson (Editors)
2009. ISBN: 978-1-60741-045-4

Marketing Food to Children and Adolescents
Nicoletta A. Wilks
2009 ISBN: 978-1-60692-913-1

Food Labelling: The FDA's Role in the Selection of Healthy Foods
Ethan C. Lefevre (Editor)
2009. ISBN: 78-1-60692-898-1

Fish Consumption and Health
George P. Gagne and Richard H. Medrano (Editors)
2009 ISBN: 978-1-60741-151-2

Milk Consumption and Health
Ebbe Lange and Felix Vogel (Editors)
2009 ISBN: 978-1-60741-459-9

Red Wine and Health
Paul O'Byrne (Editor)
2009 ISBN: 978-1-60692-718-2

Fruit Juices: Properties, consumption and Nutrition
Pauline G. Scardina (Editor)
2009 ISBN: 978-1-60741-505-3

Food and Beverage Consumption and Health Series

Fruit Juices: Properties, Consumption and Nutrition

Pauline G. Scardina
Editor

Nova Biomedical Books
New York

For permission to use material from this book please contact us:
Telephone 631-231-7269; Fax 631-231-8175
Web Site: http://www.novapublishers.com

Library of Congress Cataloging-in-Publication Data

Fruit juices : properties, consumption, and nutrition / [edited by] Pauline G. Scardina.
p. ; cm.
Includes bibliographical references and index.
ISBN 978-1-60741-505-3 (hardcover : alk. paper)
1. Fruit juices. I. Scardina, Pauline G.
[DNLM: 1. Beverages. 2. Fruit. 3. Food Preservation. 4. Nutritive Value. 5. Phytotherapy--methods. WB 430 F944 2009]
QP144.F78F78 2009
613.2--dc22

2009021732

Published by Nova Science Publishers, Inc. ✝ New York

Contents

Preface

Juice is a liquid naturally contained in fruit or vegetable tissue. Juice is prepared by mechanically squeezing or macerating fresh fruits or vegetables without the application of heat or solvents. For example, orange juice is the liquid extract of the fruit of the orange tree. Common methods for preservation and processing of fruit juices include canning, pasteurization, freezing, evaporation and spray drying. Juices are often consumed for their health benefits. For example, orange juice is rich in vitamin C, while prune juice is associated with a digestive health benefit. Cranberry juice has long been known to help prevent or even treat bladder infections, and it is now known that a substance in cranberries prevents bacteria from binding to the bladder. Fruit juice consumption overall in Europe, Australia, New Zealand and the USA has increased in recent years, probably due to public perception of juices as a healthy natural source of nutrients and increased public interest in health issues. This new important book gathers the latest research from around the globe in this field.

Chapter 1 - The best and complete comprehensive compilation all of the available thermal conductivity data for liquid food products (fruit and vegetable juices, oils, milks) and biological fluids (blood, urine, plasma) at the present time are provided. The overview of the most important methods (parallel-plate, coaxial-cylinder, and transient hot-wire) for determining the thermal conductivity of liquid foods is provided. The theoretical bases of the methods (working equations used to calculate the thermal conductivity), experimental apparatus details, constructions of the thermal conductivity cells for each method, procedures of the measurements, and uncertainty of the each technique were described. The effect of temperature and concentration on the thermal conductivity of liquid foods were studied. Various empirical, semiemprical, and theoretical models (polynomials, power, exponential, logarithmic, and their various combinations, composition, and structural models) for the thermal conductivity of liquid foods were stringently tested with new accurate measurements on plum, pear, cherry-plum, raspberry, cherry, peach, apricot, and sweet-cherry juices at temperatures from 20 to 120 °C and at pressures from 0.1 to 0.3 MPa for the concentrations from 9.8 to 60 °Brix. The accuracy, applicability, and predictive capability of the various theoretical models were studied. A new model was developed to accurately represent the combined effect of temperature and concentration on the thermal conductivity of fruit juices. Models which represent the thermal conductivity of juice relative to pure water were considered.

Chapter 2 - Recently, functional foods present in natural resources, such as fruits, vegetables, oilseeds, and herbs, have received a great attention both by health professionals and the common population for improving overall well-being, as well as in the prevention of diseases. In fact, regular consumption of fruits and vegetables is associated with reduced risks of chronic diseases such as cancer, cardiovascular disease, stroke, Alzheimer's disease, cataract and age-related functional decline.

The recent scientific investigations on cactus reported high content of some chemical constituents, which can give added value to cactus products in terms of functionality. The cactus pear (*Opuntia ficus-indica*) appears to be an excellent candidate for the inclusion in food. According to several studies, the great number of potentially active nutrients and their multifunctional properties make cactus pear perfect candidates for the production of health-promoting food and food supplements. Traditionally, it's appreciated for its pharmacological properties by the Native Americans. However, recent studies on *Opuntia* have demonstrated cactus pear fruit and vegetative cladodes to be excellent candidates for the development of healthy food.

The objective of this chapter is to present a review in terms of cactus pear juice including its nutraceutical and functional properties.

Chapter 3 - Pulsed electric fields (PEF) is a nonthermal processing technology that could be used to pasteurize fluid foods avoiding the negative effects of heat. The application of PEF to preserve fruit juices has been extensively studied in the last years. Both microbiological safety and spoilage delay can be achieved when juices are treated with PEF. Furthermore, PEF treatments have also been shown to inactivate varying amounts of several deleterious enzymes. Because of the inactivation of microorganisms and enzymes with a minimal impact on quality and nutritional properties, it is suggested that PEF is a technology of choice to obtain safe and high-quality fruit juices with a shelf-life similar to the attained with mild heat pasteurization treatments. Moreover, the combination of PEF with other food preservation techniques is currently being studied in order to further extend the shelf-life of juices. Future efforts will be devoted to successfully implement PEF processing at an industrial scale as an alternative to traditional heat processing or even as a way of improving quality of the final product by reducing heat treatment intensities.

Chapter 4 - Orange juice (*Citrus sinensis* L.) is probably the best-known and most widely consumed fruit juice all over the world, particularly appreciated for its fresh flavor and considered of high beneficial value for its high content in vitamin C and natural antioxidants such as carotenoids. Concentrations of bioactive compounds in oranges may depend on the variety, but also on the harvesting date and storage time. The aim of this work, therefore, was to determine the physical and chemical characteristics (juice/weight relationship, pH, °Brix, vitamin C, vitamin A, and carotenoids) of different varieties of orange and establish a relationship that would allow discrimination of oranges in terms of variety, harvesting date, and storage time. Three varieties of orange (Navelina, Navel, and Navel-Lane) were harvested randomly and directly in the field during their harvesting period. The harvesting was done on 3 different dates: 0 days (initial harvesting), 14 days later, and 28 days after the initial harvesting. Each of the harvested samples was stored at 4 ± 2 °C. To study the effect of storage, 3 determinations were made at 3 different times: 0 (initial), 15, and 30 days. A study was made of the evolution of the juice/weight relationship, pH, °Brix, vitamin C, vitamin A, and carotenoid profile of the different varieties of orange during harvesting and storage. The values of the juice/weight relationship, pH, ºBrix, and vitamin C were in the ranges 46.30–57.81 mL/100 g, 3.31–4.01, 10.6–12.5, and 45.58–57.79 mg/100 mL, respectively, depending on the variety, harvesting date, and storage time. Fourteen carotenoids (including *cis* forms) were determined in the oranges analyzed, and the vitamin A (RAE) concentration obtained ranged between 2.93 and 29.44. A predictive model was obtained that could be used to differentiate the orange varieties analyzed. The model was verified with the results obtained for the Navel variety of orange harvested in the following season

Chapter 5 - Antimicrobial/antiviral activity by grape (*Vitis labrusca*) and cranberry (*Vaccinium macrocarpon*) species remains an area of interest among food scientists. The purpose of this study accordingly, was to investigate the effect of pure and store-purchased grape and cranberry drinks on the infectivity/inactivation of the reovirus, a mammalian enteric infectious agent. Infectivity titrations were performed by a cell culture based immunofluorescence focus assay. Polyacrylamide gel electrophoresis was used to determine the integrity of the viral dsRNA in cell-free suspensions. Cytotoxicity testing was performed in part, using an adenylate kinase – bioluminescence assay. Animal studies employed athymic mice. Treatment of cell cultures with concentrations of 2 to 16% pure or store purchased cranberry and grape juice drinks prior to virus inoculation reduced infectivity titers by approximately one order of magnitude. Neither juice affected a monolayer toxicity. The vitamin C supplement in store-purchased cranberry juice cocktail (CJC) drink displayed no adverse effect on viral titers. A synergistic effect between store-purchased grape (CGJ) and CJC drinks was not observed. A proanthocyanidin-enriched cranberry concentrate (PACran™) of <1% reduced virus infectivity titers by ca. 95%. Reovirus dsRNA was not detected in virus-juice cell-free suspensions. Clinical disease was not apparent in mice after oral administration of juice-reovirus suspensions. Mice treated with CJC-reovirus suspensions displayed normal colon histology. These data suggest that the viral inhibitory effects may be associated with a blockage of virus receptor sites, a direct inactivation of the infectious particles *per se*, or a combination of both. *In vivo* studies supported the *in vitro* antiviral activity by grape and cranberry juices.

Chapter 6 - The production of Chinese quince fruit is very few in the world, even in Japan. It is nevertheless a unique fruit, traditionally used in folk medicine. It cannot be eaten raw owing to strong astringency and large amounts of insoluble dietary fiber. Because of this fiber, it is difficult to extract juice from this fruit. However, it is rich in pectic substances, polyphenols, organic acids, and ascorbic acid. Juice extraction by applying sucrose osmotic pressure is time consuming but effective. Boiling is also a convenient and effective way of extracting the juice and bioactive constituents such as procyanidins and soluble pectins. Some phytochemicals have been identified as active ingredients responsible for the medicinal functions of the fruit or extract. Triterpenoid compounds and polyphenols are important phytochemicals with antibiotic, anti-inflammatory, anti-viral, and anti-ulcerative properties among others. However, many aspects remain to be studied, such as the change in functional compounds during processing, mechanisms of action of functional components, and verification of the effects of these components by clinical investigations.

Chapter 7 - Viscosity of four fruit (pomegranate, pear, tangerine and lemon) juices have been measured at temperatures from 292 to 403 K and at pressures from 0.1 to 10 MPa for the concentrations from 11 to 45 °Brix. The best and complete comprehensive compilations all of the available viscosity data for liquid foods at the present time are provided. The effect of temperature, pressure, and concentration on the viscosity fruit juices were studied. The measured values of the viscosity were used to calculate the temperature, $(\partial \ln \eta / \partial T)_x$, and concentration, $(\partial \ln \eta / \partial x)_T$, coefficients for the fruit juices. Various theoretical models (polynomials, power, exponential, logarithmic, and their various combinations) for the viscosity of fruit juices were stringently tested with new accurate measurements on pomegranate, pear, tangerine and lemon juices. The applicability, accuracy and predictive capability of the various models were studied. New models were developed to accurately represent the combined effect of temperature and concentration on the viscosity of the fruit juices. Models which represent the viscosity of fruit juices relative to pure water viscosity was considered. The empirical extension of the various theoretically based models for the viscosity of aqueous solutions to the fruit juices is considered. It was found that theoretically based models originally developed for the viscosity of aqueous system can be adopted with success for fruit juices. The average absolute deviation (AAD) between measured and calculated values from these models for the viscosity of fruit juices was within 0.8 % to 2 %.

The values of the Arrhenius equation parameters (flow activation energy, E_a, and η_0) were calculated for the measured viscosities of pomegranate, pear, tangerine, and lemon juices as a function of concentration. The new viscosity models for the fruit juices are recommended for the future scientific and engineering used.

Chapter 8 - Membrane based clarification and concentration of fruit juice has become a popular unit operation in modern fruit juice processing industries. The well known membrane modules used for this purpose are tubular and spiral wound modules. Therefore, design of these modules is of utmost industrial importance. The key parameter for design of membrane modules is mass transfer coefficient. Most of the fruit juices have non-Newtonian rheology, e.g., power law, ellis fluid, etc. Till today, the mass transfer coefficient for such systems used is approximated from the corresponding relations developed for Newtonian fluids. Hence, a detailed fluid flow modeling with non-Newtonian rheology is urgently warranted. In the present work, this aspect is attempted. The expressions of the mass transfer coefficients are derived from the first principles for laminar, non-Newtonian fluid flow in a porous conduit. The effects of the permeation are incorporated quantitatively in the mass transfer coefficient from a theoretical basis. The analysis is carried out for various non-Newtonian rheologies. Effects of the operating conditions, i.e., Reynolds number, permeate flux, etc. on mass transfer coefficient are also investigated. Two flow geometries are considered. Flow through a tube and that through a rectangular thin channel, which are useful for the design of the tubular and spiral wound cross flow membrane modules. The developed relations of mass transfer coefficients would be of tremendous help to the design engineers.

Chapter 9 - This chapter discusses the effect of externally applied d.c electric field during cross-flow ultrafiltration of synthetic juice (mixture of sucrose and pectin) and mosambi (Citrus Sinensis (L.) Osbeck) fruit juice using 50000 (MWCO) polyerthersulfon membrane. Pectin, completely rejected by the membrane, forms a gel type layer over the membrane surface. Under the application of an external d.c. electric field across the membrane, gel layer formation is restricted leading to an enhancement of permeate flux. During ultrafiltration of synthetic juice, application of d.c. electric field (800 V/m) increases the permeate flux to almost threefold compared to that with zero electric field. A theoretical model based on integral method assuming suitable concentration profile in the boundary layer is developed. The proposed model is used to predict the steady state permeate flux in gel-layer governed electric field assisted ultrafiltration. A gel polarization model is also proposed incorporating continuous as well as pulsed electric field and numerically solved to quantify the flux decline and growth of the gel layer thickness. The gel layer thickness is also measured with high-resolution video microscopy and successfully compared with results from the numerical solution of the model under various operating conditions. Predictions of the model are successfully compared with the experimental results under a wide range of operating conditions.

Application of d.c. electric field during ultrafiltration of mosambi juice has resulted in significant improvement of permeate flux. A steady state gel polarization model has been applied to evaluate the gel layer concentration, effective diffusivity and effective viscosity of the juice within the concentration boundary layer, by optimizing the experimental flux data. Application of pulsed electric field is found to be more beneficial in terms of energy consumption, and equally effective in terms of flux augmentation as compared to constant field.

In: Fruit Juices: Properties, Consumption and Nutrition
Editor: Pauline G. Scardina
ISBN: 978-1-60741-505-3

Chapter 1

Effect of Temperature, Pressure and Concentration on the Thermal Conductivity of Liquid Food Products (Fruit and Vegetable Juices, Oils, Milks) and Biological Fluids: Experimental and Modeling

A.I. Abdulagatov[b], *I.M. Abdulagatov*[b,*], *M.A. Magerramov*[a], *and N.D. Azizov*[c]

[a]Azerbaijan State Economic University, Az 1001 Baku, Istiglaliayt Str. 31, Azerbaijan
[b]Institute of Physics of the Dagestan Scientific Center of the Russian Academy of Sciences, 367003 Makhachkala, Shamilya Str. 39-A, Dagestan, Russia
[c]Azerbaijan State Oil Academy, Baku, 370601, Azerbaijan

Abstract

The best and complete comprehensive compilation all of the available thermal conductivity data for liquid food products (fruit and vegetable juices, oils, milks) and biological fluids (blood, urine, plasma) at the present time are provided. The overview of the most important methods (parallel-plate, coaxial-cylinder, and transient hot-wire) for determining the thermal conductivity of liquid foods is provided. The theoretical bases of the methods (working equations used to calculate the thermal conductivity), experimental apparatus details, constructions of the thermal conductivity cells for each method, procedures of the measurements, and uncertainty of the each technique were described. The effect of temperature and concentration on the thermal conductivity of liquid foods

* Correspondence should be addressed: Email: ilmutdin@boulder.nist.gov; Fax: (303) 497-5224; Tel: (303) 497-4027

were studied. Various empirical, semiemprical, and theoretical models (polynomials, power, exponential, logarithmic, and their various combinations, composition, and structural models) for the thermal conductivity of liquid foods were stringently tested with new accurate measurements on plum, pear, cherry-plum, raspberry, cherry, peach, apricot, and sweet-cherry juices at temperatures from 20 to 120 °C and at pressures from 0.1 to 0.3 MPa for the concentrations from 9.8 to 60 °Brix. The accuracy, applicability, and predictive capability of the various theoretical models were studied. A new model was developed to accurately represent the combined effect of temperature and concentration on the thermal conductivity of fruit juices. Models which represent the thermal conductivity of juice relative to pure water were considered.

Keywords: coaxial-cylinder (steady-state) method; fruit juices; parallel-plate method; thermal conductivity; transient hot-wire method; thermal conductivity model.

1. Introduction

Thermal conductivity is an important property of liquid food products in the prediction of heat – and mass-transfer coefficients and in the design of heat- and mass-transfer equipment for food industry. As well known, fruit juices sometimes stored in large containers for later processing or blending with concentrates from other varieties of juices to obtain the best characteristics. Also in caning technologies the cans are filled with liquid concentrate and then rapidly chilled. A value of thermal conductivity is prime necessity in all problems dealing with flow of heat. Consequently, the calculation of heating or cooling times of fruit concentrates requires that the value of thermal conductivity of this substance be known.

Thermal treatments such as pasteurization, concentration, drying, cooling and others are frequently used in food processing, transportation, and storage and cooking. Therefore, knowledge of the thermal conductivity of food is important not only for the process design but also for the prediction and control of various changes occurring in food during thermal processing. To understand and control those processes which used liquid foods, it is necessary to know their thermodynamic (density, vapor pressure, activity coefficient) and transport (viscosity, thermal conductivity, and diffusivity) properties. However, the lack of reliable data over wide temperature and concentration ranges makes it necessary to estimate the missing properties by empirical and semi-empirical methods. Therefore, new accurate experimental data for thermal conductivity of liquid foods in the wide temperature and concentration ranges are needed also to improve and extend the range of validity of available estimation and correlation methods which will be capable of reproducing the experimental thermal conductivity data and develop a new more reliable prediction technique.

Modeling, optimization and automation of food processes is difficult due to complexity of the raw materials and product involved, which affect thermophysical properties such as density, viscosity, heat capacity, and thermal conductivity. Thermophysical properties of liquid foods are varying with the chemical composition, physical structure, temperature, concentration, and pressure. The thermophysical properties of fruit juices exhibit substantial changes with temperature, pressure, and concentration during processing (storage, transport, marketing and consumption, chilled, change temperature, tank farm change concentration, evaporator change concentration, see for example, Moresi & Spinosi [1] and Crandall *et al.* [2]. For this reason the thermophysical properties should be studied as a function of temperature, pressure, and concentration. The thermal conductivity and other thermophysical properties of liquid foods are also depend on another factors such as composition and soluble solids content due to: fruit type, generic characteristics, variety, ripening, place in the plant, size, plant nutritive level, agricultural practices, weather. This could explain the published data discrepancy for the same liquid food.

Many fluid foods are subjected to high temperatures (above 90 °C) and high pressure (up to 350 MPa) during pasteurization and thermal processing [3-6]. Fruit juices are also present at high temperatures and high pressures in high pressure food processing technologies during pasteurization and thermal processing and other industrial operations. The preservation temperature is about 60 to 90 °C. Last 20 years the high-pressure technology (high-pressure treatment in food preservation) was expanded to food industry. High pressure presents unique advantages over conventional thermal treatments including, application at low temperature, which improves the retention of food quality. Almost all previous thermal conductivity measurements for liquid foods were performed at atmospheric pressure, although high pressure food processing technologies need the data at moderate (3-10 MPa) and high pressures (up to 350 MPa). Very few measurements of the thermal conductivity are available in the literatures at high temperatures. Little is known about the effect of temperature, pressure, concentration, and chemical composition on the thermal conductivity of liquid foods.

Because of the wide variation across liquid food products, it is impossible to obtain the reliable thermal conductivity data for all kinds of foods from the measured data. Predictive methods for the thermal conductivity of liquid foods are needed. There are a number of models for the prediction of the thermal conductivity which is based on empirical and theoretical studies. Unfortunately, the thermophysical properties of liquid food products cannot be accurately predicted theoretically, due to their complicated physical and chemical structure. Therefore, the thermal conductivity measurements of liquid foods are also research interest. The available theoretical models for liquid foods cannot describe complex real system as they met in practice. Better prediction models can be developed based on reliable experimental information on thermal conductivity data for liquid foods. The models are required reliable thermal conductivity measurements for validation. Thus, there is great practical and theoretical interest in the study of the effect of temperature, pressure, and concentration on thermal conductivity of liquid food products at equipment operating conditions.

Other thermophysical properties such as thermal diffusivity, a, or heat capacity, C_P, can be estimated from thermal conductivity, k, measurements, according to the definition, $a = k / \rho C_P$, where ρ is the density. Therefore, the accurate thermal conductivity data are need for the independent test of the consistence and accuracy of the different kind measurements (thermal diffusivity, heat capacity, and density). However published thermal conductivity data for liquid food products are very limited. Most reported thermal conductivity data of food products are concerned with solid materials. Thus, the main purpose of this Chapter is to provide the readers with a comprehensive review on the available experimental data sets on the thermal conductivity of liquid food products, critical analyses of the estimation, correlation, and prediction methods, to select more reliable data sets and to give some preliminary recommendations for scientific and applied used. Another objective of this work was to develop new correlation and prediction models for the thermal conductivity of liquid foods as a function of temperature and concentration. Tables of the original experimental thermal conductivity data for eight fruit juices at high temperatures (up to 120 °C) are given in the Appendix. These data were used to examine the existing correlation equations and prediction techniques for the thermal conductivity of liquid food products. All of available sources of data for the thermal conductivity of liquid food products in the wide temperature and concentration ranges has been collected and estimated their reliability. The summary table with a list of information on available data sets for the thermal conductivity of liquid food products including the information about the temperature and concentration ranges, the experimental method used and references on original experimental sources will be presented.

1.1. Materials descriptions

Experimental samples 15.1, 12.2, 18.5, 14.0, 14.3, 15.1, 9.8, and 14.8 °Brix of plum, cherry-plum, apricot, pear, sweet-cherry, cherry, raspberry, and peach juices, respectively, used in this study were obtained from fresh full-ripe fruits from a plant in Baku, Azerbaijan. The natural juices were obtained by squeezing the full-ripe fruits with a laboratory screw press, eliminating the suspended solids by filtering and clarifying. Concentrated juices with various soluble solids contents were obtained from the original concentrate using a rotary glass vacuum evaporator (SPT-200, Zeamil-Horyzont, Poland) at temperature below 60 °C. The evaporation chamber was rotated at a constant rotational speed in water bath at 40°C. The soluble solids content as °Brix was measured using a universal laboratory refractometer (RLU-1, Russia) at room temperature (20 °C). In order to adjust the concentration of the juice, the concentrated juice was diluted with distilled water. The samples were stored in glass vessel at 2-4 °C (8 hours) until used for the density measurements. Microelements (potassium, calcium, magnesium, and phosphates) were determined using an atomic absorption spectrophotometer (C-115-M1, Russia). The glucose and fructose contents were determined by the method of Bertrand. The total sugar was calculated by summation of individual sugars. The pH was measured using a digital pH-meter (Kent EIL 7020, UK) at 20 °C. Total acidity was determined by potentiometric titration with NaOH 0.1 N until pH 8, monitored with pH-meter. Physical and chemical characteristics of eight fruit (pear, plum, peach, cherry-plum, cherry, raspberry, apricot, and sweet-cherry) juices are given in Table 1.

Table 1. Physico-chemical characteristics of fruit juices

Pear juice		**Cherry-plum juice**	
Soluble solids	15.2 °Brix	Soluble solids	12.2 °Brix
Pectin	0.25 %	Pectin	-
Total sugar	8.70 %	Total sugar	3.6 %
Glucose	1.43 %	Glucose	1.8 %
Fructose	6.91 %	Fructose	0.8 %
Sucrose	0.36 %	Sucrose	1.0 %
Amino acid nitrogen	0.141 %	Amino acid nitrogen	-
Tannic acid	0.0171	Tannic acid	-
Cellulose	0.90	Cellulose	-
pH	4.15	pH	3.4
Potassium	48 mg l^{-1}	Potassium	58 mg
Calcium	12 mg l^{-1}	Calcium	3.9 mg
Magnesium	3 mg l^{-1}	Magnesium	-
Phosphate	13 mg l^{-1}	Phosphate	22 mg
Ash	0.3	Ash	-
Plum juice		**Peach juice**	
Soluble solids	15.1°Brix	Soluble solids	14.8°Brix
Total sugar	10.5 %	Total sugar	9.30 %
Sucrose	3.00 %	Glucose	4.10 %
Glucose	5.20 %	Fructose	3.00 %
Fructose	2.20 %	Sucrose	2.10 %
Acidity	0.98 %	Acidity	0.60 %
Potassium*	39.0 mg	Pectin	0.30 %
Calcium*	4.10 mg	Potassium*	35.0
Magnesium*	3.50 mg	Calcium*	8.50
Phosphates*	17.0 mg	Magnesium*	9.50
pH	3.50	Phosphates*	24.0
-		pH	3.90
Cherry juice		**Raspberry juice**	
Soluble solids	9.8 °Brix	Soluble solids	15.1°Brix
Total sugar	9.43 %	Total sugar	5.50 %
Sucrose	0.24 %	Sucrose	1.20 %
Glucose	5.48 %	Glucose	1.77 %
Fructose	3.71 %	Fructose	2.50 %
Pectin	0.08 %	Pectin	0.58 %
Acidity	1.30 %	Acidity	1.10 %
Potassium*	70.0 mg	Potassium*	88.0 mg
Calcium*	8.20 mg	Calcium*	8.00 mg
Magnesium*	7.50 mg	Magnesium*	24.0 mg
Phosphates*	23.0 mg	Phosphates*	38.0 mg
pH	3.1	pH	3.70
Apricot juice		**Sweet-cherry juice**	
Soluble solids	18.5 °Brix	Soluble solids	14.3 °Brix
Total suar	-	Total sugar	-
Sucrose	6.5 %	Sucrose	0.3 %

Table 1. (Continued)

Apricot juice		**Sweet-cherry juice**	
Glucose	2.4 %	Glucose	5.3 %
Fructose	1.5 %	Fructose	4.9 %
Pectin	-	Pectin	-
Acidity	-	Potassium*	85
Potassium*	105	Calcium*	31
Calcium*	15.9	Magnesium*	-
Magnesium*	8.8	Phosphates*	19
Phosphates*	26	pH	3.8
pH	3.5		

*mg in 100 g juice

2. Thermal Conductivity

Unlike equilibrium properties (density, heat capacity, enthalpy), the experimental determination of the thermal conductivity of liquid foods encounters some difficulties because of effects caused by deviation of a system from the thermodynamic equilibrium. The temperature gradient, for example, usually induces not only thermal conductivity but convection and radiation as well. To take account of this a special technique should be developed for measuring the thermal conductivity which would minimize the effects of convection and radiation. Various methods were employed to perform measurements of the thermal conductivity of liquid food products. Most available thermal conductivity data sets for liquid foods were derived with techniques parallel-plate, coaxial-cylinder, and transient hot-wire (see Table 2). In this section these methods employed to measure the thermal conductivity of liquid foods will discussed. In general, the uncertainty of all the available experimental thermal conductivity data derived with the first two methods should be within 1 % to 2 %. The data obtained with the transient hot-wire technique are expected to be of worse uncertainty. This section presents an overview of the most important methods for determining the thermal conductivity of liquid foods. The theoretical bases of the methods (working equations used to calculate thermal conductivity), experimental apparatus details, constructions of the thermal conductivity cells for each method, procedures of the measurements, and uncertainty of the each technique will be described.

The thermal conductivity of liquids measures its propensity to dissipate energy, when disturbed from equilibrium by the imposition of a temperature gradient. For isotropic fluids the thermal conductivity, k, is defined by Fourier's law

$$Q = -k\nabla T\,, \tag{1}$$

where Q is the instantaneous flux of heat, which is the response of the medium to the instantaneous temperature gradient. In liquid foods the main source of experimental uncertainty is convection. Thermal conductivity is one of the more difficult properties to measure due to convection (Wakeham et al. [7]) and the effect of heat losses. Choi and Okos

[8], Reidy and Rippen [9], Reidy [10], Tabil [11], Jowitt et al. [12], Saravacos and Maroulis [13], and Mohsenin [14] reported extensive review of the methods used for the measurements of thermal conductivity liquid foods.

Table 2. Summary of experimental thermal conductivity data for liquid foods

Liquid foods and biological fluids	**References**	**Concentration**	**Temp. (°C)**	**Method**
Orange	Telis-Romero et al. [74]	34-69 wt. %	0.5-62	CC
Orange	Morgan [132]	58.9 , 42 °Brix	-17.8 – 32	N/A
Orange	Keller [78]	20, 40, 60 °Brix	-11 – - 42	CC
Orange, mango	Xu *et al.* [75]	34 wt %, 12.6 wt %	31-53	CC
Orange, fructose solution, sucrose solution, grape, pineapple, peach, cream	Muramatsu *et al.* [129]	10-60 wt %	10-50	THF
Coffee	Telis-Romero *et al.* [80]	49-90 wt %	30-82	CC
Caja	Tadini *et al.* [70]	8.8-49.4 °Brix	0.4-77.1	CC
Pear	Dickerson [136]	-	20	N/A
Pear	Reidy [10]	15-61 °Brix	20-80	N/A
Tomato	Choi and Okos [139]	40-95.2 °Brix	30-150	TCP
Tomato	Maslikov and Medvedev [141]	30-76 °Brix	20-60	BC
Tomato	Filkova [140]	9.5 wt %	N/A	N/A
Apple, orange, grapefruit, grape, pear	Quashou [128]	up to 60 °Brix	20-80	N/A
Apple, cherry, grape, pear, raspberry, milk	Riedel [67]	89 mass %, 8.3-10.8-64°Brix	20-80	CC
Apple, orange	Frandas and Bicanic [130]	0-70.2 °Brix	0-70	PPE
Apple, orange	Ziegler and Rizvi [131]	3.92-64 °Brix	20	TCM
Apple	Constenla [133]	12-68.5 °Brix	20-80	TCP
Apple	Muramatsu *et al.* [134]	10-45 wt %	10-50	TPM
Apple	Kolarov and Gromov [135]			PP
Passion fruit	Gratão *et al.* [66]	50.6-90.2 wt % H_2O	0.4-68.8	CC
Cherry tomato	Sweat [157]			TCP
Peach, raspberry, cherry, plum	Magerramov *et al.* [76]	9.8 – 60 °Brix	20-120	CC
Pear, sweet-cherry, apricot, cherry-plum	Magerramov *et al.* [77]	12.2-50 °Brix	20-120	CC
Celery	Lau [143]	0-30 %	-9.1-0.0	CD
Grape	Voitko *et al.* [138]	20-60 °Brix	0-20	CC

Table 2. (Continued)

Guava	Shamsudin [142]	10-40 °Brix	30 – 80	TPA
Pink guava	Zainal [137]	9, 11 °Brix	65-80	ODM
Beet	Khelemskii and Zhadan [144,145]	8-25 wt %	24.7	BC
Yellow mombin	Assis *et al.* [72]	8.8-49.4 °Brix	0.4-77.1	CC
Lemon	Pedro *et al.* [71]	38.1-90 wt %	0.3-80.6	CC
Graviola, cupuaci, acai,	Moura [158]	8.4, 11.9, 11.5 °Brix	21	DR
Reconstituted milk, skim milk, whey	Muramatsu *et al.* [148]	10-40 wt %	10-50	TPM
Reconstituted milk	Reddy and Datta [150]	40-70 mass %	35-65	TCP
Whole and skim milks1 -3.7 concentration degree (fat 0.1-11.17 %)	Fernandez-Martin and Montes [69]	8.71-40.83 mass %	5-75	CC
Whole and skimmed milk	Minim *et al.* [68]	72-92 mass %	2-71	CC
Whole and skimmed milk	Kessler [146]	NA	0-100	N/A
Whole and skimmed milk	More and Prasad [223]	37 – 72.4 mass %	40-90	PP
Cow's milk, skimmed milk, egg white, egg yolk, cod liver oil	Spells [149]	N/A	31-38	GD
Condensed milk (10 mass % fat)	Leidenfrost [159]	0.3 -1.52 concentration degree	20-60	N/A
Skim and whole (2.5 %fat) milk	Konrad [147]	20-40 °Brix	20-60	N/A
Vegetable oil-water, olive oil	Nowrey [152]	9.3-100 wt %	23.9	PP
Olive oil	Woolf [79]			CC
Human and animal blood, urine, plasma, gastric juice, egg yolk,	Poppendiek [151]	N/A	23.9-37.8	PP
Liquid egg	Coimbra *et al.* [73]	51.8 – 88.2 mass %	0-38	CC

[*]CC-concentric-cylinder method (steady-state); PPE-photopyroelectric; THF-transient heat flow method; TCP-thermal conductivity probe; TPA-thermal properties analyzer; TPM-twin probe method; PP-parallel plate; BC-bicalorimeter; GD-glass disk; CD- derived from ρ, a, and C_P data; ODM-oven drying method; TCM –thermal comparator method; DR-derived from other experimental data.

2.1. Experimental techniques

Most of the conventional techniques of thermal conductivity measurements of liquids are based on the steady-state solution of Eq.(1), *i.e.* establishing a stationary temperature difference across a layer of liquid confined between two cylinders or parallel plates (Kestin and Wakeham [15]). In recent years, the transient hot-wire technique for the measurement of the thermal conductivity of liquids has also widely been employed [16-31].

In Table 2 all available experimental thermal conductivity data sources for liquid food product are presented. As one can see from this table, all data were derived by the concentric-cylinder (steady-state); parallel plate; transient heat flow; thermal conductivity probe; photopyroelectric; bicalorimeter; and twin probe methods. Majority reported thermal conductivity data for liquid food products were measured by using the concentric-cylinder (steady-state), parallel plate, and thermal conductivity probe techniques. In this section a brief analyses of these methods is presented. The theoretical bases of the methods, and the working equations employed is presented, together with a brief description of the experimental apparatus and the measurements procedure of each technique. For a more thorough discussion of the various techniques employed, the reader is referred to relevant literature [7,15,20,32,33].

2.1.1. Parallel-plate technique

This technique for the measurement of the thermal conductivity has been used for almost a century (Todd [34]), and it has in fact been considerably improved over the years [35-55].

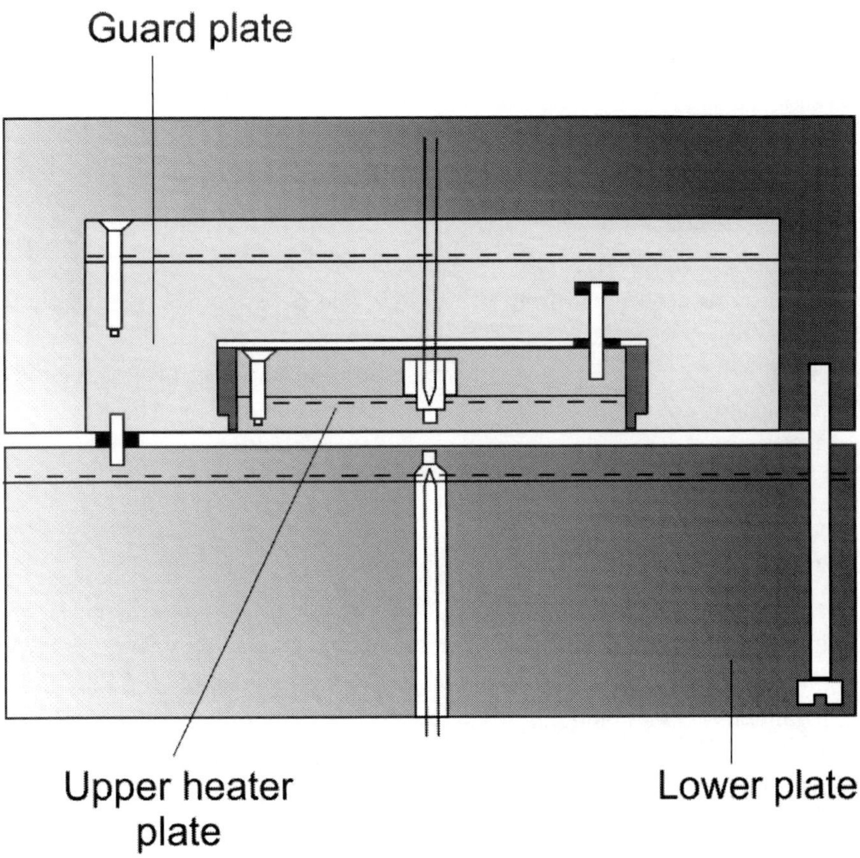

Fig. 1. Parallel-plate thermal conductivity cell by Michels *et al.* [52]

2.1.1.1. Theoretical

According to the parallel-plate technique, the fluid under investigation is confined between two horizontal plates, heated from above, so that the upper plate is at a higher temperature than the lower one (see Fig.1). Provided the two plates are maintained at constant uniform temperatures T_1 and T_2 respectively, the steady-state solution of Eq. (1) is

$$Q = k\,S\frac{(T_1 - T_2)}{d}, \tag{2}$$

where d is the thickness of the fluid layer, S is the area across which the heat flows, k is the thermal conductivity and Q represents the total amount of heat generated in the emitter. In this solution it is assumed that the thermal conductivity of the fluid is constant over the temperature difference applied, that the plate dimensions are infinite and that the heat flux is in one dimension.

In a real experiment, the measured heat flux Q_{exp} and temperature difference ΔT_{exp}, differ from the aforementioned Q and ΔT (= T_1-T_2), due to parasitic heat losses, Q_{p}, heat losses due to radiation, Q_{r}, and convective heat losses, Q_{c}. Thus

$$Q = Q_{\mathrm{exp}} - Q_{\mathrm{p}} - Q_{\mathrm{r}} - Q_{\mathrm{c}}\,. \tag{3}$$

The parasitic heat losses, Q_{p}, can be calculated (Moster *et al.* [35]) from

$$Q_{\mathrm{p}} = (c_1 + c_2 k)Q_{\mathrm{exp}} - (c_3 - c_4 k)Q_{\mathrm{s}}, \tag{4}$$

where c_i are constants determined from cell design, and Q_{s} is the heat relieved in the guard ring and plate.

The thermal conductivity cell design proposed by Moster *et al.* [47], is a good example of a cell constructed in order to minimize the effects of convection. The Rayleigh number, *Ra*, for the laminar convection is

$$Ra = Gr\,Pr = g\alpha\,\rho^2 C_{\mathrm{P}} \Delta T\,d^3 / k\eta\,, \tag{5}$$

where g is the gravitational acceleration, α is the thermal expansion coefficient of the fluid, ρ is the density, C_{p} the isobaric heat capacity, k the thermal conductivity, and η is the viscosity. For an infinite horizontal layer the critical value of the Rayleigh number, *Ra*, is 1708 [56].

If the parallel plates that bind the liquid layer deviate from the horizontal plane by angle φ then convection of the fluid can occur. The values of the convective heat loss, Q_{c}, can then be calculated from the de Groot theory [57,58] as

$$Q_{\mathrm{c}} < Ra\,l \sin\varphi\, \Delta T / 720\,. \tag{6}$$

This expression is valid at $d/l << 1$, where l denotes the diameter of the upper plate. It follows, from Eq. (5) and (6), that the convective heat loss, Q_c, is proportional to ΔT^2. Therefore, any deviation from the linearity of Q_c vs. ΔT, can be regarded as an indication of the presence of convection. In practice, the presence of convection can be checked by measuring the thermal conductivity at various temperature differences ΔT. The presence of convection will show as a dependence of the thermal conductivity on this temperature difference. The effects of convection can be made negligibly small by ensuring horizontality and employing a small distance d. The uncertainty in thermal conductivity measurement due to convection in a layer between two parallel plates is given by [52]

$$\delta k = \beta \frac{d\, Ra \sin\varphi}{180\pi D}, \tag{7}$$

where D is the diameter of the hot plate, and β is the constant (<1).

A correction for the temperature difference can be expressed as

$$\Delta T = \Delta T_{\mathrm{exp}} - \Delta T_{\mathrm{s}} - \Delta T_{\mathrm{a}}, \tag{8}$$

where ΔT_{s} is a correction connected with the temperature nonuniformity in the plates, and ΔT_{a} is the correction for the temperature drop at the surfaces of both upper and lower plates (the accommodation effect). The values of these corrections can be estimated as [35]

$$\Delta T_{\mathrm{s}} = C_{\mathrm{g}} k \, \Delta T_{\mathrm{exp}}, \tag{9}$$

$$\Delta T_{\mathrm{a}} = 2\left(\frac{2-0.83\alpha}{\alpha}\right)\sqrt{\frac{2\pi\kappa T}{m}}\frac{k}{C_{\mathrm{P}}+C_{\mathrm{V}}}\frac{\Delta T_{\mathrm{exp}}}{Pd}, \tag{10}$$

where C_{g} is a constant, α is the accommodation coefficient, P is the fluid's pressure, and C_{V} is the isochoric heat capacity. It is apparent from Eq. (10) that $\Delta T_{\mathrm{a}} \approx P^{-1}$, and therefore, the accommodation correction is important at low pressures only. The values of α depends on the nonideal behavior of thermal exchange between the plate surface and the fluid under study. For a detailed discussion of the parallel-plate technique, the reader is referred to the review by Sirota [59].

2.1.1.2. Experimental

In order to perform accurate measurements of the thermal conductivity of liquids under high pressures (up to 100 MPa) and high temperatures (up to 650 K), a parallel-plate apparatus was developed by Amirkkhanov and Adamov [36] and Amirkhanov *et al.* [37]. This instrument was further improved by Abdulagatov and Magomedov [38-49]. The thermal conductivity measurement system consists of a thermal-conductivity cell, a high-pressure vessel, a liquid thermostat, dead-weight pressure gauge, a water-to-oil separator, containers for degassed water and solution, and backing pump. A schematic diagram of the experimental cell construction developed by Abdulagatov and Magomedov [38-49] for high temperature and high pressure thermal conductivity measurements is schematically shown in Fig. 2. The thermal-conductivity cell consists of three plates: guard plate-1, upper (hot) plate-2, and lower plate-5. The guard plate is surrounded by a guard heater-4. The thermal-conductivity cell has a cylindrical form with a 21 mm height and 90 mm diameter. The thickness d of the gap between the upper and lower plates is fixed by supports-10. The upper plate has a diameter of 68.05 mm. The lower plate has a thickness of 9 mm. The cell is made from stainless-steel. The fluid surrounds the cell and fills the gap between upper and lower plates. The gap between the guard and the upper plates is 1 mm and filled with glass fiber. Differential thermocouples-6 are used for the measurement of the temperature difference ΔT between the upper and lower plates. The temperature of the upper and the lower plates is measured with a chrome l – cope l thermocouple-9 with a precision of 0.02 K. The cell described above was used in conjunction with an automatic Wheatstone bridge-19. The thermal-conductivity cell is mounted inside a high-pressure vessel which is placed in the liquid thermostat.

2.1.1.3. Working equation and uncertainty

The thermal conductivity k of the fluid was calculated from Eq. (2), employing measurements of the heat Q transmitted across the solution layer, the temperature difference ΔT between the upper and lower plates, the thickness of the solution layer d and the effective area of the upper plate S. The dimensions S and d of the thermal-conductivity cell entered in the working equation need some corrections in order to account for the effect of their changes due to the applied temperature and pressure. The cell constant (d/S) has also to be corrected for thermal expansion and compression. The effect of pressure is negligibly small in the pressure range of the experiments (up to 100 MPa) since the entire cell was under pressure. The uncertainty of the cell constant determination was 0.3 %. The uncertainty of the power Q_{exp} (amount of electrical energy released by the heater) measurements, was less than 0.08 %. The uncertainty in the temperature difference ΔT_{exp} was less than 0.14 %. The correction for parasitic heat flow was of the order of 0.003 %. Taking into account the uncertainties of temperature, pressure, and concentration measurements, the total experimental uncertainty in the thermal conductivity is estimated to be less than 1.6 %.

At low temperatures T = 313 K the values of Q_r at ΔT = 0.5 K is 0.0617 W which is considerably less than values of heat Q = 7.5121 W, transmitted across the fluid layer. To reduce the values of Ra, a small gap distance d = 301.0±0.1 μm was employed by Abdulagatov and Magomedov [38-49], while the temperature difference ΔT employed in the measurements was 1 K. In this way, it is possible to minimize the risk of convection.

Another version of the parallel-plate apparatus was developed by Yusufova *et al.* [60,61], Pepinov and Guseynov [62-65]. The parallel-plate thermal conductivity cell employed these authors is schematically shown in Fig. 3. The construction of the cell is the same with that employed by Sirota *et al.* [50] and Sirota [59]. The thermal conductivity cell consisted of (see Fig. 3) a hot-2 and cold-17 plate made from stainless steel; guard plate-5 made from cooper; guard ring-21; guard heaters-6 and 7; main heater-1; thermocouples-15 and 16. The hot and cold plates are connected with a metallic ring-19. The working surface of the plates was machined flat within 0.2 mm and polished. The gap between the plates was adjusted with three packing washers-11 (diameter 4 mm). The temperature gradient between plates was within 0.5 to 1.5 K. The temperature difference between main and guard heaters were between 0.00 and 0.03 K. The plate distance was 0.85 mm. The uncertainty of the thermal conductivity measurements with this instrument is 1.5 to 2.0 %.

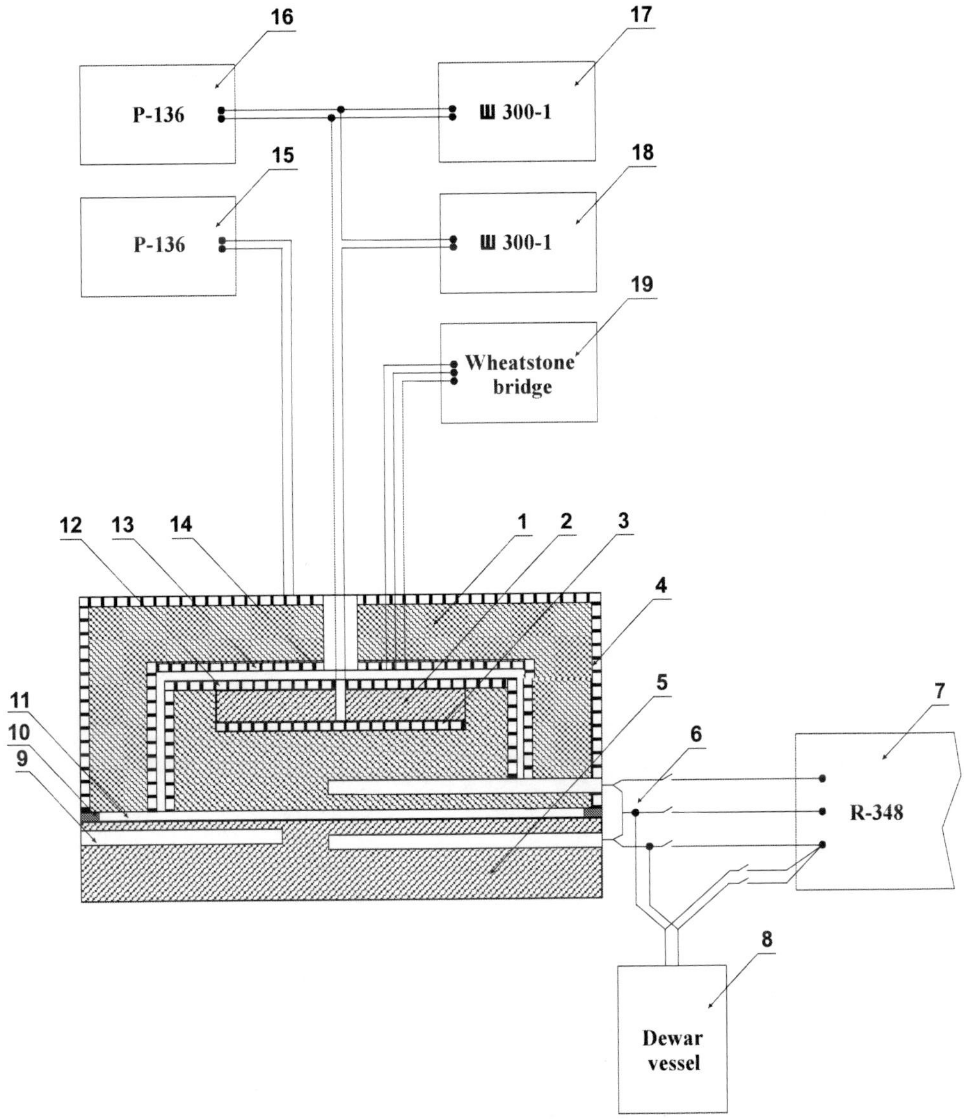

Fig. 2. Guarded parallel-plate thermal conductivity cell (Abdulagatov and Magomedov [38]) : 1-guard plate; 2-upper (hot) plate; 3-inner heater; 4-guard heater; 5- lower (cool) plate; 6- differential thermocouple; 7- direct current potentiometer (R-348, a rated uncertainty of 0.002 %); 8- Dewar vessel; 9-absolute thermocouple; 10- supports; 11- fluid layer; 12 and 14 - arms of the Wheatstone bridge; 13- glass-fiber layer; 15 and 16- stabilized sources of direct current (P-136, a rated uncertainty of 0.02%); 17 and 18- digital potentiometer (Ш 300-1, a rated uncertainty of 0.07 %); 19- Wheatstone bridge (a rated uncertainty of 0.001 K).

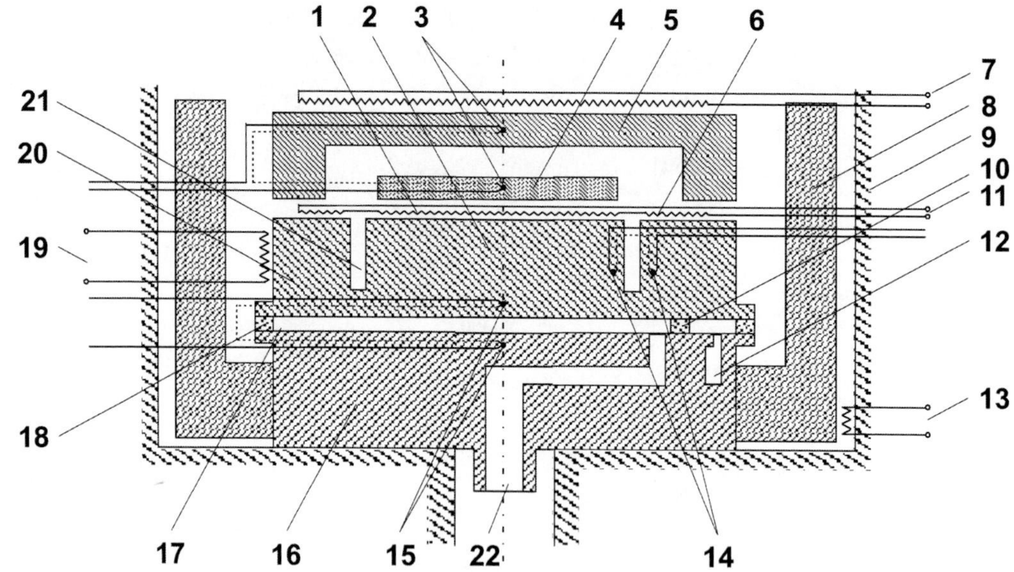

Fig. 3. Parallel-plate high temperature and high pressure thermal conductivity cell, developed by Yusufova *et al.* [60,61] and Pepinov and Guseynov [62,65]. 1-Main heater; 2- hot plate; 3-differential thermocouple; 4- plate; 5- guard plate; 6- and 7-guard heaters; 8-tumbler; 9-high pressure vessel; 10-spirali of the main and guard heaters; 11-washers; 12-contact with washer; 13-heater; 14-differential thermocouple; 15- and 16-thermocouples; 17-cold plate; 18-connecting piece; 19- jointing ring; 20-heater; 21-guard ring; 22-gap; 23-channel.

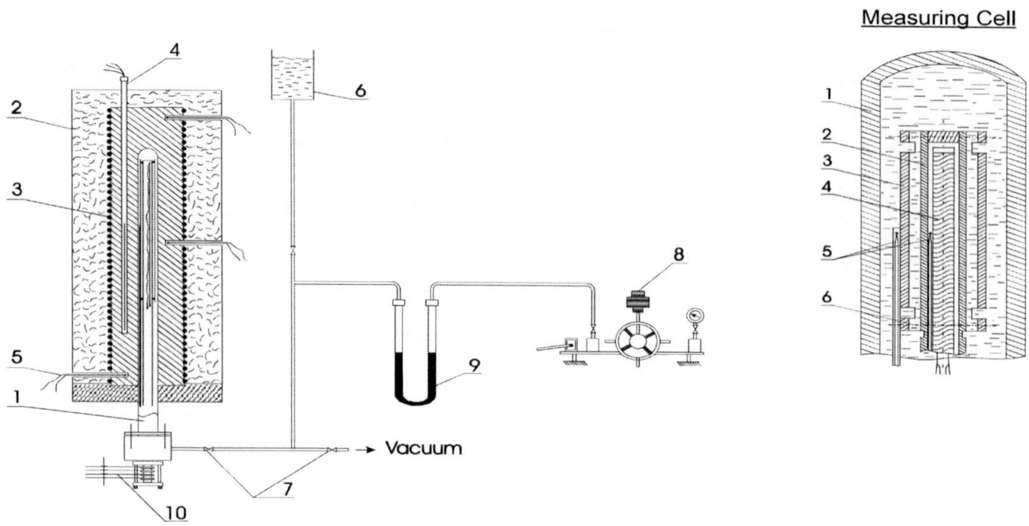

Fig. 4. Schematic diagram of the experimental apparatus and experimental cell for measuring the thermal conductivity of liquids at high temperatures and high pressures by the coaxial cylinders method (Abdulagatov *et al.* [91-93]). High-pressure autoclave-1; thermostat-2; heater-3; PRT-4; thermocouple-5; filling tank-6; set of valves-7; dead-weight pressure gauge (MP-600)-8; separating U-shape capillary tube-9; electrical feedthrough-10. Measuring cell: Autoclave-1; inner cylinder-2; outer-cylinder-3; microheater-4; thermocouples-5; axial alignment screws-6.

2.1.2. Coaxial-cylinder technique

The coaxial-cylinder technique was successfully employed for the measurement of the thermal conductivity of liquid food products by many authors [66-80], liquids, and aqueous solutions [82-86]. In Table 2, 15 out of 43 published data sets for fruit juices employed this technique. The coaxial-cylinder technique is a steady-state method which measures the heat exchange by conduction between two concentric cylindrical surfaces separated by a small gap filled with the fluid sample, each of these surfaces being maintained at constant temperature. This technique was successfully employed to measure the thermal conductivity of pure liquids and aqueous solutions. The method was considerably improved by Le Neindre *et al.* [87-89]. The thermal conductivity experimental cell developed by Le Neindre *et al.* [87-89] is schematically shown in Fig. 5.

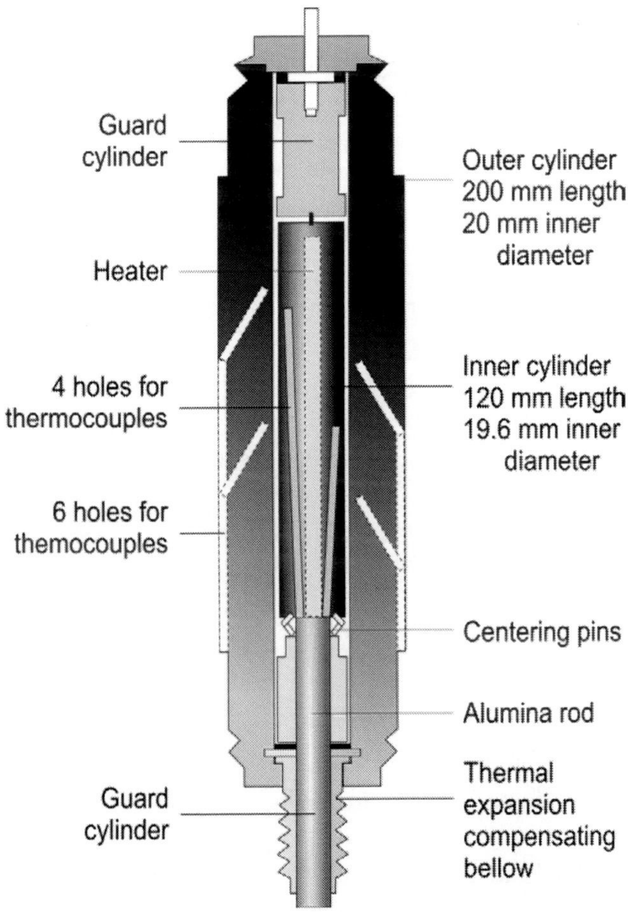

Fig. 5. Coaxial-cylinder cell developed by Le Neindre [87-89].

2.1.2.1. Theoretical

In this technique, the fluid is placed in a ring-shaped gap between two coaxial cylinders with a common vertical axis. According to the ideal model, a thin layer of a homogeneous fluid with a uniform thermal conductivity, k, is enclosed between two coaxial cylinders of length l. If a heat flux is uniformly generated in the inner cylinder and propagates radially through the fluid under study, to the outer cylinder in steady state conditions, the temperatures of the inner and outer cylinders will be T_1 and T_2 respectively. The thermal conductivity is determined as a function of these two temperatures and the amount of heat, Q, released by the inner cylinder, as

$$Q = \frac{2\pi l k}{\log(d_2 / d_1)}(T_1 - T_2). \tag{11}$$

In the above relation, d_1 is the external radius of the inner cylinder; and d_2 is the internal radius of the external cylinder. The ends of the cylinders can be made in different shapes: flat, conical or spherical.

When measuring the thermal conductivity with this technique, some corrections should be made for: 1. radiation-induced heat transfer (radiative correction); 2. parasitic heat transfer from the inner to the outer cylinder through a central solid pintle, electric wires, and thermocouples; 3. convective heat transfer; and 4. effects of possible temperature jumps at the interface between the liquid layer and the cylinder surface.

The correction for radiation is usually calculated by the Stefan-Boltzmann law

$$Q_r = 4\pi R^2 \sigma T_L^3 \left(\frac{1}{\varepsilon_U} - \frac{1}{\varepsilon_L} - 1 \right) \Delta T . \tag{12}$$

The radiation absorption in the liquid is negligibly small. Le Neindre *et al.* [89] employed silver cylinders with perfectly polished surfaces to reduce the heat transfer by radiation (see Fig. 5). The emissivity of these cylinders was small and Q_r estimated from Eq. (12) is negligible by comparison with the heat transfer by conduction.

The convective heat transfer, Q_c, can be calculated from the relation [90]

$$Q_c = Ra \frac{\pi d_1}{720} k \Delta T , \tag{13}$$

where Ra is the Rayleigh number defined in Eq. (5), d_1 is the radius of the inner cylinder; and ΔT is the temperature difference between the cylinders. In most experimental cells, the radius of the inner cylinder is about 0.01 m and the gap between cylinders is between 0.2 and 0.4 mm. The corrections for heat losses through the solid parts of the cell are determined by calibrating with measurements on standard fluids, for which the thermal conductivity is well known.

2.1.2.2. Experimental

The coaxial-cylinder apparatus and the thermal conductivity cell employed by Abdulagatov *et al.* [91,92] and Abdulagatov and Azizov [93], to measure the thermal conductivity of aqueous solutions at temperatures up to 591 K, is schematically shown in Fig. 4. The main part of the apparatus consisted of a high-pressure autoclave-1, thermostat-2, and thermal conductivity cell. The thermal conductivity cell consisted of two coaxial cylinders: inner (emitting) cylinder-2 and outer (receiving) cylinder-3. The cylinders were made from stainless steel and located in a high pressure autoclave. The deviation from concentricity was 0.002 cm or 2 % of the sample layer. The temperature in the thermostat was controlled with heater-3. The temperature differences between various sections (levels) of the copper block were within 0.02 K. The important dimensions of the thermal conductivity cell are: OD of the inner cylinder is $d_1 = (10.98 \pm 0.01)\times10^{-3}$ m. ID of the outer cylinder is $d_2 = (12.92 \pm 0.02)\times10^{-3}$ m. The length of the measuring section of the inner cylinder (emitter) is $l = (150 \pm 0.1)\times10^{-3}$ m. The gap between cylinders (thickness of the liquid gap) was $d = (0.97 \pm 0.03)\times10^{-3}$ m. The choice of this gap represents a compromise between decreasing convection and accommodation effect. The acceptable value for the thickness of the liquid layer d is between 0.5 and 1 mm. The optimal value ratio of the length l to the diameter of the inner cylinder d_1 should be $l/d_1 = 10$ to 15.

In the cell, the heat was generated in the micro-heater-4 which consists of an isolated constantan wire of 0.1 mm diameter. A micro-heater was mounted inside the inner cylinder (emitter) which was closely wound around a surface of a 2 mm diameter ceramic tube and isolated with high temperature lacquer.

To reduce the values of the Rayleigh number, Ra, a small gap distance between cylinders $d = (0.97 \pm 0.03)\times10^{-3}$ m was used. This way the risk of convection was minimized. Convection could develop when the Ra exceeds a certain critical value Ra_c, which for vertical coaxial cylinders is about 1000 (Gershuni [94]). The absence of convection can be verified experimentally by measuring the thermal conductivity with different temperature differences ΔT across the measuring gap and different power Q transferred from inner to outer cylinder. Since heat transfer by radiation is proportional to $4T^3\Delta T$, we would expect radiation losses to substantially increase as a function of the cell temperature. This kind of correction is included in the calibration procedure. The emissivity of the walls was small and Q_{rad}, estimated by Eq. (7) is negligible ($\approx$ 0.164 W) by comparison with the heat transfer (13.06 W) by conduction in the temperature range up to 600 K. This thermal conductivity apparatus was used to measure the thermal conductivity of fruit (peach, raspberry, cherry, plum, pear, sweet-cherry, apricot, and cherry-plum) juices (Magerramov *et al.* [76,77]). The results are presented in Appendix.

2.1.2.3. Working equation and uncertainty

The thermal conductivity of the sample at a given temperature and pressure for this method is calculated from Eq. (11), as

$$k = \frac{Q \log(d_2 / d_1)}{2\pi l \Delta T}, \qquad (14)$$

where $Q = Q_{meas} - Q_{los}$ is the amount of heat transferred by conduction alone across the sample layer between the cylinders. Q_{meas} is the amount of heat released by the calorimetric micro-heater, while Q_{los} is the amount of heat losses through the ends of the measuring cell (end effect). Equivalently, $\Delta T = \Delta T_{meas} - \Delta T_{corr}$. The values of Q and ΔT are measured indirectly and some corrections are necessary. As however it is difficult to estimate the values of the Q_{los} and ΔT_{corr} by calculation, they are estimated by measuring the thermal conductivity of standard liquids, such as water, whose thermal conductivity is very well known (IAPWS standard, Kestin *et al.* [95]). Typically, the amount of heat flow Q and the temperature difference ΔT were found to be 13.06 W and 3.5 K, respectively, while the estimated value of Q_{los} is about 0.05 W, which is negligible (0.38 %). Taking into account all corrections, the final working equation for the thermal conductivity for this instrument can be rewritten as

$$k = A\frac{Q_{meas} - Q_{los}}{\Delta T_{meas} - \Delta T_{corr}}, \qquad (15)$$

where $A = \ln(d_2 / d_1)/2\pi l$ is the cell constant which can be determined either from its geometrical characteristics, or by means of a calibration technique using thermal conductivity data for a reference fluid (pure water, IAPWS, Kestin *et al.* [95]). The values of the cell constant determined in these two ways are 0.1727 m^{-1} and 0.1752 m^{-1}, respectively.

After a careful analysis of the uncertainties all of the quantities (Abdulagatov *et al.* [91]) entering Eq. (15), it is estimated that the combined relative uncertainty in the thermal conductivity measurements was 2 %.

Another version of this technique was developed by Eldarov *et al.* [96-103] and Abdullaev *et al.* [104-113]. Three versions of a coaxial cylinder instrument were employed by Eldarov *et al.* [96-103] to measure the thermal conductivity of aqueous solutions. In the first version, the instrument was composed of a 150 mm-stainless steel-inner cylinder and a 120 mm-length copper-outer cylinder with a 0.5 mm gap between cylinders. In the second version of the cell, the heater was inserted into melted tin in the inner cylinder. This arrangement reduced the heat loss generated in the inner cylinder and resulted in the accurate measurement of the temperature difference between the cylinders due to the excellent thermal contact between the heater and inner cylinder. Cylinders were made out of stainless steel, the length of the measuring part of the cylinder was 120 mm, and the gap between cylinders was 0.4 mm. In the third version the inner cylinder was filled with melted silver solder up to 125 mm from the bottom. The length and gap between the cylinders were 150 mm and 0.35 mm, respectively. All three versions of the measuring thermal conductivity cells were used to check how measured values of k depends on the ratio $\Delta T / \delta$, where δ is the distance between the cylinders. The apparatus and design of the coaxial-cylinder cell used by Eldarov *et al.* [96-103] is shown in Fig. 6. Outer diameter of the internal cylinder was 8.301±0.001 mm, and the inner diameter of the outer cylinder was 9.602±0.001 mm. The length of the measuring part of the cell was 215 mm. The total uncertainty in thermal conductivity measurement in this instrument is estimated to be 1.33 to 2.2 %.

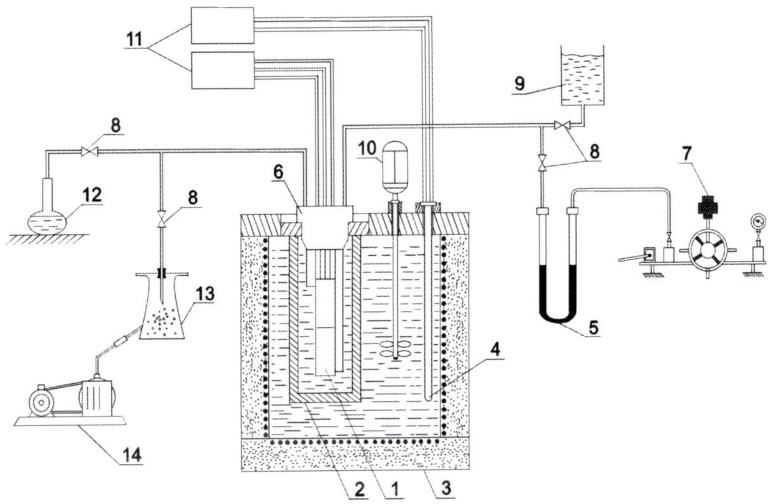

(a)

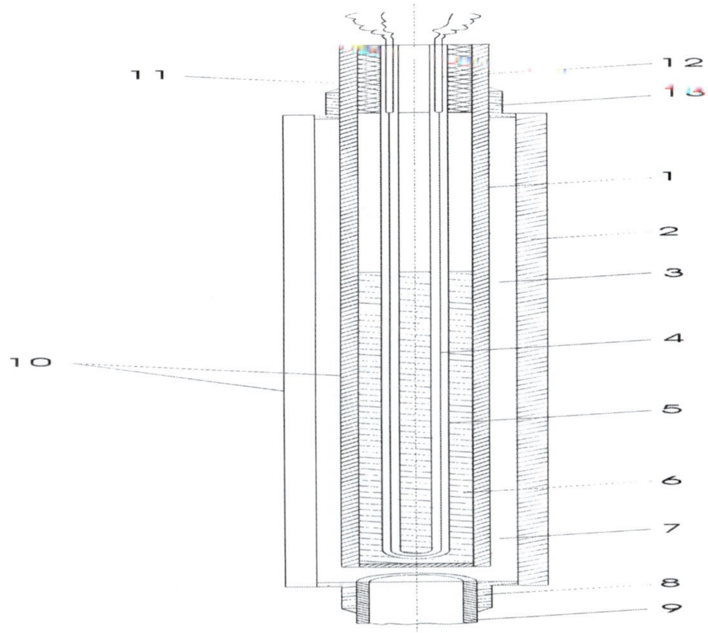

(b)

Fig. 6. Experimental apparatus (a) and experimental cell (b) for the high temperature and high pressure thermal conductivity measurements, developed by Eldarov [96-103]. (a): 1-Thermal conductivity cell; 2-autoclave; 3-liquid thermostat; 4-PRT; 5-U-shaped separated vessel; 6-lid; 7- hydraulic press; 8-high pressure valves; 9-sample; 10-mixer; 12-indicating tank; 13-separated flask; 14-vacuum pump. (b): 1-Inner cylinder; 2- outer cylinder; 3-annular gap between the cylinders; 4-heater; 5-U-shaped quartz tube; 6-melted tin; 7-sprocket; 8-thin wall bushing; 9-filling tube; 10-differential thermocouples; 11-asbestos plug; 12-copper wires; 13- bushing.

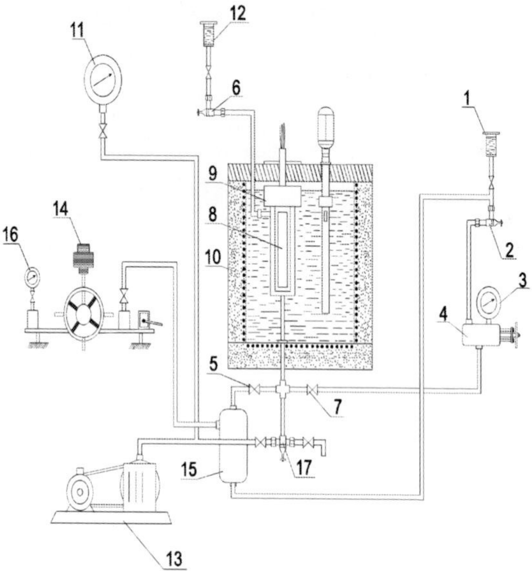

(a)

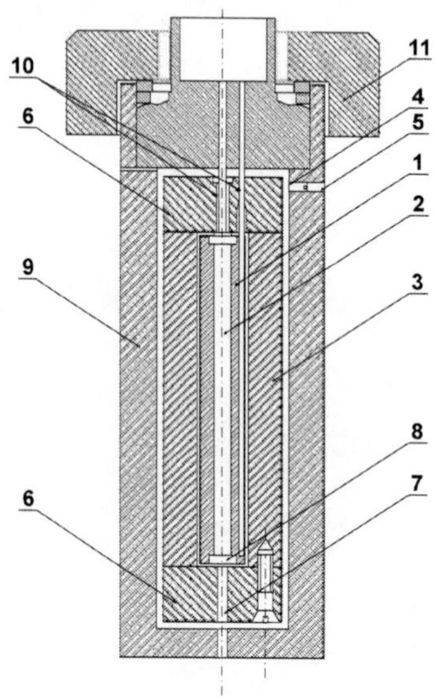

(b)

Fig. 7. Experimental apparatus (a) and experimental cell (b) for the thermal conductivity measurements of aqueous solutions at high temperatures, developed by Safronov *et al.* [114] and Grigor'ev [115,116]. (a): 1-Glass vessel with sample; 2-valve; 3-manometer; 4- hydraulic press; 5-, 6-, 7-valves; 8-thermal conductivity cell; 9-high pressure autoclave; 10-liquid thermostat; 11-vacuum-gauge; 12-glass vessel with sample; 13-vacuum pump; 14- dead-weight pressure gauge (manometer MP-2500); 15-separating vessel; 16-manometer. (b): 1-Inner cylinder; 2-heater; 3-outer cylinder; 4-centering body; 5-screws; 6-flat covers; 7-filling hole; 8-textolite standoff insulator; 9-autoclave; 10-scrolls; 11-jointing ring.

A schematic diagram of the thermal conductivity instrument employed by Safronov *et al.* [114] and Grigor'ev [115,116] is shown in Fig. 7. It consisted of a thermal conductivity cell-8 which was immersed in a high-pressure autoclave-9, a liquid (spindle oil) thermostat (0.09

m^3) -10, the system for create and measure pressure (hydrostatic press-4 and manometer-14, MP-2500), and four (3-main and 1 regulating) heaters and a thermo-regulator. The thermostat temperature was controlled with uncertainty of 0.02 °C. The thermal conductivity cell consisted of two coaxial chromium-plated cylinders (inner-1 and outer-3). The length of the inner cylinder was 199.890±0.001 mm and its diameter was 19.989 ±0.01 mm. The ID of the outer cylinder was 20.963±0.005 mm. The cell constant A was calculated using a geometrical constant of the cell as

$$A^{-1} = 2\pi\left[\frac{l + \Delta l}{\ln(d_2 / d_1)} + \frac{d_1 + \Delta d^2}{4\delta_T}\right], \tag{16}$$

where d_1 the diameter of the inner cylinder; d_2 the inner diameter of the outer cylinder; l is the length of the inner cylinder; Δl the changes of the cylinder length; Δd the changes of the cylinder diameter; δ_T the gap between end face of the inner cylinder and end covers. The value of A calculated by Eq. (16) was found to be equal to 0.0364166 m^{-1}. The value of A was also calculated by using the dielectical constants of vacuum (ε_v) and air (ε_a) and electrical capacity C of the gap between cylinders as

$$A^{-1} = \frac{\varepsilon_V \varepsilon_a}{C}. \tag{17}$$

The value of A calculated with Eq. (17) is 0.0362582 m^{-1}. The uncertainty in thermal conductivity measurements for this instrument is within 1.3 to 2.2 %.

Yata *et al.* [117-120] used a vertical coaxial-cylinder instrument with guard cylinders to measure the thermal conductivity of pure water and aqueous CH_3OH and $C_3H_4F_4O$ solutions at high temperatures. The details of the construction of the thermal conductivity cell are given by Yata *et al.* [117]. Schematic representation of the apparatus and thermal conductivity cell is given in Fig. 8. The gap between the inner and outer cylinders is 0.9 mm. Increasing the width of the gap results in an increase in the accuracy of the measurements, but at the same time, convection in the fluid layer is apt to occur. The geometrical dimensions of the cell are: OD of inner cylinder is 19.170±0.0015 mm; length of the inner cylinder is 120.000±0.002 mm; ID of the outer cylinder is 21.002±0.0015 mm; OD of the outer cylinder is 33.311±0.002 mm; and the length of the outer cylinder is 199.780±0.002 mm. In the cell heat is generated in the inner heater 5. The inner cylinder-1 and the guard cylinders -3 and -4 are separated by thin mica spacers-9, and connected by six alumina pieces-10. The inner cylinder is connected to the outer cylinder-2 by six alumina pins-12 and brass screws-11. At the top and bottom of the cell the alumina insulators -7 and -8 are fitted to the outer cylinder with a brass screw -13. Eleven sheathed copper–constantan thermocouples -6 are employed for the temperature measurements.

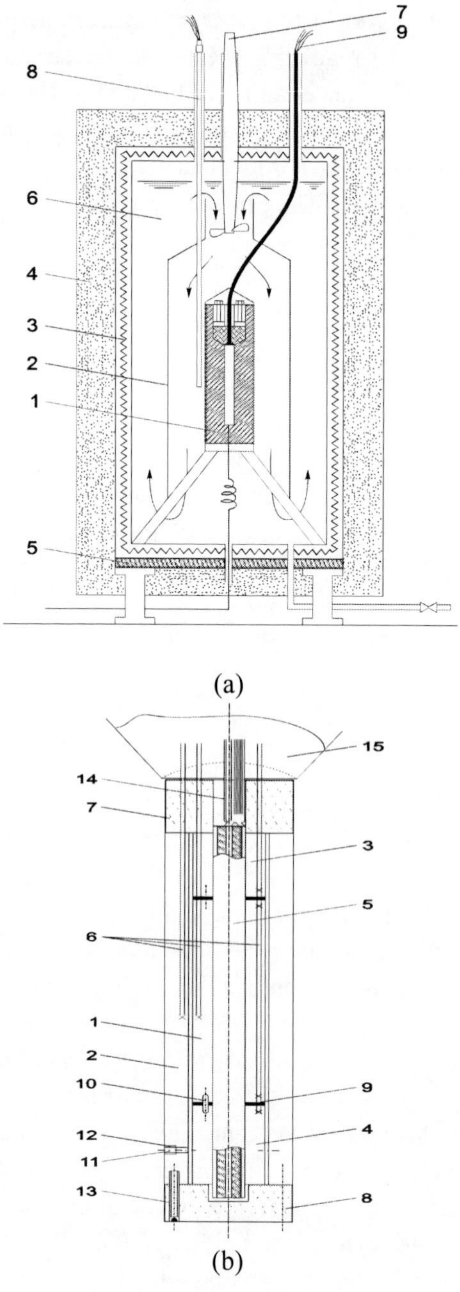

Fig. 8. Thermal conductivity apparatus and coaxial-cylinder cell, developed by Yata et al. [117-120]. (a): 1-High pressure vessel; 2-fluid separator; 3-heater; 4-heat insulator; 5-support table for bath; 6-heat transfer fluid (water or glycerin); 7-screw propeller; 8- standard resistance thermometer; 9-thermocouples and heaters. (b): 1-Inner cylinder; 2- outer cylinder; 3- upper guard cylinder; 4-lower guard cylinder; 5- inner heater; 6-thermocouples; 7- upper alumina insulator; 8-lower alumina insulator; 9-mica spacer; 10-alumina piece; 11-brass screw; 12-alumina pin; 13-brass screw; 14- compensative heater; 15-top closure of high pressure vessel.

After correcting for radiation and minimizing convective heat loss, the uncertainty in the heat transferred was about 0.2 %. Equivalently, the uncertainty in the experimental temperature rise was estimated to be less than 0.6 %. The uncertainty in the geometrical constant *A*, was estimated to be 1.1 % and thus the total uncertainty in thermal conductivity measurements was less than 2 %.

2.1.3. Transient hot-wire technique

2.1.3.1. Theoretical

A transient thermal conductivity measurement is one in which a time-dependent perturbation, in the form of a heat flux, is applied to a fluid initially at equilibrium. The thermal conductivity is obtained from an appropriate working equation relating the observed response of the temperature of the fluid to the perturbation. In an actual instrument the perturbing heat flux is applied by means of electrical dissipation in a thin, cylindrical wire as a step function. In this case the wire is itself used as the thermometer to monitor the temperature rise of the fluid at its interface. In such a case, it can easily be shown that for a cylindrical wire of radius r_o, and for small values of the term $(r^2/4at)$,

$$\Delta T(r_o,t) = \frac{q}{4\pi k}\left[\ln\left(\frac{4at}{r_o^2\gamma}\right)+\left(\frac{r_o^2}{4at}\right)+\ldots\right] \tag{18}$$

where $\Delta T(r_o, t)$ is the transient temperature rise of the fluid at the wire surface, k and a the thermal conductivity and thermal diffusivity of the fluid, respectively, q the heat input power per unit length, and $\gamma = 0.577216$ is the Euler-Mascheroni constant. In the ideal model, Eq. (18) describes the temperature rise of the wire in contact with the fluid at its surface. In practice a real instrument departs from the ideal model in a number of respects and analytical corrections have been developed (Healy *et al.* [121]; Assael *et al.* [16]) for the departure of a practical instrument from the ideal one. The two major additive corrections to Eq. (18) that need to be applied in practice are: a. the heat capacity correction, significant only at short experimental times, and b. the outer boundary correction, significant only at long experimental times.

The application of this methodology to liquids and gases at moderate pressures has provided many reliable thermal-conductivity data over the last two decades. Unfortunately, the analytical corrections proposed by Healy *et al.* [121] proved to be inadequate (Assael *et al.* [18]) for the description of experiments in the gas phase at low densities, where fluids exhibit exceedingly high thermal-diffusivity values.

To overcome these difficulties, a numerical finite element method was proposed by Assael *et al.* [18], in order to solve the complete set of energy-conservation equations that describe the heat-transfer experimental processes. The choice of this particular numerical method was dictated by the high accuracy the method exhibits in computational heat transfer problems. Hence, two coupled partial differential energy-conservation equations, one for the wire and one for the fluid, with appropriate boundary conditions, were solved.

In practice, experimental means are employed to yield a finite segment of a wire that behaves as if it were part of an infinite wire. This allows the numerical solution of the differential equations to be used iteratively to determine the thermal conductivity and diffusivity of the fluid that yields the best match between the experimental and calculated temperature rise of this finite segment of wire.

2.1.3.2. Experimental

Since the technique was first employed in 1931 (Stahlane and Pyk [122]) to measure the thermal conductivity of powders, there have been significant improvements in the practical realization of the technique. In modern instruments the wire sensor acts both as the heat source and as a thermometer. Rapid development of analogue and digital equipment as well as of computer-driven data-acquisition systems, have meant that precise measurements of transient electrical signals can be made quickly. Thus, it has become possible to measure the resistance change taking place in the hot wire as a consequence of its temperature rise with a precision better than 0.1%. Furthermore, instead of a single wire, two wires identical in all respects except for length are employed (see Figs. 9 and 10). This allows a practical and automatic means of compensating for the finite length of the wires. For electrically insulating fluids, platinum has usually been employed as the heating wire and sensing thermometer because of its chemical stability and resistance/temperature characteristics. In order to allow measurements of electrically conducting fluids, tantalum wires are often employed, because upon electrolytic oxidation, tantalum forms tantalum pentoxide on its surface, which is an electrical insulator. Together with a more systematic approach to the theory it has been possible to provide instruments with an uncertainty of 0.5 %.

2.1.3.3. Working equation and uncertainty

In the modern transient hot-wire instruments, operated for zero time to 5 s, with a resolution of 20 μs, the analytic working equation has been substituted by the FEM solution of the two coupled differential energy-conservation equations already discussed previously. As discussed above, in the modern instruments, composed of two-wires coupled to a fast bridge, the uncertainty attained is of the order of 0.5%.

A transient hot-wire instrument was employed by DiGuilio *et al.* [123,124], Bleazard *et al.* [125], and Bleazard and Teja [126] to measure the thermal conductivity of aqueous solutions at temperatures up to 493 K and up to the saturation pressure. The thermal conductivity cell constructed by Bleazard *et al.* [125] is schematically shown in Fig. 11. The thermal conductivity cell consisted of a fine pyrex (or borosilicate glass) capillary filled with liquid mercury (or gallium) to serve as the insulated hot-wire from the liquid. The hot-wire cell was made by forming a U shaped tube of Pyrex (2 mm ID by 4 mm OD). A tungsten wire, inserted into each end of the U tube, served as electrical leads. The other parts of the apparatus were a Wheatstone bridge, a data acquisition system, and a constant temperature bath. The mercury thread acted as the resistance in one arm of the Wheatstone bridge. Thermal conductivity measurements were made by placing the pyrex cell in a pressure vessel filled with the sample. The temperature rise was determined from the increased resistance of the wire. The uncertainty of the measurements estimated by the authors was 2 %. Since however, only a one-wire arrangement, contained within a glass, was employed, it is most unlikely that this is a reasonable estimate.

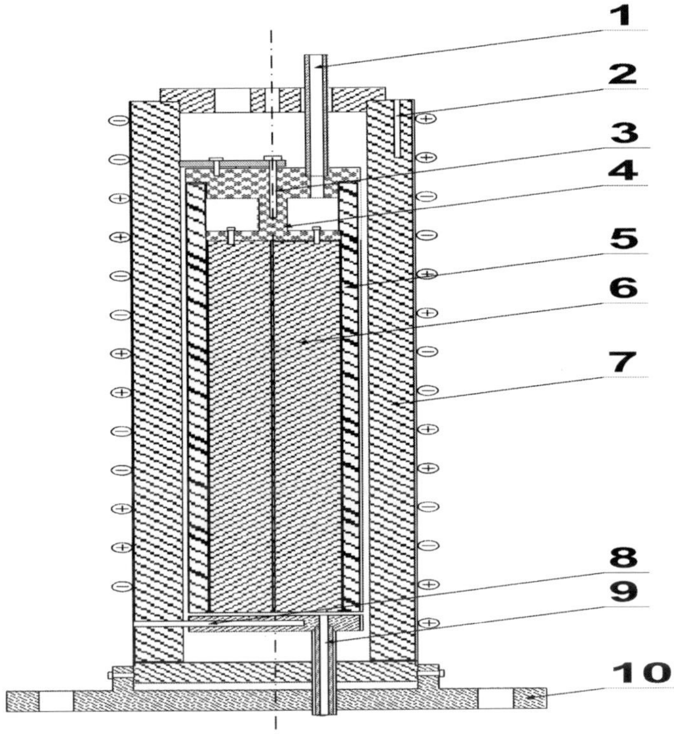

(a)

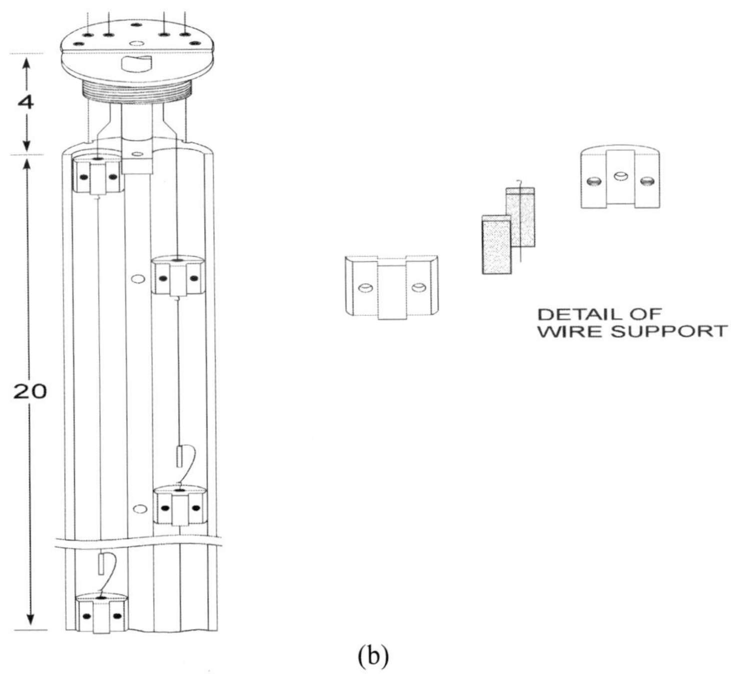

(b)

Fig. 9. The thermal conductivity vessel assembly (a) and hot-wire cell (b), developed by Assael *et al.* [17]. (a): 1- Liquid vent; 2- temperature controller thermocouple; 3- top thermometer; 4- cell top; 5- supporting vessel; 6-cell; 7-thermostat enclosure; 8-bottom thermometer; liquid inlet; 10-base stand.

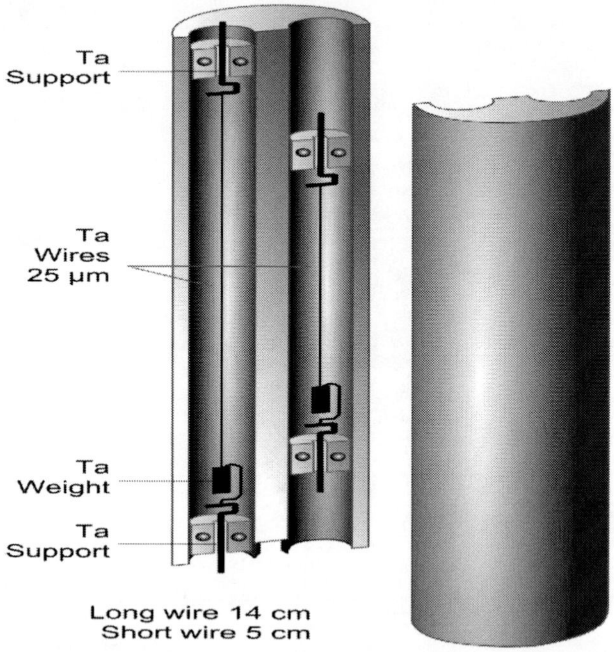

Fig. 10. Wires with weights arrangement, developed by Assael *et al.* [17,18] for the measurement of electrically conducting liquids.

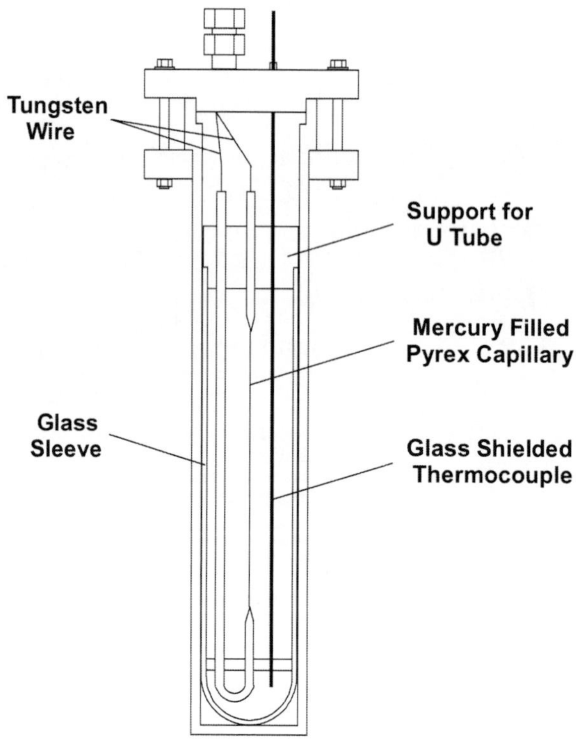

Fig. 11. Liquid metal hot-wire thermal conductivity cell and accompanying pressure vessel, developed by Bleazard *et al.* [125].

Nagasaka and Nagashima [23] developed the apparatus for precise and absolute measurements of the thermal conductivity of electrically conducting liquids using the transient hot-wire method. In this apparatus, a metallic wire coated with a thin electrical insulation layer has been used as a heating element and a resistance thermometer instead of a bare metallic wire. The effects on the thermal conductivity measurement caused by the thin insulation layer are negligibly small. The usability of the method for electrically conducting liquids has been tested to measure the thermal conductivity of aqueous NaCl solutions (Nagasaka and Nagashima [23]). The uncertainty of the measurement was estimated 0.5 %. Nagasaka *et al.* [24,25] and Kawamata *et al.* [127] used this technique for the measurement of the thermal conductivity of aqueous KCl and LiBr solutions at high temperatures (up to 473 K) and high pressures (up to 40 MPa). The schematic diagram of the high pressure vessel together with hot-wire cell developed by Kawamata *et al.* [127], Nagasaka and Nagashima [23], and Nagasaka *et al.* [24,25] is shown in Fig. 12. The main frame of the hot-wire cell consist of a titanium plate 5 mm in thickness -3 on which semicircular sintered alumina discks-10 are fastened on both sides. The hot-wire -9 is made up of a 25 μm-diameter tantalum wire (99.95 % purity) and a tantalum pentoxide (Ta_2O_5) insulation layer about 0.18 μm thick. Two hot wires differing only in their lengths (about 180 and 80 mm), are employed in order to compensate the end effects. Four electrical leads for each wire are brought out through terminals -5.

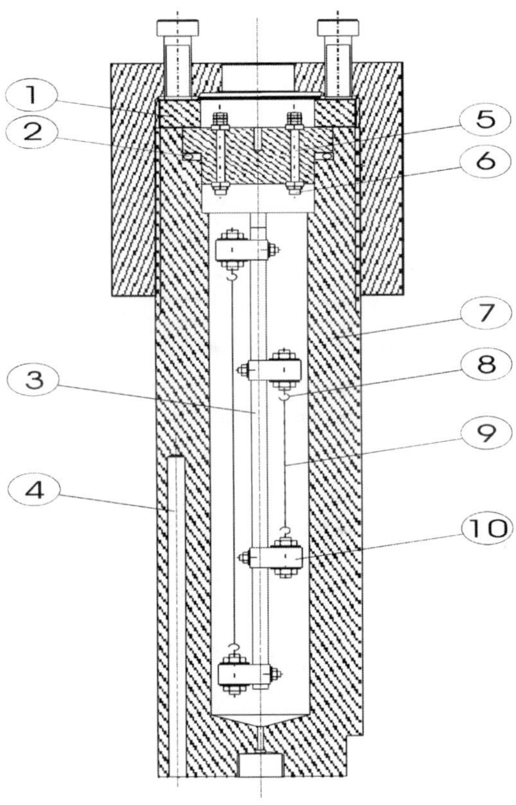

Fig. 12. Pressure vessel with hot-wire assembly, developed by Nagasaka and Nagashima [23] and Nagasaka *et al.* [24,25]. 1-Thrust ring; 2-PTFE ring; 3-titanium plate; 4-thermometer well; 5- terminal; 6-PTFE seal; 7- pressure vessel; 8-platinium hook; 9-tantalum wire; 10-alumina disc.

3. Experimental Thermal Conductivity Data for Liquid Food Products

This section aims to provide the readers with a review of the available experimental data sets on the thermal conductivity of liquid foods, to present a critical analysis of the estimation, correlation, and prediction methods, to select the most reliable models and to propose preliminary recommendations.

A survey of the literature reveals the scarcity of reliable experimental thermal conductivity data for liquid foods. The summary all of the available thermal conductivity data sets of liquid foods are given in Table 2. In this table, the authors and the method employed are given together with the temperature and concentration ranges. Table 2 provides, to our knowledge, the largest and the most useful collection (the best and most comprehensive compilation) all of the available thermal conductivity data for liquid foods at the present time.

Orange juice: Eight datasets were found [128,129,130,74,131,75,132,78] for orange juice. These thermal conductivity data were obtained by using the various (concentric cylinders, transient heat flow, thermal conductivity probe) techniques. The maximum temperature range of the measurements is 80 °C.

Apple juice: Seven datasets were found [128,133,67,134,130,131,135] for apple juice. Five different methods (concentric cylinders, parallel plate, twin probe method, thermal conductivity probe, and photopyroelectrc) were used to measure the thermal conductivity of apple juice. The maximum temperature range was 80 °C.

Pear juice: Fife datasets were found [128,136,10,67,77] for pear juice reported by different research groups. Most data were measured with concentric cylinder method in the range of temperature from 20 to 120 °C. The measurements by Magerramov *et al.* [40] were performed at pressures slightly above atmospheric pressures (about 0.3 MPa at temperatures above 100 °C).

Grape juice: Four datasets were reported for grape juice by the various authors [128,67,129,138]. Concentric cylinders and transient heat flow methods were employed to mesure thermal conductivity of grape juices. The measurements were made at temperatures from 20 to 80 °C and concentrations up to 64 °Brix.

Tomato juice: Three datasets were found [139,140,141] for tomato juice. The thermal conductivity probe and bicalorimeter techniques were employed to obtain these data. The measurements were carried out at maximum temperature of 150 °C and at concentrations up to 95.2 °Brix.

Raspberry juice: Only two datasets were found [67,76] for raspberry juice. Both data sources were obtained with the concentric cylinder technique in the temperature range from 20 to 120 °C and at concentrations up to 64 °Brix.

Cherry juice: Two datasets [67,76] were found for cherry juice. These data were measured with concentric cylinder methods. The maximum temperature was 120 °C.

Peach juice: Two datasets were found [76,129] peach juice.

Lemon, Plum, Mango, Apricot, Caja, Guava, Peanapple, Passion fruit, Grapefruit juices: Only one data source was found for these juices [66,70,71,76,77,128,129,142].

Vegetable (Celery, Beet) juices: One dataset was found for these juices [143-145].

Whole milk: Five datasets [68,69,146,147,223] were found for whole milk.
Skimmed milk: Three datasets [147-149] were found for skimmed milk.
Reconstituted milk: Two datasets [148,150] were found for reconstituted milk.
Egg yolk: Two datasets [149,151] were found for egg yolk.
Olive oil: Two datasets [79,152] were found for olive oil.

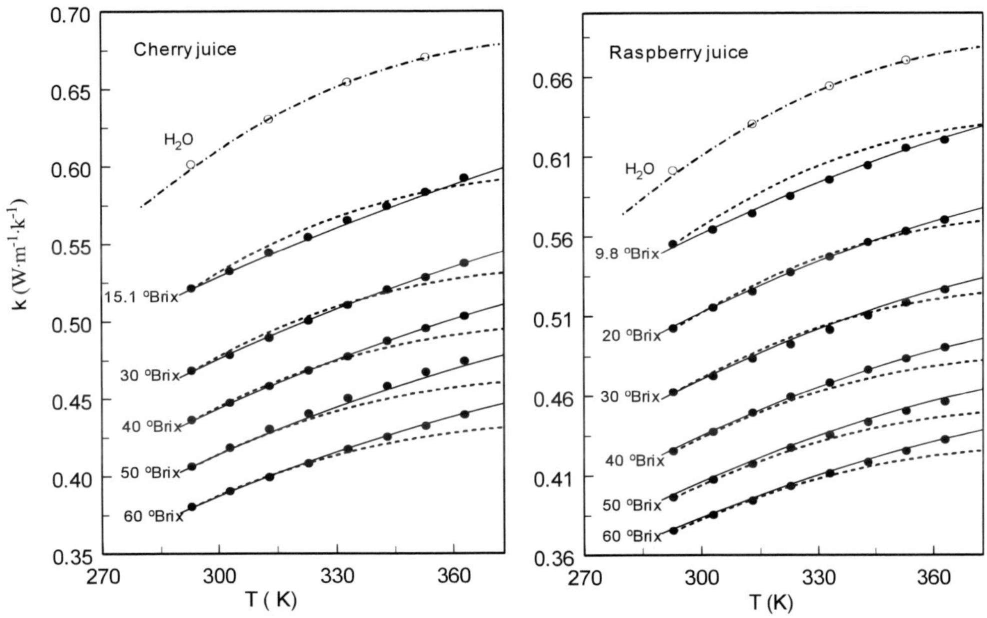

Fig. 13. Measured values of thermal conductivity *k* of cherry and raspberry juices as a function of temperature *T* along selected constant concentrations. (–· – · – · –), pure water (IAPWS, Kestin *et al.* [95]; (– – – –), Model-20; (——), Model-A.

Unfortunately the direct comparison different data sources for the same liquid food is difficult and some time no sense because thermal conductivity of liquid foods essentially depends on composition and soluble solids content due to fruit type, generic characteristics, variety, ripening, place in the plant, size, plant nutritive level, agricultural practices, weather. These factors are one of the reasons of the reported data discrepancy for the same liquid food (see below Figs. 17-23).

Some selected experimental thermal conductivity data for fruit juices as an example are shown in Figs. 13 to 16 in the $k-T$ and $k-x$ projections together with values for pure water calculated with IAPWS formulation (Kestin *et al.* [95]). These figures show the typical temperature and concentration dependency of thermal conductivity of fruit juices.

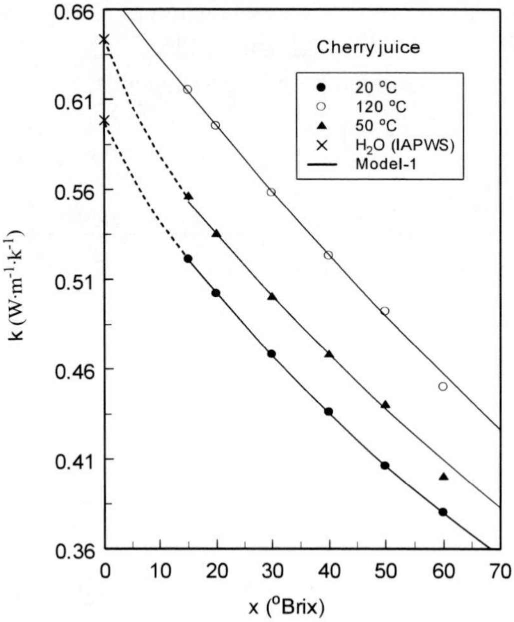

Fig. 14. Measured values of thermal conductivity k of cherry and raspberry juices as a function of concentration x along selected isotherms. (– – – –), extrapolation to zero concentration (pure water).

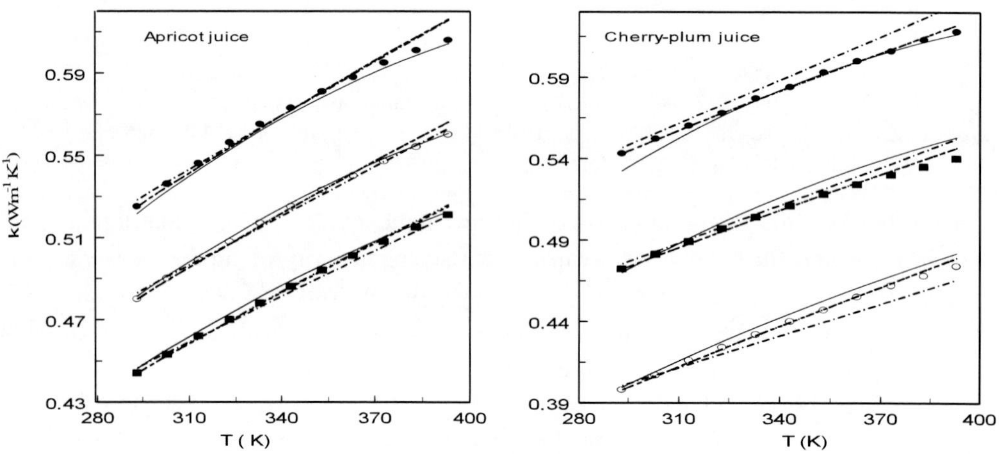

Fig. 15. Comparison measured and calculated with various models values of the thermal conductivity of juices. **Apricot juice**: •, 18.5 °Brix; ○, 30 °Brix; ■, 40 °Brix, **cherry-plum**: •, 12.2 °Brix; ■, 30 °Brix; Δ, 50 °Brix, (———), Model-A; (–· – · – · –), Model-B; (–··· –··· –··· –), Model-C; (– – – –), Model-D.

Previously the available experimental thermal conductivity data for liquid foods have been extensive reviewed by various authors [8,9,12-14,128,156]. Most existing thermal conductivity measurements for fruit juices are at moderate temperatures (up to 60-80 °C) and limited concentration range (up to 60 °Brix). Telis-Romero *et al.* [74] reported measured thermal conductivity data for orange juice for concentrations from (0.34 to 0.69) wt fractions of water content at temperatures from (0.5 to 62) °C. The measurements were made with concentric cylinder method. The measured values of the thermal conductivity were fitted as a linear function of temperature and water content. The authors found that the water content exhibited a greater influence on the thermal conductivity than temperature. Sweat and Haugh [157] used a probe method to measure the thermal conductivity of cherry tomato at room temperature. Constenla *et al.* [133] reported the thermal conductivity data for apple juice as a function of concentration and temperature in the range from (20 to 90) °C and at concentrations between (12 and 70) °Brix. The thermal conductivity data for tomato juice over wide temperature range from (30 to 150) °C and at concentrations between (40 and 95.2) mass % were reported by Choi and Okos [139]. The measurements were made by using line heat source probe technique. Recently, Gratão *et al.* [66] reported the thermal conductivity of passion juice. These measurements were made using the concentric-cylinder technique in the concentration range from (0.506 to 0.902) fraction of water content and at temperatures from (0.4 to 68.8) °C. The results were presented using a simple linear polynomial function of temperature and concentration. Reidy [10] reported a few data points for pear juice at two temperatures of (20 and 80) °C and at three concentrations 15, 40, and 61 °Brix. Riedel [67] also reported the thermal conductivity data for grape, apple, pear, cherry, and raspberry juices at temperature of (20 and 80) °C and at concentrations between 8.3 and 61 °Brix. Measurements have been made by using concentric-cylinder method. Muramatsu *et al.* [129,134] measured the thermal conductivity of several fruit juices (apple, grape, orange, pineapple, peach) and reconstituted and skim milks at temperatures from (10 to 50) °C and solid content between (10 and 60) wt %. The measurements were made with heat probe method. The method based on the transient heat flow technique using twin probes. This is relative method and can be provide high accuracy thermal conductivity measurements. The measured thermal conductivity data were represented as a function of temperature and total solid content. The observed values of the thermal conductivity were compared with the values predicted with structural models (series, parallel, and random). Coaxial cylinders technique was applied by Minim *et al.* [68] to accurate measure the thermal conductivity of liquid food (whole and skimmed milk, and partially skimmed milk) in the temperature range from (2 to 71) °C. The measured data were represented as function of water and fat content and temperature. Fernandez-Martin and Montes [69] employed coaxial cylinder technique for the measurements of thermal conductivity of skim and whole milks with fat content of 0.1-11.73 % and grade concentration within 1 to 3.7 at temperatures from (5 to 75) °C. The measured data were satisfactory fitted to a quadratic function of temperature. The authors found that the thermal conductivity increase with temperature increasing, but the rate of changes was decreasing with increase in either temperature or total solid content.

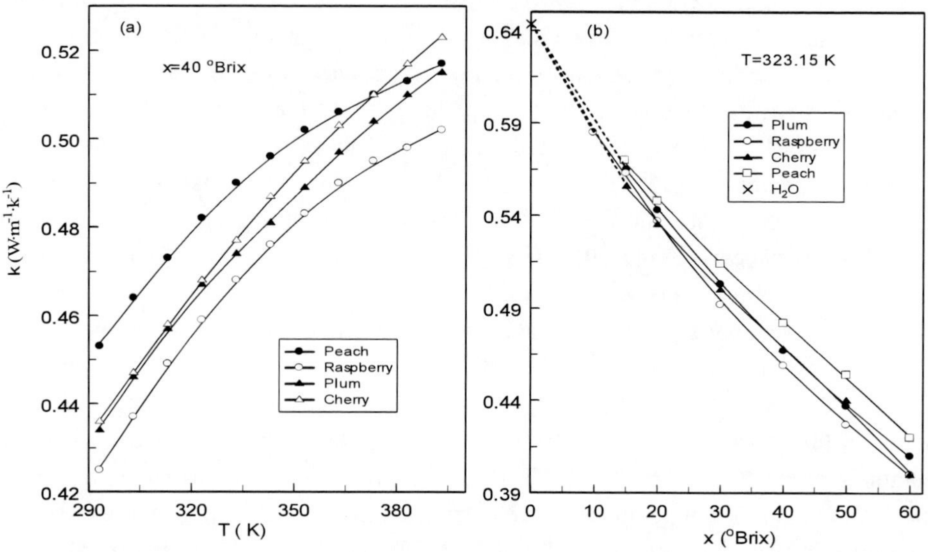

Fig. 16. Comparison of the temperature and concentration dependences of the measured values of thermal conductivity k of various juices.

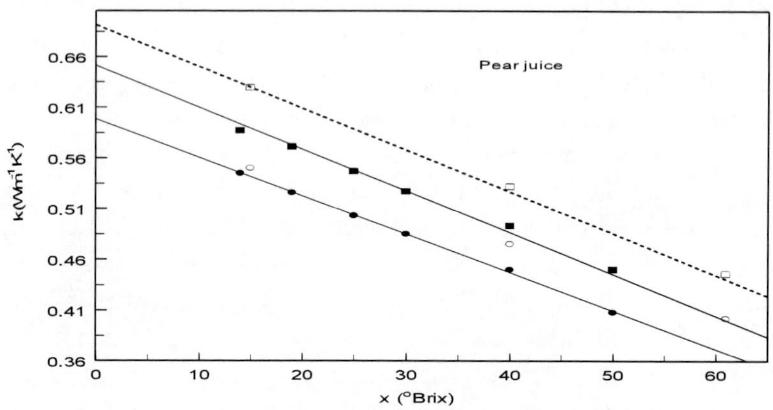

Fig. 17. Comparison present thermal conductivity results for pear juice with those reported by Reidy [10] at two selected temperatures 293 and 353 K. ●, 293 K (this work); ○, 293 K (Reidy [10]); ■, 353 K (this work); □, 353 K (Reidy [10]); Solid curves are calculated with Model-I.

Tadini *et al.* [70] reported thermal conductivity data for caja juice between 8.8 and 49.4 °Brix and at temperatures from (0.4 to 77.1) °C using coaxial cylinders method. The results were fitted to the polynomial type equation. The photopyroelectric (PPE) method was developed by Frandas and Bicanic [130] in order to measure the thermal conductivity of fruit juices (orange and apple) in the temperature range from (0 to 70) °C and between 0 and 80 °Brix. The method consists of the measurement of the sample temperature increase due to absorption of radiation by using a pyroelectric sensor placed in thermal contact with the sample. The results were compared with predictive models from the literature. Shamsudin *et al.* [142] reported thermal conductivity data for guava juice at concentrations between 10 to

40 °Brix and at temperatures from (30 to 80) °C. Measurements were performed by using the thermal properties analyzer (type KD2) which based on the line heat source method. Pedro *et al.* [71] are employed concentric cylinders technique to measure the thermal conductivity of lemon juice for the concentration from 0.381 to 0.9 wt fractions and at temperatures from (0.3 to 80.6) °C. The measured results were presented as a function of temperature and water content. The line heat source method was employed by Reddy and Datta [150] to measure of the thermal conductivity of milk between concentrations of 40 and 70 mass % and temperatures of (35 and 65) °C. Assis *et al.* [72] also used concentric cylindrical cell to measure thermal conductivity of yellow mombin juice at temperatures from (0.4 to 77.1) °C and at concentrations between 8.8 and 49.4 °Brix. The cell was calibrated with pure water. The results were presented as a linear function of temperature and concentration. Coimbra *et al.* [73] used steady state technique to measure the thermal conductivity of liquid egg with concentrations from 51.8 to 88.2 mass % at temperatures between (0 and 38) °C. Measured thermal conductivity data were presented as a linear function of temperature and water content. The thermal conductivity data of celery juice were reported by Lau *et al.* [143] in the low temperature range from (0 to -9.1) °C for the concentrations from 0 to 30 wt %. These data were calculated with ρ, a, and C_p measurements. Ziegler and Rizvi [131] are reported thermal conductivity data for two fruit juices apple, orange, and for milk. The method used by these authors is thermal comparator method. This method can be used for rapid and accurate measurements of the thermal conductivity of liquid foods. Xu *et al.* [75] used concentric cylinder method to measure the thermal conductivity two fruit (mango and orange) juices with concentrations (34 and 12.6) wt % solids content. The inner cylinder is stationary and the outer rotated to study the effect of shear rate on the measured values of the thermal conductivity.

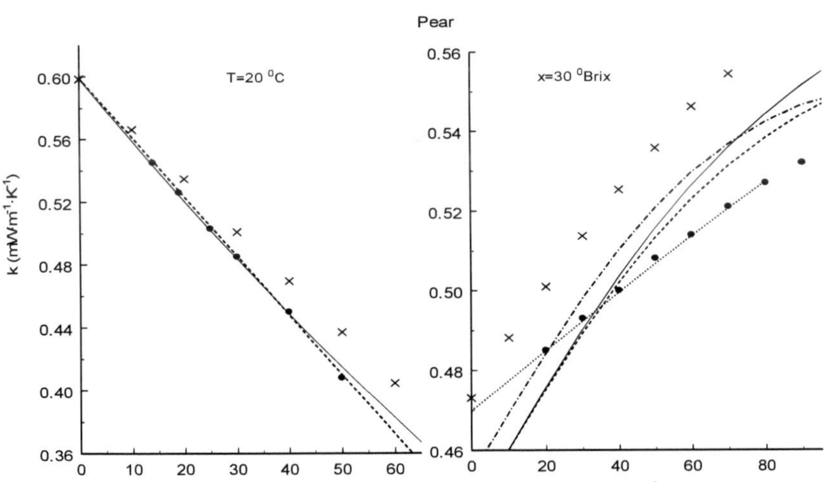

Fig. 18. Measured and predicted values of thermal conductivities of pear juice as a function of concentration (left) and temperature (right). (•), Magerramov *et al.* [77]; (×), Riedel [67]; (———), Maxwell model (Eq. 39); (– – – – –), first order arithmetic mean (parallel model, Eq. 43); (—·—·—·—), Model-20; (· · · · · ·), this work (Model-21).

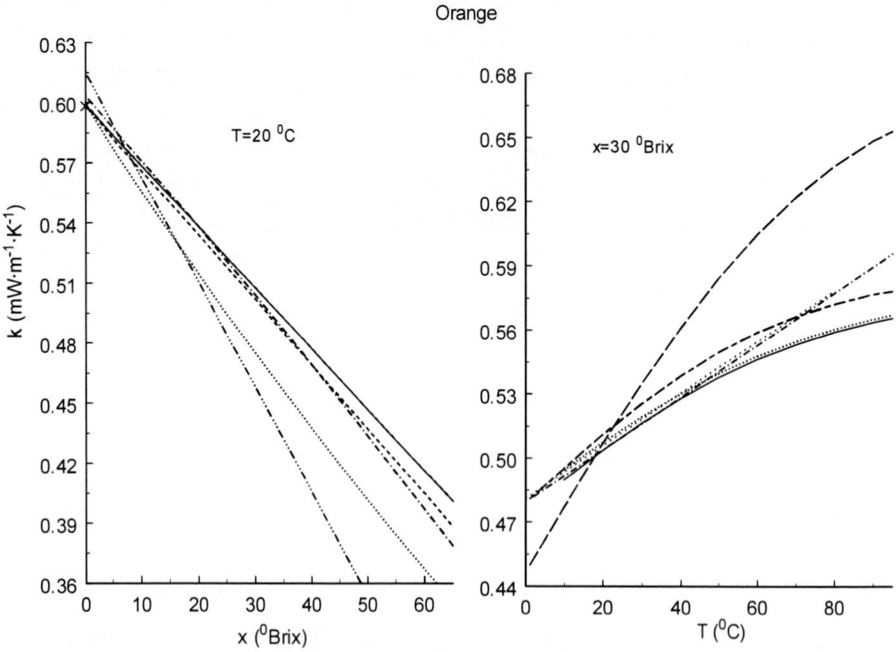

Fig. 19. Thermal conductivity of orange juice as a function of concentration predicted from various models. (———), first order arithmetic mean (parallel model, Eq. 43); (· · · · · ·), Maxwell model (Eq. 39); (–· – ·– ·–), Muramatsu *et al.* [129]; (– – – – –), Cheng and Torquato [202]; (———), Frandas and Bicanic [130]; (–···–···–···–), Telis-Romero *et al.* [74]; (— — — — —), Model-20; (……), this work (Model-21).

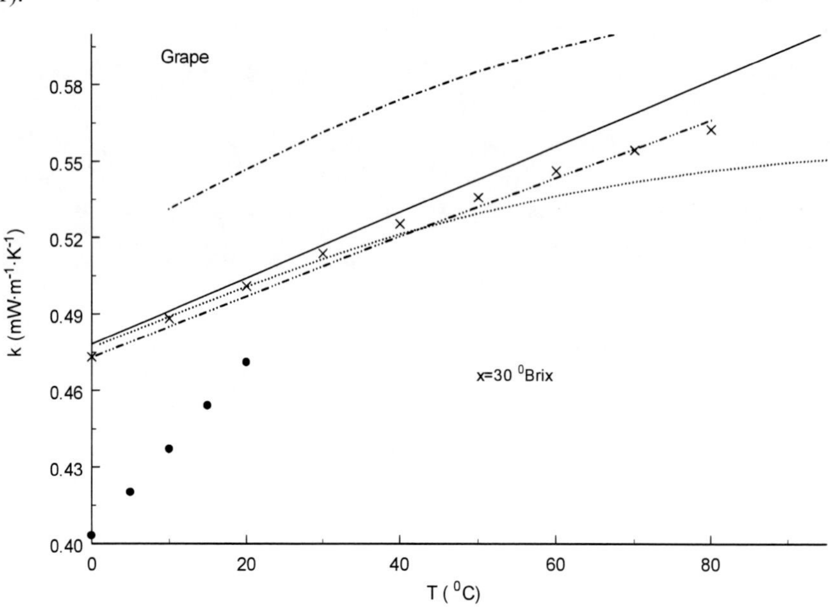

Fig. 20. Measured thermal conductivities of grape juice together with the values calculated from various predictive models. (•),Voitko *et al.* [138]; (×), Riedel [67]; (–·–·–·–·–), Frandas and Bicanic [130]; (———), Muramatsu *et al.* [129]; (–···–···–···–), this work (Model-21); (· · · · · ·), Maxwell model (Eq. 39).

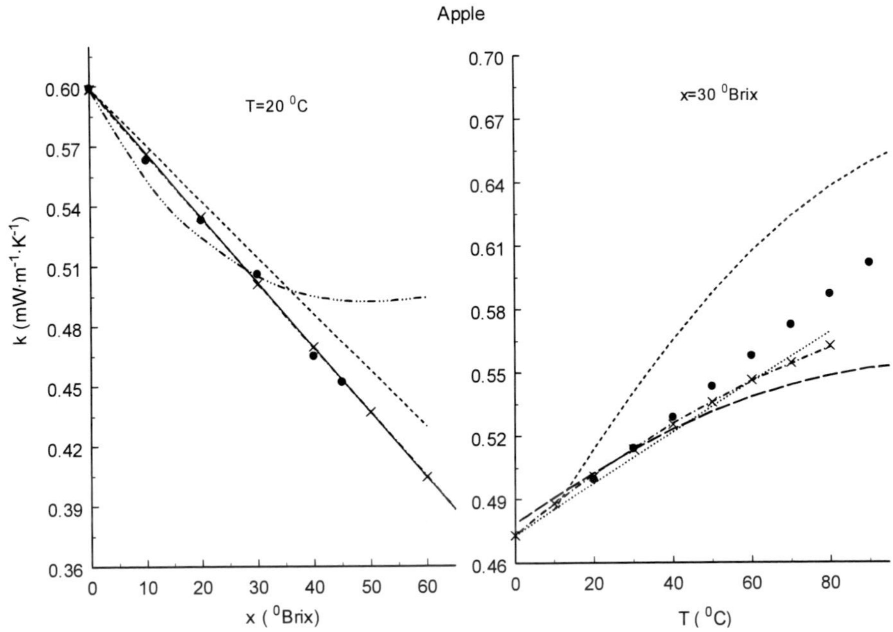

Fig. 21. Measured thermal conductivities of apple juice together with the values calculated from various predictive models. (•), Muramatsu *et al.* [134]; (×), Riedel [67]; (———), first order arithmetic mean (parallel model, Eq. 43); (– – – –), Frandas and Bicanic [130]; (–···–···–···–), Waff [188] model (Eq. 50); (· · · · · ·), this work (Model-21); (———), Maxwell model (Eq. 39); (–·–·–·–), Cheng and Torquato [202].

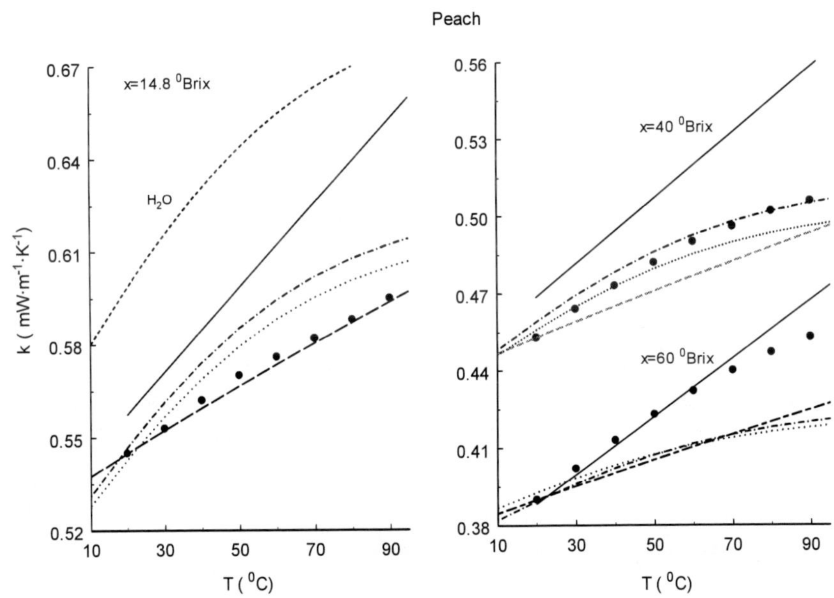

Fig. 22. Measured thermal conductivities of peach juice together with the values calculated from various predictive models. (•), Magerramov *et al.* [76]; (———), Muramatsu *et al.* [129]; (-------), pure H_2O (Kestin *et al.* [95], IAPWS); (–·–·–·–), Frandas and Bicanic [130]; (———), this work (Model-21); (· · · · · ·), Maxwell model (Eq. 39).

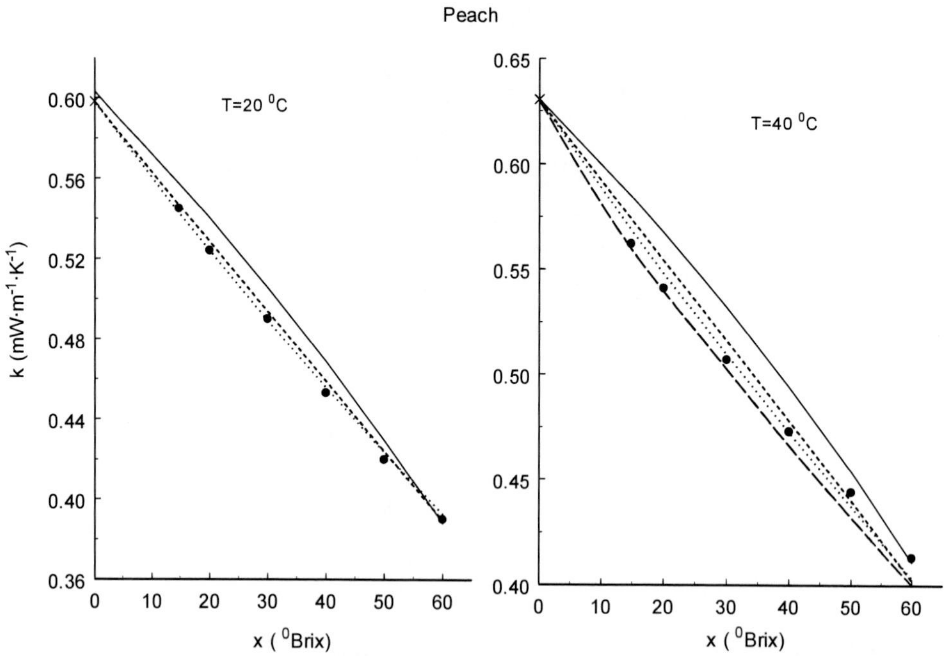

Fig. 23. Measured thermal conductivities of peach juice together with the values calculated from various predictive models. (•), Magerramov *et al.* [76]; (———), Muramatsu *et al.* [129]; (×), pure H_2O (Kestin *et al.* [95], IAPWS); (– – – – –), Frandas and Bicanic [130]; (———), this work (Model-21); (· · · · · ·), Maxwell model (Eq. 39).

Poppendiek *et al.* [151] are reported thermal conductivity data for some biological fluids (human and animal bloods, human plasma and urine, gastric juice, and egg yolk. Measurements were made using parallel plate method. The thermal conductivity cell consists of two highly conductive plates. The heat source is composed of two flat electrical heating elements with a null heat flow meter inserted between them. The electrical powers for the two heaters were so adjusted that the heat flow through the null heat flow meter was zero. Therefore, all the heat generated in the bottom heater was forced to flow through the cell containing the biological specimen. The measured results were used to develop predicting method on the basis of chemical composition. The method based on postulate that the small particles are uniformly distributed in a second component and that volume of all particles is small compared to the total. The thermal conductivity for cherry, raspberry, plum, peach, pear, sweet-cherry, apricot, and cherry-plum juices over wide range of temperature and concentration were reported recently by Magerramov *et al.* [76,77] at temperatures between (20 and 120) °C and at concentrations up to 60 °Brix using a coaxial-cylinder (steady-state) technique. At temperatures above 100 °C the measurements were made at pressures about 0.3 MPa (slightly above vapor pressure). This technique has been previously used for accurate measurements on other liquids (water and aqueous solutions) at high temperatures and high pressures (Abdulagatov *et al.* [91-93]).

3.1. Temperature dependence

Figures 13, 15, 16 (left), 18 (right), 20, 21 (right), and 22 demonstrate the typical effect of temperature on the thermal conductivity various fruit juices. Figure 16 (left) compare the temperature dependence of the thermal conductivity of a series of fruit juices at the selected concentration of 40 °Brix. This figure demonstrates the effect of nature of the fruit juice on the temperature dependence of the thermal conductivity. As one can see from this figure, the peach juice has the highest observed values of the thermal conductivity among other fruit juices at the same thermodynamic (T,x) conditions, while raspberry juice exhibit the lowest value of the thermal conductivity. This is can be explain due to the effect of chemical compositions (water, protein, fat, ash, carbohydrate, fiber content) of the fruit juices on the thermal conductivity.

The thermal conductivity of juices affected up to (11-18 % for pear; 16-21 % for sweet cherry; 14-19 % for cherry plum; 15-17 % for apricot; 12-18 % for peach; 15-22 % for plum; 15-18 % for raspberry; and 18-20 % for cherry juices) by the temperature at temperatures from 20 to 120 °C and concentration from 10 to 60 °Brix. For pure water at the same temperature range the thermal conductivity changes up to 14 %. The measured values of thermal conductivity were used to calculate the temperature coefficient, $\beta_T = \left(\partial \ln k / \partial T\right)_x$, for the some selected juices. The derived values of β_T are shown in Figure 24 (left) as a function of temperature for various constant concentrations and as a function of concentration (Fig. 24 right). The rate of temperature changes at low temperatures is higher than at high temperatures. Figures 13 and 15 also demonstrate how the behavior of the temperature dependence of the thermal conductivity of fruit juices depends on concentration. At low concentrations the curvature of the $k-T$ curves is higher than at high concentrations. The value of temperature coefficient of thermal conductivity, $\left(\partial \ln k / \partial T\right)_x$, at low temperatures (about 1.47×10^{-3} K^{-1}) is almost two times higher than at high temperatures (about 0.66×10^{-3} K^{-1}). At low concentrations the curvature of the $k-T$ dependence is more essential than at high concentrations. The temperature coefficient is slightly changes (almost constant) with concentration changing (see Fig. 24 right).

3.2. Concentration dependence

Figures 14, 16 (right), 17, 18 (left), 19 (left), 21 (left), and 23 demonstrate the effect of concentration on the thermal conductivity of fruit juices at various fixed temperatures. As one can see from these figures, the thermal conductivity of fruit juices monotonically decreased (almost linearly) with concentration. A small curvature of the $k-x$ curves at high concentrations is exhibit. Thermal conductivity considerably decreases (up to 38-48 %) with concentration at low temperatures (20 °C) and up to 35-43 % at high temperatures (120 °C).

Measured thermal conductivity data for some fruit juices are compared with the values reported by various authors from the literature (see Figs. 17 to 23). Figure 17 compare the experimental values of the thermal conductivity for pear juice with the data reported by Reidy [10]. The agreement between our results and the values reported by Reidy [10] for pear juice is within 6 to 9 % at high temperature 80 °C (our result systematically lowers than Reidy [10] data), while at low temperatures (20 °C) the difference is about 1.5 to 5 %. Differences are about 4-7 % were found between the present data and the data reported by Riedel [67] for pear juice (see Fig. 18). Good agreement within 4-5 % was observed between the data by Riedel [67] and Muramatsu *et al.* [129] for grape juice. Excellent agreement shows between the data reported by the same authors for apple juice (see Fig. 21). The deviations between the present results and the data reported by Muramatsu *et al.* [129] for peach juice are within 4-10 % (see Fig. 22) at low concentrations, while the excellent agreement within 1-2 % is observed at high concentration. This is probably due to the difference of the chemical compositions of the juice samples by the authors. For example, it is well known that the thermal conductivity of juices is significantly affected by the chemical compositions (water, protein, fat, ash, carbohydrate, fiber content). Since the chemical compositions of liquid foods are imperfect, the comparison reported thermal conductivity data for the same fruit juice some time is incorrect.

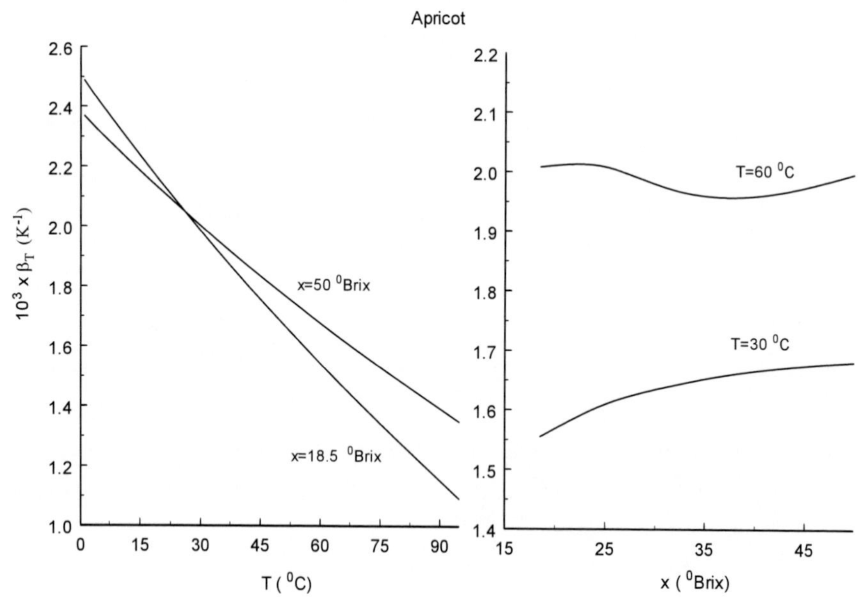

Fig. 24. Temperature coefficient of the thermal conductivity of apricot juices as a function of temperature (left) and concentration (right) at two selected constant concentrations and constant temperatures derived from experimental data by Magerramov *et al.* [77].

4. Thermal Conductivity Models. Prediction and Correlation Techniques

The comprehensive review of the correlation, prediction, and estimation techniques for the thermal conductivity of liquid foods are reported in the works by several authors Cuevas and Cheryan [153], Sweat [160], Becker *et al.* [161], Frandas and Bicanic [130], Peacock [162], Bhumbla *et al.* [163], Choi and Okos [8,164], and Heldman and Singh [165]. Based on the experimental data many empirical and semi-empirical models for the prediction of thermal conductivity of liquid foods have been proposed by various authors (Riedel [67]; Kolarov and Gromov [135]; Sweat [154,157,160], Miles *et al.* [166], Choi and Okos [8,164], Saravacos and Maroulis [13], and Mattar *et al.* [224]). A number of correlation equations have been developed in the literature to calculate and predict the thermal conductivity of liquid foods as a function of temperature and concentration (see Table 3). Table 3 provides correlations and prediction models which were frequently used to calculate the effect of concentration and temperature on the thermal conductivity of liquids and liquid mixtures including liquid food materials. These models previously were successfully used to correlate experimental thermal conductivity data for aqueous systems and were examined by various authors. We used the experimental thermal conductivity data for some fruit juices to examine most of them for their applicability, accuracy, and predictive capability. Due to lack of theoretical background of the temperature and concentration dependences of the thermal conductivity for liquids (aqueous solutions) and liquid foods the empirical and semi-empirical correlation equations and prediction techniques are often used in the literature (see for example, Millat *et al.* [167], Aseyev [168], Horvath [169], Reid *et al.* [170], Saravacos and Maroulis [13], and Abdulagatov *et al.* [182]). In this work we studied the applicability of the various theoretical and empirical models for the thermal conductivity of aqueous solutions as a function of temperature and concentration for fruit juices and their predicting capabilities. Here we will briefly review the empirical and semi-empirical correlation and prediction models which were used to describe the effect of temperature and concentration on the thermal conductivity of aqueous systems and test results their applicability for the fruit juices.

Table 3. Summary of the models used for the correlation of the thermal conductivity of fruit juices and aqueous solutions

Functional Form of the Models		Reference
Empirical Correlation Models		
N	**Temperature dependency models at *x*=constant**	
1	$k(T) = a_0 + a_1T + a_2T^2$	Choi and Okos [139], Telis-Romero *et al.* [80], Magerramov *et al.* [76,77]
2	$k(T)=k(298)[1+\alpha(T-298.15)]$	Magerramov *et al.* [76,77]
3	$(k/k_0) = A(T/T_0)^n$, $n=2/3$	Magerramov *et al.* [76,77]
4	$k(T,x)/k_0(x) = A + Bt$	
Concentration dependency models at *T*=constant		
5	$k(x) = a+bx+cx^2$	Magerramov *et al.* [76,77], Ziegler and Rizvi [131]
6	$k(x) = a_0 + a_1x$	Kolarov and Gromov [135]

Table 3. Continued

	Functional Form of the Models	Reference
Combined models (Temperature and concentration dependency models)		
7	$k(T,x)=\sum_{i=0}^{2}\sum_{j=0}^{2}a_{ij}\Delta T^{j}x^{i}$, $\Delta T=T-273.15$	Ramires and Nieto de Castro [171,172]
8	$k(T,x)=a_0+a_1x+a_2x^2+b_0T+b_1T^2+c_0xT$	Reddy and Datta [150]
9	$k(T,x)=a_0+a_1x+a_2T$	Pedro *et al.* [71], Coimbra *et al.* [73], Gratão *et al.* [66], Maslikov and Medvedev [141]
10	$k(T,x)=a_1x+a_2T$	Assis *et al.* [72], Hermans [174], Tadini *et al.* [70]
11	$k(T,x)=a_0+a_1x+a_2x^2+b_1T$	Alloush *et al.* [175], Magerramov *et al.* [76,77]
12	$k(T,x)=a_1xT+a_2x+a_3T+a_4$, $k(T,x)=a_1x^2T+a_2x^2+a_3xT+a_4x+a_5T+a_6$	Muramatsu *et al.* [129,134]
13	$k(T,x)=c_1+c_4x+(c_2+c_5x)T+(c_3+c_6x)T^2$	Magerramov *et al.* [76,77]
14	$k(T,x)=(b_0+b_1T_r+b_2T_r^2)(1+a_1x+a_2x^2)$	Magerramov *et al.* [76,77]
15	$k(T,x)=[a_0+a_1T+a_2T^2](b_0+b_1x)$	Riedel [67,179], Peacock [162]
16	$k(T,x)=(b_0+b_1x)+(b_2+b_3x)T+(b_4+b_5x)T^2$	Fernandez-Martin and Montes [69]
17	$k=[a_0+a_1T_{fp}+a_2T_{fp}^2+a_3T][a_4+a_5(100-x)]$	Lau *et al.* [143]
Models which represent the thermal conductivity of liquid foots relative to pure water		
18	$k(x)=k_W+a_1x$	Magerramov *et al.* [76,77]
19	$k(x)=k_W+a_1x+a_2x^2$	Magerramov *et al.* [76,77]
20	$k(x)=k_W(1+a_1x+a_2x^2)$	Magerramov *et al.* [76,77], Chiquillo [176], Losenicky [177]
21	$k(T)=k_{sol}(293)[k_W(T)/k_W(293)]$	Magerramov *et al.* [76,77]
22	$k=k_S+[(\rho_P/\rho_W)k_W-(\rho_P/\rho_W)k_S]x_W$	Bhumbla *et al.* [163]
23	$k=k_w(a+bx+ct)/(a+ct)$	White *et al.* [178]
24	$k(t,x)=k_w(t)[1-(a_0+a_1t+a_2t^2)x-(c_0+c_1t+c_2t^2)x^2]$	Yusufova *et al.* [60], Pepinov and Guseynov [62,65]
25	$k(T,x)=[k_W-(k_W-k_S)x_S](a+bT+cT^2)$	Frandas and Bicanic [130]
26	$k(T,x)=k_W(T)[1-(a_0+a_1T+a_2T^2)x-(c_0+c_1T+c_2T^2)x^2]$	Magerramov *et al.* [76,77]

Functional Form of the Models		Reference
27	$k(T,x)=k_w(T)\left[1-A(x+Bx^3)\right]-CTx$	Magerramov *et al.* [76,77]
28	$k(T,x)=k_W(T)\,[1\text{-}a(x+2\times10^{-4}x^3)]-2\times10^{-8}Tx$	Magerramov *et al.* [76,77]
29	$k=(k_w\rho/\rho_w)(a_0+a_1x_w)$	Telis-Romero *et al.* [80], Gratão *et al.* [66]
Empirical Prediction Models		
30	$k(T)=k_{sol}(T_0)\,[k_W(T)/k_W(T_0)]$	Vargaftik and Osminin [173], Riedel [179]
31	$(k/k_0(x))=(T/T_0)^n$, where n=2/3 (theory), for most juices n is whitin 0.4 to 0.7	Magerramov *et al.* [76,77]
32	$k=k_S+(k_W-k_S)x_W$	Choi and Okos [8]
33	$k=k_S+[(\rho_P/\rho_W)k_W-(\rho_P/\rho_W)k_S]x_W$	Bhumbla *et al.* [163]
Composition Models		
34	$k=a_0x_w+a_1x_c+a_3x_f+a_4x_p$	Sweat [154,160]
35	$k=a_0+a_1x_w+a_2x_f+a_3T$	Minim *et al.* [68]
36	$k=a_0x_w+a_1x_p+a_2x_c+a_3x_f+a_4x_a$	Choi and Okos [139]
37	$k=\sum_{i=1} K_ix_i^v,\ x_i^v=x_i^w/\rho_i/\sum_{i=1} x_i^w/\rho_i,$ $K_i=a_1+a_2T+a_3T^2,\ \rho_i=c_1+c_2T$	Choi and Okos [8]
38	$k=a_0x_w+a_1x_p+a_2x_c+a_3x_f$	Dominguez *et al.* [180]

* where x_w, x_c, x_f, x_p, and x_a concentration of water, carbohydrate, fat, protein, and ash, respectively; T_{fp} freezing point; x_i^w is the weight fraction of component i (protein, lipids, etc.), x_i^v is the estimated volume fraction.

4.1. Empirical and semi-empirical models

4.1.1. Concentration dependence models

The most often use models for the concentration dependence of thermal conductivity of aqueous solutions and liquid foods are given in Table 3. Model-18 (or 6) (linear relation) is commonly used for the concentration dependence of the thermal conductivity of aqueous solutions and liquid foods [66-68,70-72,76,77,80,134,135,129,141,143,160,162,179,180]. But, as Figs. 14 and 16 (right) shows, the linear dependence of the thermal conductivity for some fruit juices (raspberry, plum, cherry, and peach) is valid only at low concentrations (below 30 °Brix). Probably this is depending on chemical composition of the juice (juice nature). At high concentrations the quadratic term Model-19 (or 5) is required to accurate describe the experimental thermal conductivity data (Ziegler and Rizvi [131]). Figure 25 shows concentration dependence of the relative thermal conductivity (k_{juice}/k_W-1) of raspberry and plum juices versus of concentration x for two selected temperatures. As one can see from this figure, $(k_{juice}/k_W - 1)$ is varies almost linearly with concentration x only in the range up to 30 °Brix and is almost independent of temperature (a function of concentration only). This is means that the temperature dependence of the thermal conductivity of juices governing by the temperature dependence of the thermal conductivity of pure water. At higher concentrations, the nonlinear behavior (quadratic term) of concentration dependence of the thermal conductivity is observed, $(k_{sol}/k_W - 1) = a_1 x + a_2 x^2$ (see Model-20).

4.1.2. Temperature dependence models

A number of correlation equations have been developed in the literature to calculate and predict the thermal conductivity of liquid foods as a function of temperature (Fernández-Martin and Montes [69], Cuevas and Cheryan [153], Choi and Okos [139], Constenla *et al.* [133], Telis-Romero *et al.* [74], and Gratão *et al.* [66]). Several widely used models for the temperature dependence of the thermal conductivity are shown in Table 3 (Models 1 to 4). These models have been successfully used previously to correlate experimental thermal conductivity data for aqueous solutions as well. Here we examined the applicability of these models for the thermal conductivity of fruit juices. The Model-1 (quadratic polynomial in temperature T, see Table 3) was used by many authors [38-49,76,77,80,139,169,181] to represent experimental thermal conductivity data of liquids and liquids mixtures in the wide temperature and concentration ranges. Model-2 (linear temperature dependence) is applicable only in the limited temperature range (basically at low temperatures, Assael *et al.* [18,19]).

4.1.3. Combined effect of temperature and concentration

Different models were proposed by various authors to represent the combined effect of temperature and concentration on the thermal conductivity of liquid foods and aqueous solutions (see Models-7 to 17, Table 3). Model-7 reproduced concentration and temperature effects on the thermal conductivity of aqueous systems in the wide temperature and concentration ranges within accuracy of ±0.6 %. Models 8 to 17 are the different combinations of polynomial functions of temperature and concentration. All of them were successfully used previously for the description of thermal conductivity of aqueous solutions. In this work we developed different models to describe the combined effect of temperature and concentration on the thermal conductivity of fruit juices.

Model-A. The effects of temperature and concentration on thermal conductivity of fruit juices can be combined by taking into account the concentration dependence of the parameters $a_0(x)$, $a_1(x)$, and $a_2(x)$ in the Model-1 (see Table 3) as quadratic functions

$$a_0(x) = c_1 + c_2 x + c_3 x^2, \tag{19}$$

$$a_1(x) = c_4 + c_5 x + c_6 x^2, \tag{20}$$

$$a_2(x) = c_7 + c_8 x + c_9 x^2, \tag{21}$$

Model-A was applied to the present experimental thermal conductivity data for some fruit juices. The derived values of coefficients c_i are given in Table 4. The AAD (%) between measured and calculated values for peach, plum, raspberry, cherry, pear, sweet-cherry, apricot, and cherry-plum juices are: 0.07 (R^2=0.9991), 0.18 (R^2=0.9906), 0.20 (R^2=0.9902), 0.13 (R^2=0.9946), 0.1 (R^2=0.9893), 0.2 (R^2=0.9951), 0.22 (R^2=0.9906), and 0.19 (R^2=0.9879), respectively.

Table 4. The values of parameters c_i (Eqs. 19 to 21) for fruit juices (Model-A)

Juice	Peach	Plum	Raspberry	Cherry
c_1	0.5888×10^{0}	0.5905×10^{0}	0.5835×10^{0}	0.5601×10^{0}
c_2	-4.2108×10^{-3}	-5.6132×10^{-3}	-6.0697×10^{-3}	-4.4534×10^{-3}
c_3	6.7985×10^{-6}	2.8382×10^{-5}	3.7629×10^{-5}	1.7796×10^{-5}
c_4	1.9662×10^{-3}	1.0869×10^{-3}	1.2492×10^{-3}	1.0573×10^{-3}
c_5	-8.1694×10^{-5}	6.2466×10^{-6}	1.2418×10^{-5}	1.4187×10^{-5}
c_6	1.2627×10^{-6}	-5.919×10^{-8}	-2.323×10^{-7}	-1.9678×10^{-7}
Juice	Peach	Plum	Raspberry	Cherry
c_7	-4.8206×10^{-7}	-1.3729×10^{-6}	-2.4189×10^{-6}	-9.4700×10^{-7}
c_8	-7.3754×10^{-8}	-8.8027×10^{-8}	-1.1036×10^{-7}	-8.9423×10^{-8}
c_9	-2.9782×10^{-10}	1.0639×10^{-9}	1.61845×10^{-9}	9.1168×10^{-10}

Model-B. In food products, water is a major component and its thermal conductivity is a function of temperature. The models which are representing the thermal conductivity of liquid foods relative to the pure water thermal conductivity are presented in Table 3 (Models 18 to 29. The present experimental thermal conductivity data for some selected fruit juices were also fitted to the Model-19 (see Table 3). The derived equations for the fruit juices are:

$$k = k_w(T) - 5.30\times10^{-3}x + 2.50\times10^{-5}x^2 \text{ for plum juice, } (R^2=0.9005) \tag{22}$$

$$k = k_w(T) - 5.78\times10^{-3}x + 3.34\times10^{-5}x^2 \text{ for raspberry juice, } (R^2=0.9901) \tag{23}$$

$$k = k_w(T) - 4.65\times10^{-3}x + 1.35\times10^{-5}x^2 \text{ for cherry juice, } (R^2=0.9083) \tag{24}$$

$$k = k_w(T) - 4.69\times10^{-3}x + 1.65\times10^{-5}x^2 \text{ for peach juice, } (R^2=0.8965) \tag{25}$$

where the equation for the thermal conductivity of pure water is

$$k_W(T) = 0.566 + 1.86\times 10^{-3}T - 7.363\times 10^{-6}T^2 . \tag{26}$$

In this model the temperature dependence of the thermal conductivity of fruit juices is represented through the thermal conductivity of pure water, $k_W(T)$. This model reproduces the present experimental thermal conductivity data for peach, plum, raspberry, and cherry juices within (AAD) 1.19, 0.68, 1.09, and 1.52 %, respectively.

Model-C. Another Model-20 (modification of the Model-B) was applied to the same thermal conductivity data of the fruit juices. This model was previously successfully used for aqueous solutions (see, for example, Horvath [169] and Abdulagatov *et al.* [182]). The results are given below

$$k = k_w(T)(1 - 8.8\times 10^{-3}x + 5.1\times 10^{-5}x^2) \text{ for plum juice, } (R^2{=}0.9945) \tag{27}$$

$$k = k_w(T)(1 - 7.2\times 10^{-3}x + 2.7\times 10^{-5}x^2) \text{ for peach juice, } (R^2{=}0.9895) \tag{28}$$

$$k = k_w(T)(1 - 8.7\times 10^{-3}x + 4.3\times 10^{-5}x^2) \text{ for raspberry juice, } (R^2{=}0.9916) \tag{29}$$

$$k = k_w(T)(1 - 8.5\times 10^{-3}x + 4.5\times 10^{-5}x^2) \text{ for cherry juice, } (R^2{=}0.9852) \tag{30}$$

$$k = k_w(T)(1 - 7.9\times 10^{-3}x + 3.75\times 10^{-5}x^2) \text{ for pear juice, } (R^2{=}0.9791) \tag{31}$$

$$k = k_w(T)(1 - 8.4\times 10^{-3}x + 4.29\times 10^{-5}x^2) \text{ for sweet cherry juice, } (R^2{=}0.9811) \tag{32}$$

$$k = k_w(T)(1 - 8.72\times 10^{-3}x + 4.87\times 10^{-5}x^2) \text{ for cherry-plum juice, } (R^2{=}0.9882) \tag{33}$$

$$k = k_w(T)(1 - 7.54\times 10^{-3}x + 2.75\times 10^{-5}x^2) \text{ for apricot juice, } (R^2{=}0.9699) \tag{34}$$

The accuracy (AAD, %) for the Model-C are 0.82, 1.16, 0.90, 1.44, 1.04, 1.3, 1.06, and 0.93, respectively for peach, plum, raspberry, cherry, pear, sweet-cherry, apricot, and cherry-plum juices. The comparison between experimental and calculated with Models A, B, and C is showed in Fig. 15. As one can see, the multi-parametric Model-A is best represents the present experimental thermal conductivity data, but the extrapolation and prediction capabilities of the Models -B and -C are better than Model-A. Moreover, according the Models-B and C the thermal conductivity difference, $k(T,x) - k_W(T)$, and reduced thermal conductivity, $k(T,x)/k_W(T)$-1, are almost independent of the temperature (function of concentration only, see also Fig. 25). This is means that the temperature dependence of the thermal conductivity of juice can be represented through the thermal conductivity of pure water as a function of temperature. Therefore, Models-B and C are allow to predict the values of thermal conductivity of juices at any temperature just by knowing the concentration dependence of $k(T_0, x)$ at a fixed (or reference) isotherm T_0. This makes it much easier to predict the temperature dependence of the thermal conductivity of juices.

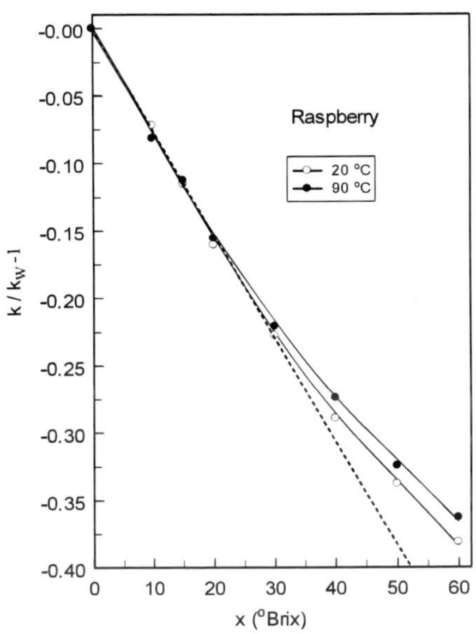

Fig. 25. Relative thermal conductivity, $(k_{juice} / k_W - 1)$, of raspberry and plum juices as a function of concentration x at two fixed temperatures Magerramov *et al.* [76].

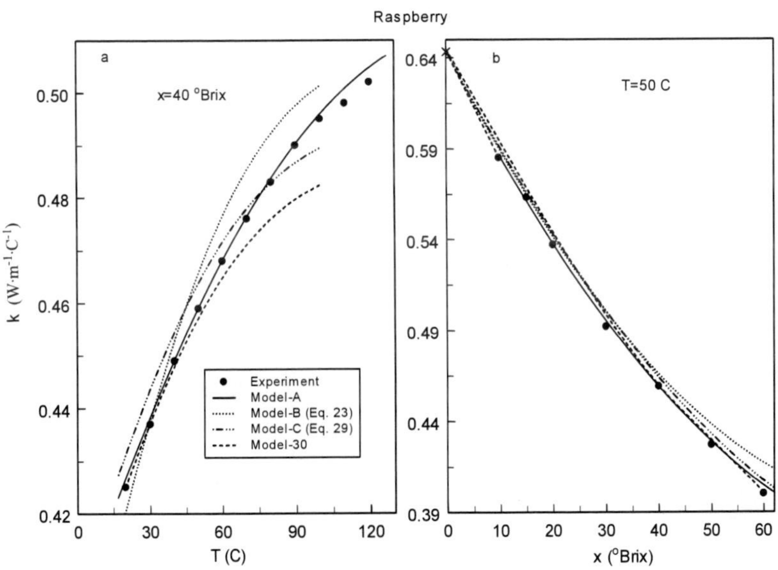

Fig. 26. Comparison measured and calculated values of the thermal conductivity of raspberry juice using various models Magerramov *et al.* [76].

Model-D: Model-3 (see Table 3) with concentration dependent parameters $A(x)$ and $n(x)$ can be also used to represent the combined effect of temperature and concentration on the thermal conductivity of fruit juices, where $k_0(x)$ is the thermal conductivity of juice as a function of concentration along the constant reference temperature of $T_0 = 293.15$ K

$$k_0(x) = k_w(T_0) - 3.7888 \times 10^{-3} x + 1.59 \times 10^{-7} x^2 \text{ for pear juice,} \quad (35)$$

$$k_0(x) = k_w(T_0) - 5.0826 \times 10^{-3} x + 2.3106 \times 10^{-5} x^2 \text{ for sweet-cherry juice,} \quad (36)$$

$$k_0(x) = k_w(T_0) - 4.3357 \times 10^{-3} x + 1.2778 \times 10^{-5} x^2 \text{ for apricot juice,} \quad (37)$$

$$k_0(x) = k_w(T_0) - 4.6340 \times 10^{-3} x + 1.2718 \times 10^{-5} x^2 \text{ for cherry-plum juice,} \quad (38)$$

where $k_w(T_0) = 0.5985$ W m^{-1} K^{-1} is the thermal conductivity of pure water at T_0=293.15 K. Figure 27 shows the plot of (k/k_0) *vs.* (T/T_0) for the two selected fruit juices at various concentrations. As one can see from this figure, the temperature dependence of (k/k_0) at temperature up to 336 K is almost linear. The measured thermal conductivities for juices were fitted to the Model-D by using the lowest temperature (293.15 K) and corresponding thermal conductivity data as reference values T_0 and k_0. The values of the *A* and *n* were evaluated for each juice as a function of concentration (see Table 5).

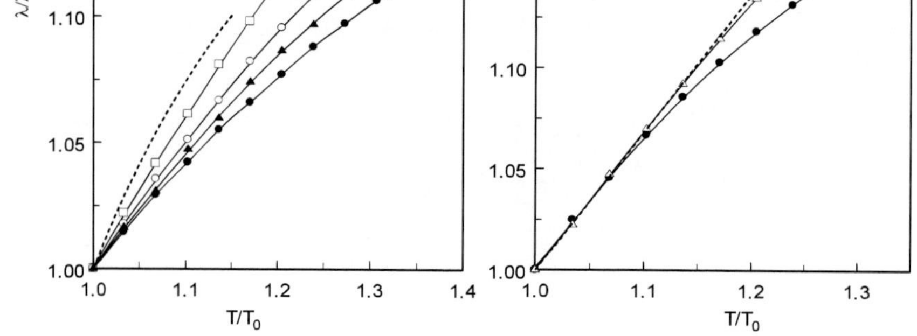

Fig. 27. Relative thermal conductivity, (k/k_0), of pear and sweet-cherry juices as a function of relative temperature (T/T_0) along various fixed concentrations. Pear juice: ●, 14 °Brix; ▲, 30 °Brix; ○, 40 °Brix; □, 50 °Brix; (– – – –), pure water (IAPWS calculation, Kestin *et al.* [95]); Sweet-cherry juice: ●, 14.3 °Brix; ○, 50 °Brix.

Table 5. The values of parameters $\ln A$ and *n* as a function of concentration (Model-D) for fruit juices

Juice	Pear					
Concentration	14 °Brix	19 °Brix	25 °Brix	30 °Brix	40 °Brix	50 °Brix
$\ln A \times 10^2$	0.38238	0.61277	0.32143	0.38678	0.46807	0.34865
n	0.36829	0.38580	0.41977	0.41000	0.44782	0.56293
Juice	Apricot					
Concentration	18.5 °Brix	25 °Brix	30 °Brix	35 °Brix	40 °Brix	50 °Brix
$\ln A \times 10^2$	0.64735	0.66449	0.40881	0.43615	0.27709	0.39896
n	0.48987	0.51812	0.52559	0.53729	0.54640	0.54536
Juice	Cherry-plum					
Concentration	12.2 °Brix	18 °Brix	24 °Brix	30 °Brix	40 °Brix	50 °Brix
$\ln A \times 10^2$	0.18041	0.47329	0.39646	0.46882	0.45136	0.37181
n	0.44757	0.44585	0.45119	0.45844	0.51719	0.50760
Juice	Sweet-cherry					
Concentration	14.3 °Brix	20 °Brix	27 °Brix	35 °Brix	45 °Brix	50 °Brix
$\ln A \times 10^2$	0.96425	0.79707	0.64021	0.41472	0.69675	0.31254
n	0.52013	0.51072	0.55043	0.55497	0.61836	0.64744

Model-D with parameters presented in Table 5 reproduced experimental thermal conductivity data of juices within 0.36 % to 0.75 %.

As one can see from Table 5, the values of A for each juice are close to unity, A=1.0 (varying for various juices from 1.0018 to 1.0083), therefore, this parameter can be assigned a common value of 1.0 for all juices at any concentrations. The concentration dependence of the parameter n is given in Table 10 for the fixed values of parameter A=1. As this table shows, the values of parameter n are very small changes with concentration. Therefore, this parameter can be also assigned a common value for any concentrations without losing the accuracy in describing of the experimental thermal conductivity data. The value of n for pear, sweet-cherry, apricot, and cherry – plum juices are 0.4525, 0.6219, 0.52099, and 0.56923 respectively. This is means that the thermal conductivity of a juice can be predicted just by knowing the thermal conductivity k_0 at a reference temperature T_0 at fixed n for each juice.

Model-E: At temperatures up to 336 K the values of (k/k_0) can be represent as linear function of temperature (see Model-4, Table 3 and Fig. 27). The values of adjusting parameters A and B for each juice are given in Table 6. This model reproduced the experimental thermal conductivity data within 0.70, 0.73, 0.90, and 0.60 %, for pear, sweet-cherry, apricot, and cherry - plum juices, respectively. However, to increase the accuracy of the model at high temperatures (above 336 K) the quadratic term Ct^2 is required. As one can see from the Table 6, the values of parameter A are almost unity, (varying for various juices from 1.0018 to 1.0083). Therefore, this parameter can be assigned a common value (A=1.0) for any concentrations without losing accuracy of the thermal conductivity calculation. Only one adjustable parameter B in this model is need to accurate calculate the temperature dependence of the thermal conductivity fruit juices.

Table 6. The values of parameters A and B (Model-E) for fruit juices

Juice	A	B
Pear	0.9792	1.304×10^{-3}
Sweet-cherry	0.9738	1.750×10^{-3}
Cherry-plum	0.9742	1.633×10^{-3}
Apricot	0.9729	1.667×10^{-3}

The accuracy (AAD, %) for the Models A to E described above for each juice is given in Table 7. The comparison between experimental and calculated values with Models A to E is shown in Fig. 15. As one can see from Table 7, the multi-parametric Model-A is best represented the present experimental thermal conductivity data, but the predicting capability of the Model-D is much better than others. Moreover, in this model the minimum experimental thermal conductivity information at a reference temperature is needed to predict the values of the thermal conductivity of juices at high temperatures. The accuracy of the Models-C and D is very close. The Model-D can be recommended to calculate the combined effects of the temperature and concentration on the thermal conductivity of juices over wide ranges of temperature and concentration just using the values of thermal conductivity at reference temperature T_0.

Table 7. The AAD (%) between measured and calculated values of thermal conductivities of fruit juices for various models

Juice	Pear	Sweet-cherry	Cherry-plum	Apricot
Model-A	0.10	0.20	0.22	0.19
Model-B	1.04	1.30	1.06	0.93
Model-C	0.60	0.65	0.75	0.36
Model-D	0.70	0.73	0.90	0.60
Model-E	0.64	0.69	0.80	0.38

Table 8 provides the results of the test of various combined models for the thermal conductivity of selected fruit juice (pear juice). As one can see from this table, best result is achieved for the four-parametric Model –IV. Among one-parametric models which are represent the thermal conductivity of juice relative to pure water values best representation of the experimental thermal conductivity data was observed for the Model-IX. The Model-VIII can be used to predict the temperature dependence of the thermal conductivity of juice just by using the single data point at reference temperature T_0=293 K, $k_{juice}(T_0, x)$.

Model -13 (see Table 3) (multi-parametric correlation model) was also applied to the present experimental thermal conductivity data for fruit juices to study of the combined effect of temperature and concentration on thermal conductivity. The derived values of coefficients c_i are given in Table 9. The AAD between measured and calculated values for pear, sweet-cherry, apricot, and cherry-plum juices are 0.1, 0.2, 0.22, and 0.19 %, respectively.

Table 8. Comparison accuracy and predictive capability of various combined models for the thermal conductivity of pear juice (a_i parameters of the models)

	1	2	3	4	5	S
Model-I,	$k(T,x)=k_W(T)\,[1-(a_1+a_2T)x-(a_3+a_4T)x^2]$					
a_i	-3.8795×10^{-3}	-1.21×10^{-5}	-8.256×10^{-5}	3.4×10^{-7}	-	0.340×10^{-4}
Model-II,	$k(T,x)=k_W(T)\,[1-a_1(x+2\times10^{-4}x^3)]-2\times10^{-8}Tx$					
a_i	0.00994867	-	-	-	-	0.666×10^{-3}
Model-III,	$k(T,x)=k_W(T)[1-a_1(x+a_2x^3)]-a_3Tx$					
a_i	0.0088695	5.359×10^{-5}	-2.74×10^{-6}	-	-	0.462×10^{-4}
Model-IV,	$k(T,x)=a_1+a_2x+a_3x^2+a_4T$					
a_i	0.409025	-3.802×10^{-3}	1.93×10^{-6}	6.51×10^{-4}	-	0.598×10^{-5}
Model-V,	$k(x)=k_W+a_1x$					
a_i	-4.3475×10^{-3}	-	-	-	-	0.154×10^{-3}
Model-VI,	$k(x)=k_W+a_1x+a_2x^2$					
a_i	-5.2597×10^{-3}	2.338×10^{-5}	-	-	-	0.840×10^{-4}
Model-VII,	$k(x)=k_W(1+a_1x+a_2x^2)$					
a_i	0.96649	-5.747×10^{-3}	2.93×10^{-6}	-	-	0.313×10^{-4}
Model-VIII,	$k(T)=k_{juice}(T_0,x)\,[k_W(T)/k_W(T_0)]$					
a_i	-	-	-	-	-	-
Model-IX,	$(k/k_0)=(T/T_0)^n$, $k_0(293,x)$, $T_0=293.15$ K					
a_i	n=0.44251	-	-	-	-	0.326×10^{-4}
Model-X,	$k(T)=k(293,x)[1+a_1\,(T-293.15)]$					
a_i	0.001411	-	-	-	-	0.354×10^{-4}

Table 9. The values of parameters c_i for fruit juices (Model-13)

Juice	Pear	Sweet-cherry	Cherry-plum	Apricot
c_1	0.5794×10^{0}	0.5468×10^{0}	0.5468×10^{0}	0.5592×10^{0}
c_2	9.6237×10^{-4}	1.5230×10^{-3}	1.5230×10^{-3}	1.4307×10^{-3}
c_3	-2.7390×10^{-6}	-4.8318×10^{-6}	-4.8318×10^{-6}	-3.9099×10^{-6}
c_4	-3.7520×10^{-3}	-3.3525×10^{-3}	-3.3525×10^{-3}	-3.3103×10^{-3}
c_5	-7.5953×10^{-7}	-9.3931×10^{-6}	-9.3931×10^{-6}	-1.0422×10^{-5}
c_6	2.2198×10^{-8}	6.3587×10^{-8}	6.3587×10^{-8}	5.3053×10^{-8}

Table 10. The values of parameter *n* as a function of concentration (*A*=1.0, Model-3)

Juice	Pear					
Concentration	14 °Brix	19 °Brix	25 °Brix	30 °Brix	40 °Brix	50 °Brix
N	0.38656	0.41508	0.43513	0.42848	0.47018	0.57959
Juice	Apricot					
Concentration	18.5 °Brix	25 °Brix	30 °Brix	35 °Brix	40 °Brix	50 °Brix
N	0.54594	0.57590	0.56254	0.57727	0.57187	0.58188
Juice	Cherry-plum					
Concentration	12.2 °Brix	18 °Brix	24 °Brix	30 °Brix	40 °Brix	50 °Brix
n	0.46370	0.48614	0.48672	0.50036	0.55760	0.63143
Juice	Sweet-cherry					
Concentration	14.3 °Brix	20 °Brix	27 °Brix	35 °Brix	45 °Brix	50 °Brix
n	0.50124	0.57767	0.60619	0.59277	0.68067	0.67300

4.2. Prediction Models

4.2.1. Empirical prediction models

Here we examined the applicability of empirical prediction models (see Table 3) for the thermal conductivity of fruit juices. The Model-20, $k(T)=k_{sol}(T_0)\,[k_W(T)/k_W(T_0)]$, where T_0 is the reference temperature and $k_{sol}(T_0)$ and $k_W(T_0)$ are the thermal conductivity of solution or liquid food at T_0, and $k_W(T)$ is the thermal conductivity of pure water, is preferable to use for the prediction of the temperature dependence of thermal conductivity of solution at fixed composition (Riedel [179]; Vargaftik and Osminin [173]). This model can predict the thermal conductivity of solutions or liquid foods just by knowing the thermal conductivity k_0 of solution at a reference temperature T_0 and pure water thermal conductivity $k_W(T)$ as a function of temperature. This model was applied for the thermal conductivity measurements of fruit juices. The comparison between the predictions and the present experimental results for thermal conductivity of cherry and raspberry juices is shown in Fig. 13 (dashed lines). The agreement between predicted and measured values of thermal conductivity is about (0.25 to 1.5) % at high concentrations and (0.7 to 1.5) % at low concentrations. This model can be recommended for future use to predict the temperature dependence of the thermal conductivity of fruit and vegetable juices. This makes it easier to predict the thermal conductivity of fruit juices just by knowing the thermal conductivity k_0 at a reference temperature T_0 (usually at room temperature) and well-known pure water thermal conductivity data [95].

Model-21 (see also above) is allow to predict the thermal conductivity of liquid foods just by knowing the thermal conductivity k_0 at a reference temperature T_0 at fixed value of n. For most pure liquids the value of n is constant (2/3≈0.67, theoretical value) (Klaas and Viswanath [183]). The values of n for some real liquid juices (pear, sweet-cherry, apricot, and cherry – plum juices) are 0.4525, 0.6219, 0.52099, and 0.56923 respectively. Probably the values of parameter *n* are depend on chemical composition of the juice (or nature of the juice) and should be predicted from chemical composition data. Choi and Okos [8] prediction model (Model-22) allow calculating the thermal conductivity of liquid foods by knowing the pure water values of thermal conductivity and the thermal conductivity of juice components (k_S).

4.2.2. Composition models

The several techniques of determination of the thermal conductivity of liquid foods from the chemical composition were developed in the literature. For example, some composition models (see Table 3) for the thermal conductivity of liquid food products were proposed by Miles *et al.* [166], Sweat [154,160], Rahman [184], and Bálint [221]. Composition model proposed by Sweat [154] predict the thermal conductivity of liquid food with satisfactory results. Composition models are not including temperature effect and geometry (structural properties) of the component mixing. Usually, it is valid at room temperature 25 °C. The composition models have their shortcomings in that the resulting models may be applicable only to the particular suite of liquid food being investigated.

4.2.3. Structural models

The measurement of thermal conductivity of liquid food products are time consuming and costly. It is, therefore, accurate theoretically based predictive models are very important. For many food engineering and scientific applications the relationship between thermal conductivity and concentration is needed. Concentration of juices is the most important parameter affecting its thermophysical properties, but their relationship to concentration is poorly understood. Increasing concentration leads in general to a decrease in thermal conductivity (see Figs. 14, 16-19, 21, 23), but in detail, the microstructure of the solid dispersed particles (chemical components) is important, *i.e.* the size, shape and distribution as well as the conditions in the contact area of the connecting particles. Most models are only valid for low-concentration.

4.2.3.1. Theoretical backgrounds. Mechanism of heat transfer in liquid – solid suspended systems

Most available thermal conductivity models are empirical and cannot be used for accurate prediction. The majority empirical models have their shortcomings in that the resulting models may be applicable only to the particular suite of liquid food being investigated. The theoretical models are based on the mechanism of heat transfer applicable (heat transfer theory) to simplified the structure of the solid-fluid system. There is still a lack of detailed knowledge of how the heat is transferred through liquid foods, and in particular, at the transitions solid-liquid surfaces and interfaces at the solid-liquid-solid. Preferably, one would use a theoretical model to describe the physics (physical nature) of heat conduction, but sufficiently reliable models have not yet beet developed, and empirical modifications of the equations are needed. Liquid food products are a heterogeneous mixture of numerous suspended (randomly dispersed) solid particles forming a non-continuous phase and fluid component (water as a continue fluid). Particular fruit juices might be composed of water, ash, carbohydrates, fat, and protein (Watt and Merril [185]). The accurate thermal conductivity of the composites is needed to predict the thermal conductivity of liquid foods. The thermal conductivity is depending also on size, shape, and distribution of the dispersed particles. Nonideal behavior of thermal exchange between the solid particles surface and the liquid phase due to temperature drop at the surfaces of both solid particles and liquid phase (transitions surfaces and interfaces at the liquid-solid-liquid and solid-solid interfaces) is created additional sources of the thermal resistance of the solid-liquid system. It is difficult exactly take into account the effect (or contribution) of transition surface and interfaces on the total thermal conductivity of the liquid-solid system.

Main difficulties in developing theoretical models to predict the thermal conductivity of liquid food products are the complexities of the structures and composition. Due to irregularity of the microstructures, accurate theoretical prediction of the thermal conductivity of liquid foods is rather difficult and some time impossible. Existing prediction methods are based on certain simplifications such as particles (spherical or cylindrical) dispersed, simple cubic in a conducting medium (liquid), *etc.* [81,186-209]. Even with a well defined microstructure, the problem remains complex due to the existence of the interface (particle-particle, particle-liquid) resistance. Semi-empirical approach is the only practical way of predicting the thermal conductivity of liquid food products. A large number of theoretical models have been developed for the prediction of thermal conductivity of multiphase systems. Some selected and widely used theoretical models for the thermal conductivity of liquid food products as a function of temperature, concentration and thermal conductivity of solid particles are given below. The thermal conductivity of for spherical particles suspended in a continue fluid phase can be predicted with first Maxwell model [186]

$$\frac{k}{k_f}=\left[\frac{2x+(3-2x)r}{3-x+xr}\right], \tag{39}$$

where $r=(k_S/k_f)$, k_S is the thermal conductivity of suspended particles; x is the void fraction of the discontinuous phase. This relation (Maxwel [186]) is valid at small concentrations, x. Discontinues component is assume in the macro level. Eucken [187] reported the first modification of the Maxwell's model

$$\frac{k}{k_S}=\frac{1+2x\varepsilon}{1-x\varepsilon}, \tag{40}$$

where, $\varepsilon=\dfrac{1-r}{2r+1}$. Other modifications of the Maxwell's model in the improved form are given below together with models based on the mixing-law

$$k=k_f\left[\frac{1-2kx+kF}{1+kx+kF}\right], \quad \text{extended Maxwell's model,} \tag{41}$$

$$k = \left(k_f - k_S\right)/\left(k_S + 2k_f\right);\ F = 1.65\left[\left(k_S - k_f\right)/\left(k_S + 4k_f/3\right)x^{10/3}\right], \quad (42)$$

$$k_{max} = xk_f + \left(1 - x\right)k_S \text{ ,first order arithmetic mean (parallel model)}, \quad (43)$$

$$\frac{k}{k_f} = x + \left(1 - x\right)r - \frac{x\left(1 - x\right)\left(1 - 2r + r^2\right)}{3\left[x + \left(1 - x\right)r\right]}, \text{ second order arithmetic mean}, \quad (44)$$

$$k = k_f^x k_S^{(1-x)} \text{ or } \frac{k}{k_f} = r^{(1-x)}, \text{ first order geometric mean}, \quad (45)$$

$$\frac{k}{k_f} = exp\left[\left(1 - x\right)ln\,r + \frac{x\left(1 - x\right)}{6}\left(ln\,r\right)^2\right], \text{ second order geometric mean}, \quad (46)$$

$$\frac{k}{k_f} = \frac{1}{x + \left(1 - x\right)r} + \frac{2x\left(1 - x\right)\left(1 - 1/r\right)}{3\left[x + \left(1 - x\right)/r\right]}, \text{ second order harmonic mean (Brown [217])}, \quad (47)$$

$$k_{min} = \left[\frac{\left(1 - x\right)}{k_S} + \frac{x}{k_f}\right]^{-1}, \text{ first order harmonic mean (series model)}, \quad (48)$$

$$\frac{k}{k_f} = \left[\frac{2r^2\left(1 - x\right) + \left(1 + 2x\right)r}{\left(2 + x\right)r + 1 - x}\right],$$ second Maxwell model for random distributed spherical fluid-filled voids, (49)

$$k = \left[\left(1 + x\right)k_f + 2\left(1 - x\right)k_S\right]\left[2 + x + \left(1 - x\right)k_f/k_S\right]^{-1},$$ for a spherical assemblage, solid cubic grains Waff [188], (50).

In the present work these models were applied for thermal conductivity of fruit juices. The results for some selected fruit juices are presented in Figs. 17 to 23. In these models the thermal conductivity of liquid foods is a function of thermal conductivity of constitutes (thermal conductivity of solid dispersed particles k_S and continue fluid (water) k_w) and concentration x.

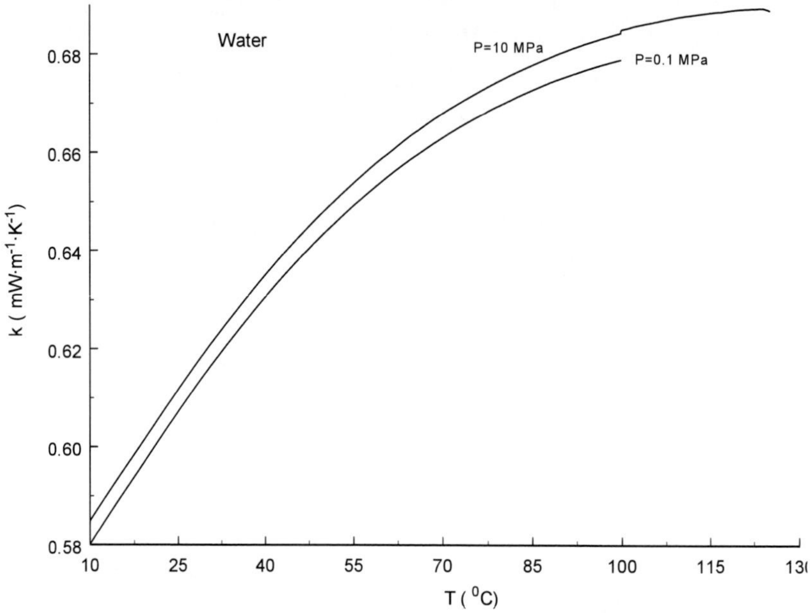

Fig. 28. Temperature dependence of the thermal conductivity of water along various selected isobars calculated with IAPWS formulation (Kestin *et al.*, [95]).

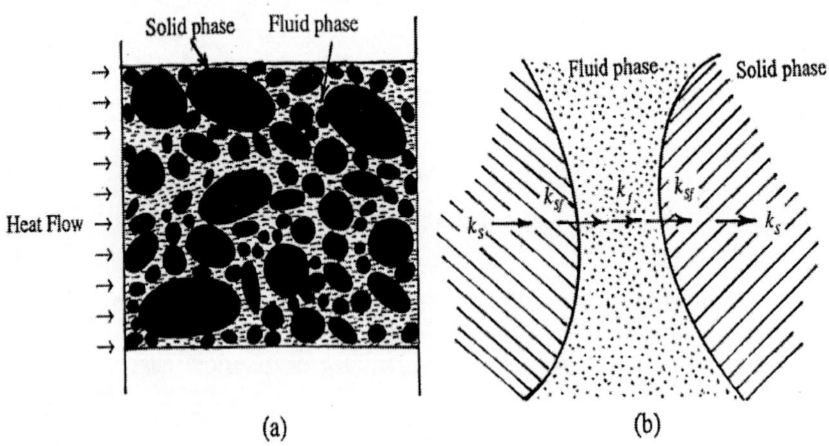

Fig. 29. Schematic model of heat transfer in solid – liquid system.

Mixing-law models (parallel, series, first and second order geometric, second order arithmetic and harmonic means models) were used by many authors to estimate the thermal conductivity of liquid food products. These models combine the values of the thermal conductivity of the solid particles (k_S) with the conductivity of the continued liquid phase (k_w) on the basis of concentration, *i.e.* representing the concentration dependency of the thermal conductivity of liquid –solid suspended systems relative to components constituting the liquid food product (k_S and k_w). It is reasonable to assume that the structural models (Eqs. 39-50) discussed above are holds at any fixed temperatures. The temperature dependence of the thermal conductivity can be considered through temperature dependencies of the $k_S(T)$ and $k_w(T)$. These models are of a general character and can be used for all types of liquid food products. These models are based on using various ways of averaging thermal conductivity of components (solid particles k_S and liquid k_w) with respect to their volume fractions, such as geometric mean model or fabric model. Although mixing-rules less stringent than Maxwell-law models, provide convenient predictions for the physical limits of the thermal conductivity. The physical limits for the thermal conductivity of the solid-particles suspended systems are very well established (see Eqs. 43 and 48, Fig. 31). Mixing-law models do not take into account the structural characteristics of liquid food products; therefore, they are limited applicability.

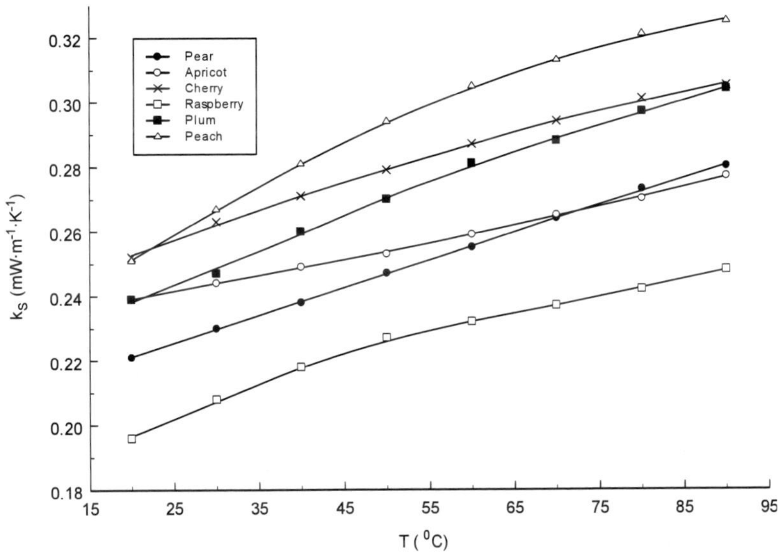

Fig. 30. Temperature dependence of $k_S(T)$ for some selected fruit juices.

The thermal conductivity is most sensitive to interface geometry if the solid-fluid conductivity ratio is large. The predictive capability of the models essentially depends on how they representing of the microstructure of the juice. The thermal conductivity of small to modest solid-fluid conductivity ratio (k_S / k_w) media can be predicted with reasonable accuracy, while our understanding of heat conduction in large solid–fluid conductivity ratio still is incomplete. Based on the fact that a liquid food is composed of solid suspended particles and continue liquid phase, many researches (see for example [153,129,134,151,163,161,210-212]) have developed the models for prediction of the thermal conductivity from concentration and solid and fluid thermal conductivity data. In developing these models, it was basically assumed that the process of transferring heat in liquid foods involves the following: (1) heat conduction through solid suspended particles; (2) heat conduction through the contact region between solid particles (protein, fat, carbohydrate, dietary fiber, ash, and miner content); and (3) heat conduction through fluid (water). Thus, the thermal conductivity in liquid food is a result of conduction in the solid, contact region, and fluid phases (see schematic Fig. 29).

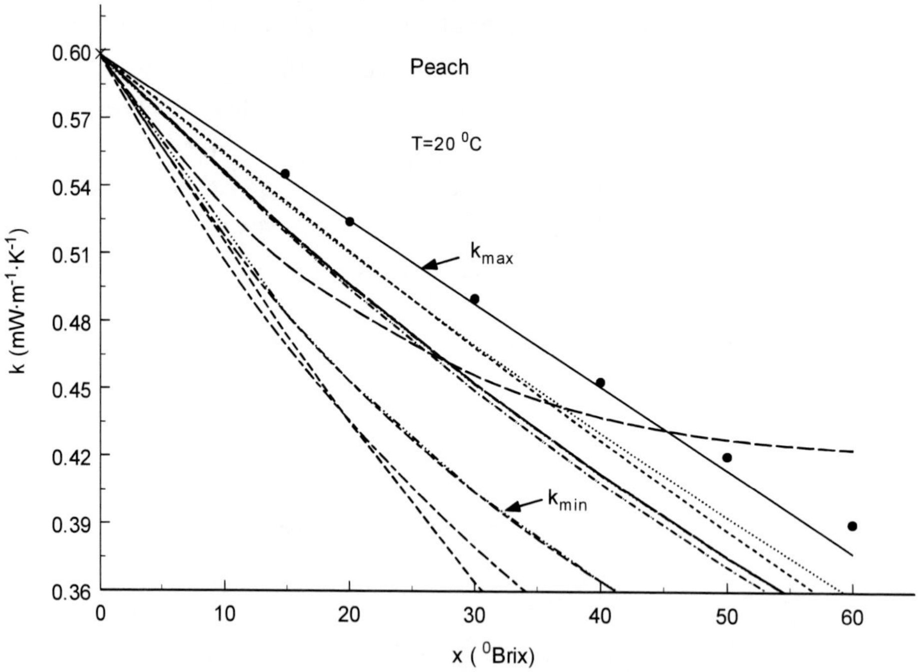

Fig. 31. Thermal conductivity of peach juice as a function of concentration predicted from various theoretical models together with measured values. (•), experiment (Magerramov *et al.* [76]); (———), first order arithmetic mean (parallel model, Eq. 43); (· · · · · ·), Maxwell model (Eq. 39); (–· – ·– ·–), first order geometric mean (Eq. 45); (------), second order geometric mean (Eq. 46); (— — —), Rzhevskii and Novik [219] model; (–··–··–··–), Ziman [218] model; (— — — — —), second order harmonic mean (Brown [217], Eq. 47); (– – – – –), Lichtencker and Rother [216] model; (.......), Waff [188] model (Eq. 50).

In order to develop the theoretical equation for thermal conductivity, the heat transfer through a dispersed medium can be considered at in a manner analogous to an electrical circuit made up of the following resistances: (a) resistance to conduction of heat through solid particles; (b) contact resistance between solid particles and between solid and liquid contact surface area; (c) resistance to conduction through fluid phase where solid particles suspended. How these resistances contribute to the total resistance (or conductance) of a natural liquid food is the main problem of the prediction techniques of the thermal conductivity of liquid food products.

The Maxwell model (see above Eq. 39) restricted to large concentrations. This model is appropriate for the low concentrations (x<20 %). Maxwell considered dilute suspension of solid particles in continue liquid phase. When the values of $\left(k_S / k_w\right)$ is large, these models give large different results between measured and predicted values. According to the relation for thermal conductivity of dispersions of spheroids (Fricke [189]), the spherical particles are caused the minimum changes in thermal conductivity (see also Fig. 31). The prediction capability of the Fricke's model is good (within 5-6 %). Maxwell model restricted to small concentration of solid particles and at large values of $\left(k_S / k_w\right)$ ratio becomes equal to Waff

[188] model. Eucken [187] first modified Maxwell's equation (see Eq. 40). At $(k_S / k_w) \to \infty$ Eucken's model reduced to Buntebarth and Schopper [213].

The results of application of some models to the thermal conductivity data for fruit juices are given in Figs. 18 through 23, and 31. In these figures the wide used structural thermal conductivity models predictions are plotted and compared with the present measurements for peach, pear, apple, orange, and grape juices. The predictive capability of the models strongly depends on the solid-liquid conductivity ratio (k_S / k_w). Aichlmayr and Kulacki [214] reviewed and classified all of the available theoretical models for the thermal conductivity into three different groups: 1. Small solid-fluid conductivity ratio ($1 \leq k_S / k_w \leq 10$); 2. Intermediate solid-fluid conductivity ratio ($10 \leq k_S / k_w \leq 10^3$); 3. Large solid-fluid conductivity ratio ($10^3 \leq k_S / k_w$). In the present work we studied the applicability and predictive capability of the various models for the thermal conductivity of liquid foods with small solid-fluid conductivity ratio, $(k_S / k_w) \approx 0.2\text{-}0.3$.

Three commonly used, basic mixing-law models (see above Eqs. 39-50) are the arithmetic mean, geometric mean, and harmonic mean. The harmonic and arithmetic mean models are based on parallel and series arrangements of the components relative to the direction of heat flow (the electric field analogy). The values of thermal conductivity estimated by these models are assumed as the upper ($k_{\max}$, Eq. 43, first order arithmetic mean, parallel model), and lower ($k_{\min}$, Eq. 48, first order harmonic mean) limits of the thermal conductivity for a liquid foods of given composition (see Fig.31). *Hashin and Strickman* [215] modified the boundary of the mixing-law models

$$k_{\min} = k_w + \frac{1-x}{[1/(k_S - k_w)] + x/3k_w} \text{ and } k_{max} = k_S + \frac{x}{[1/(k_w - k_S)] + (1-x)/3k_S}. \tag{51}$$

The geometric mean model (Eq. 45) gives an intermediate value of the arithmetic and harmonic means. Figure 31 shows the comparison between the measured values of the thermal conductivity and the values of $k_{\max}$ and $k_{\min}$ predicted with various models. Our experimental result is very close (deviation within 0.1-0.2 %) to the $k_{\max}$ predicted with Eq. 43 (first order arithmetic mean). Therefore, the arithmetic mean model is the most realistic of these models for liquid foods. The minimum values of the predicted thermal conductivity, $k_{\min}$ with geometric model lower than $k_{\min}$ by Walsh and Decker [222], while $k_{\max}$ predicted by arithmetic model is higher than $k_{\max}$ by Walsh and Decker [222] model. Walsh's model for the thermal conductivity considerable narrowing the boundary between $k_{\max}$ and $k_{\min}$.

Majority of predicted values of thermal conductivity by various models are lower than measured values. For example, the value of thermal conductivity predicted by Lichtenecker and Rother [216] and second order harmonic mean (Brown [217]) models lower than the present results by 14-35 %, while the models by Ziman [218] and Buntebarth and Schopper [213] are lower by 12-25 %. Two models Maxwell (Eq. 39) and second order arithmetic mean (Eq. 44) are predict the thermal conductivity of liquid foods which is agree with the measured values within 1.5 to 7 %. The second order geometric mean (Eq. 46) and Rzhevskii and Novik [219] models are predicts the thermal conductivity within 5-10 %. Deviation within 7 % was found between the measured and predicted by Waff [188] (Eq. 50).

4.2.3.2. Thermal conductivity of continue phase

In order to apply the structural models (see above Eqs. 41 to 50) to predict the thermal conductivity of liquid-solid suspended systems the accurate thermal conductivity data of continued phase (water) and suspended phase (solid particles) are require. In order to calculate the thermal conductivity of the pure water at high temperatures and at atmospheric pressures we used the internationally accepted (International Association for the Properties of Water and Steam, IAPWS standard) reference data reported by Kestin *et al.* [95]. The thermal conductivity of water at atmospheric pressure as a function of temperature can be also calculated with the simplified equation by (Nieto de Castro *et al.* [220])

$$k_w(T) = -0.76825 + 2.24957(T/298) - 0.874095(T/298)^2 . \qquad (52)$$

The maximum deviation of the experimental data employed, from the Eq. (52) is 1.1 %. This equation is valid at temperatures from 274 to 360 K. In order to calculate of the thermal conductivity of pure water at high temperatures (from 251.17 to 1275.00 K) and at high pressures (up to 1000 MPa) the IAPWS formulation Kestin *et al.* [95] was used. Figure 28 shows the thermal conductivity of water as a function of temperature along the two selected constant pressures calculated with IAPWS formulation Kestin *et al.* [95]. As this figure shows, thermal conductivity of water at high pressures (above atmospheric pressure) monotonically increase with temperature increasing up to 420-470 K (depending on pressure), goes through the maximum and then decrease at high temperatures.

4.2.3.3. Thermal conductivity of non-continuous phase

The thermal conductivity of fruit juices is influenced by not only the water content but also the chemical compositions of the suspended solid particles *i.e.* the protein, fat, carbohydrate, dietary fiber, and miner content. Consider a fruit juice with two components, water and solid (dissolved or suspended particles, see Fig. 29). The major liquid food components are carbohydrates (dextrose, lactose, sugar, and starch), fiber (cellulose and pectin), and salts. The accurate thermal conductivity data for major food components (such as protein, fat, carbohydrate, fiber, and ash) are reported by Choi and Okos [8] and Saravacos and Maroulis [13] as a function of temperature. The predictive capability of the structural models essentially depends on the accuracy of thermal conductivity of solid particles. Rahman [184] proposed correlation equation for the temperature dependence of the thermal conductivity of major food components (protein, gelatin, carbohydrate, starch, sucrose, fat, fiber, ash)

$$k_S = b_0 + b_1 T + b_2 T^2 + b_3 T^3 . \tag{53}$$

However, the thermal conductivity of some components (for example protein, carbohydrate) depends on their chemical and physical form. Therefore, the temperature dependence of the thermal conductivity of liquid food products strongly depends on chemical composition of the liquid foods. Since the chemical components of liquid food materials are imperfect, the solid particle thermal conductivity can be estimated from experimental $k - x$ curves at each measured constant temperature using linear extrapolating procedure low concentration data to the concentration of 100 %. The axis intercept is equal to the values of $k_S(T)$. The derived values of $k_S(T)$ for some fruit juices were fitted to the following correlation equation (see also Fig. 30 and Table 11)

$$k_S(T) = a_0 + a_1 T . \tag{54}$$

Table 11. Thermal conductivity (W m^{-1} K^{-1}) of dispersed solid particles k_S (fractions) as a function of temperature

T, K	Pear	Apricot	Peach	Plum	Raspberry	Cherry
293.15	0.221	0.239	0.251	0.239	0.196	0.252
303.15	0.230	0.244	0.267	0.247	0.208	0.263
313.15	0.238	0.249	0.281	0.260	0.218	0.271
323.15	0.247	0.253	0.294	0.270	0.227	0.279
333.15	0.255	0.259	0.305	0.281	0.232	0.287
343.15	0.264	0.265	0.313	0.288	0.237	0.294
353.15	0.273	0.270	0.321	0.297	0.242	0.301
363.15	0.280	0.277	0.325	0.304	0.248	0.305
Coefficients of Eq. (54)						
$a_1 \times 10^2$	-2.8203	8.1989	-6.3955	-4.2082	-1.2637	2.9623
$a_2 \times 10^3$	0.8508	0.5331	1.0924	0.9609	0.7270	0.7675

As one can see from Table 11, the values of k_S at 20 °C for all studied juices varied within 0.221-0.252 W/(m·K). These values of k_S are very close to the values reported by Constenla *et al.* [133] and Riedel [67] for sucrose (0.209 W/(m·K)) and glucose (0.214 W/(m·K)). For orange and apple juices the value of k_S is 0.294 W/(m·K) and 0.317 W/(m·K), respectively (Frandas and Bicanic [130]). This is still good agreement; because the experimental values of k_S include not only sucrose and glucose, but the effective thermal conductivity from all solid particles (protein, fat, carbohydrate, fiber, and ash *etc.*). The values of $k_S(T)$ can be also estimated from components of a juice, especially protein, fat, carbohydrate (dextrose, lactose, sugar, and starch), fiber (cellulose and pectin), salt, and ash. Since ash and sucrose has relative significantly larger thermal conductivity than the other components (0.35-0.45 $W \cdot m^{-1} \cdot K^{-1}$) the ash and sucrose content is the dominant factor in the thermal conductivity of the liquid foods. Most liquid foods contain a predominance of ash and sucrose.

The mechanism of heat transfer in liquid food products is complicated by the irregularity of the microstructure. In most liquid foods, heat is propagated by the thermal conductivity through the suspended solid particles and continued liquid phase (water). In general, the total thermal conductivity in multiphase materials depends on the thermal conductivity of each phase, the fractions of the phases, and the way in which the phases are distributed (structure). The distribution of the phases includes theirs size, shape, orientation, continuity relative to the heat flow direction. There are a number of models for the prediction of the thermal conductivity which are based on theoretical studies (see above). The theoretical models are based on the mechanism of heat transfer applicable (heat transfer theory) to simplified geometries of the liquid-solid system. The difficulty with these models is the degree of simplification necessary to obtain a solution. There is still a lack of detailed knowledge of how the heat is transferred through liquid food products, and in particular, at the transitions surfaces and interfaces at the liquid-solid-liquid and solid-solid interfaces (see Fig. 29). Preferably, one would use a theoretical model to describe the physical nature of mechanism of the heat conduction, but sufficiently reliable models have not yet beet developed, and empirical modifications of the equations are needed.

5. Conclusions

Comprehensive compilations all of the available thermal conductivity data for liquid food products (fruit and vegetable juices, oils, milks) and biological fluids are provided. The comprehensive review on the available experimental data sets on thermal conductivity liquid foods in the wide temperature and concentration ranges, critical analyses of the estimation, correlation, and prediction methods, to select more reliable data sets and to give some preliminary recommendations for scientific and applied used is provided.

The combined effect of temperature and concentration on the thermal conductivity of liquid foods was studied. New correlation and prediction models for the thermal conductivity of liquid food products were developed. The applicability and predictive capability of the various theoretical models used previously for aqueous solutions and solid particles suspended systems to describe the effect of temperature and concentration on thermal conductivity was examined. It was found that the prediction Model-20, $k(T) = k_{sol}(T_0)\,[k_W(T)/k_W(T_0)]$, can be adopted satisfactorily for fruit juices. The AAD between measured and calculated from predicting model for the thermal conductivity of juices were within 0.2 to 1.5 %. Therefore, minimal experimental information is needed to predict the thermal conductivity of juices as a function of temperature and concentration. The thermal conductivity of juices can be calculate just by knowing the single thermal conductivity $k_{sol}(T_0)$ of juice at a reference temperature T_0=20 °C and pure water data $k_W(T)$. This makes it much easier to predict the thermal conductivity of fruit juices.

Model-A to C can be recommended to accurate represent experimental thermal conductivity data for fruit juices in wide temperature and concentration ranges.

The simple model for the predicting of combined effect of temperature and concentration on the thermal conductivity of fruit juices was developed. It was found that the prediction Model-D, $k(T,x)/k(T_0,x)=(T/T_0)^n$, developed in this work can be adopted with satisfaction. The AAD between measured and calculated values from predicting model for the thermal conductivity of juices were within 0.36 to 0.8 %. The thermal conductivity of juices can be predicted just by knowing the thermal conductivity k_0 at a reference temperature T_0. This makes it easier to predict the thermal conductivity of fruit juices. The structural models based on the mixing-law and Maxwell-law can be also successfully used to predict the thermal conductivity of liquid food products. Best result can be archived by using the first order arithmetic mean (parallel model) model with accurate knowing the solid particles (protein, fat, carbohydrate, dietary fiber, and miner content) thermal conductivity (k_S).

Appendix

Experimental Thermal Conductivity Data for Fruit Juices

Table 1. Experimental thermal conductivity (W m^{-1} K^{-1}) of pear juice as a function of temperature and concentration

T (K)	14°Brix	19°Brix	25°Brix	30°Brix	40°Brix	50°Brix
293.15	0.545	0.526	0.503	0.485	0.450	0.408
303.15	0.553	0.535	0.511	0.493	0.458	0.417
313.15	0.561	0.543	0.519	0.500	0.466	0.425
323.15	0.568	0.551	0.526	0.508	0.473	0.433
333.15	0.575	0.558	0.534	0.514	0.480	0.441
343.15	0.581	0.565	0.540	0.521	0.487	0.448
353.15	0.587	0.571	0.547	0.527	0.493	0.456
363.15	0.593	0.576	0.553	0.532	0.499	0.462
373.15*	0.598	0.581	0.559	0.538	0.504	0.469
383.15*	0.603	0.585	0.564	0.542	0.508	0.476
393.15*	0.607	0.589	0.568	0.547	0.513	0.481

Table 2. Experimental thermal conductivity (W m^{-1} K^{-1}) of sweet-cherry juice as a function of temperature and concentration

T (K)	14.3°Brix	20°Brix	27°Brix	35°Brix	45°Brix	50°Brix
293.15	0.525	0.505	0.480	0.454	0.415	0.401
303.15	0.538	0.516	0.491	0.464	0.426	0.410
313.15	0.549	0.527	0.501	0.473	0.436	0.420
323.15	0.560	0.537	0.511	0.482	0.445	0.429
333.15	0.570	0.546	0.521	0.491	0.454	0.438
343.15	0.579	0.555	0.529	0.498	0.462	0.447
353.15	0.587	0.563	0.537	0.507	0.471	0.455
363.15	0.594	0.569	0.545	0.514	0.478	0.463
373.15*	0.601	0.576	0.552	0.522	0.485	0.470
383.15*	0.607	0.582	0.558	0.528	0.492	0.478
393.15*	0.612	0.586	0.564	0.534	0.498	0.484

Table 3. Experimental thermal conductivity (W m^{-1} K^{-1}) of cherry-plum juice as a function of temperature and concentration

T (K)	12.2°Brix	18°Brix	24°Brix	30°Brix	40°Brix	50°Brix
293.15	0.543	0.518	0.495	0.472	0.434	0.398
303.15	0.552	0.527	0.504	0.481	0.443	0.407
313.15	0.560	0.536	0.512	0.489	0.451	0.416
323.15	0.568	0.545	0.520	0.497	0.460	0.424
333.15	0.577	0.553	0.528	0.504	0.467	0.432
343.15	0.584	0.560	0.535	0.511	0.474	0.440
353.15	0.593	0.568	0.542	0.518	0.481	0.447
363.15	0.600	0.573	0.548	0.524	0.488	0.455
373.15*	0.606	0.580	0.554	0.530	0.494	0.462
383.15*	0.613	0.585	0.560	0.535	0.500	0.468
393.15*	0.618	0.590	0.565	0.540	0.505	0.474

Table 4. Experimental thermal conductivity (W m^{-1} K^{-1}) of apricot juice as a function of temperature and concentration

T (K)	18.5°Brix	25°Brix	30°Brix	35°Brix	40°Brix	50°Brix
293.15	0.525	0.498	0.480	0.461	0.444	0.415
303.15	0.536	0.509	0.490	0.471	0.453	0.424
313.15	0.546	0.519	0.499	0.480	0.462	0.432
323.15	0.556	0.529	0.508	0.489	0.470	0.440
333.15	0.565	0.538	0.517	0.497	0.478	0.448
343.15	0.573	0.546	0.525	0.505	0.486	0.455
353.15	0.581	0.554	0.533	0.513	0.494	0.462
363.15	0.588	0.562	0.540	0.520	0.501	0.469
373.15*	0.595	0.568	0.547	0.527	0.508	0.476
383.15*	0.601	0.574	0.554	0.534	0.515	0.481
393.15*	0.606	0.580	0.560	0.540	0.521	0.487

Table 5. Experimental thermal conductivity (W m^{-1} K^{-1}) of peach juice as a function of temperature and concentration

T, K	14.8 °Brix	20°Brix	30°Brix	40°Brix	50°Brix	60°Brix
293.15	0.545	0.524	0.490	0.453	0.420	0.390
303.15	0.553	0.534	0.497	0.464	0.432	0.402
313.15	0.562	0.541	0.507	0.473	0.444	0.413
323.15	0.570	0.548	0.514	0.482	0.454	0.423
333.15	0.576	0.555	0.521	0.490	0.461	0.432
343.15	0.582	0.562	0.528	0.496	0.467	0.440
353.15	0.588	0.568	0.535	0.502	0.475	0.447
363.15	0.595	0.575	0.541	0.506	0.480	0.453
373.15*	0.600	0.580	0.547	0.510	0.484	0.457
383.15*	0.605	0.585	0.553	0.513	0.488	0.460
393.15*	0.610	0.590	0.556	0.517	0.490	0.462

Table 6. Experimental thermal conductivity (W m^{-1} K^{-1}) of plum juice as a function of temperature and concentration

T, K	15.1°Brix	20°Brix	30°Brix	40°Brix	50°Brix	60°Brix
293.15	0.535	0.511	0.469	0.434	0.405	0.380
303.15	0.546	0.524	0.481	0.446	0.417	0.389
313.15	0.555	0.533	0.492	0.457	0.427	0.401
323.15	0.565	0.543	0.503	0.467	0.437	0.411
333.15	0.573	0.550	0.510	0.474	0.445	0.421
343.15	0.583	0.559	0.517	0.481	0.452	0.430
353.15	0.590	0.566	0.526	0.489	0.462	0.437
363.15	0.597	0.575	0.532	0.497	0.468	0.445
373.15*	0.605	0.582	0.540	0.504	0.475	0.453
383.15*	0.611	0.588	0.545	0.510	0.481	0.459
393.15*	0.617	0.593	0.550	0.515	0.486	0.465

Table 7. Experimental thermal conductivity (W m^{-1} K^{-1}) of raspberry juice as a function of temperature and concentration

T, K	9.8 °Brix	15°Brix	20°Brix	30°Brix	40 °Brix	50 °Brix
293.15	0.555	0.529	0.502	0.462	0.425	0.396
303.15	0.564	0.541	0.515	0.472	0.437	0.407
313.15	0.574	0.553	0.525	0.483	0.449	0.417
323.15	0.585	0.563	0.537	0.492	0.459	0.427
333.15	0.595	0.574	0.547	0.501	0.468	0.435
343.15	0.604	0.584	0.556	0.510	0.476	0.443
353.15	0.615	0.591	0.563	0.518	0.483	0.450
363.15	0.620	0.599	0.570	0.526	0.490	0.456

Table 7. Continued

T, K	9.8 °Brix	15°Brix	20°Brix	30°Brix	40 °Brix	50 °Brix
373.15*	0.629	0.605	0.577	0.533	0.495	0.461
383.15*	0.634	0.611	0.582	0.539	0.498	0.466
393.15*	0.640	0.615	0.587	0.545	0.502	0.469

Table 8. Experimental thermal conductivity (W m^{-1} K^{-1}) of cherry juice as a function of temperature and concentration

T, K	15.1 °Brix	20°Brix	30°Brix	40 °Brix	50°Brix	60 °Brix
293.15	0.521	0.502	0.468	0.436	0.406	0.380
303.15	0.532	0.513	0.478	0.447	0.418	0.390
313.15	0.544	0.524	0.489	0.458	0.430	0.399
323.15	0.554	0.535	0.500	0.468	0.440	0.408
333.15	0.565	0.544	0.510	0.477	0.450	0.417
343.15	0.574	0.553	0.520	0.487	0.458	0.425
353.15	0.583	0.562	0.528	0.495	0.467	0.432
363.15	0.592	0.571	0.537	0.503	0.474	0.439
373.15*	0.600	0.579	0.544	0.510	0.481	0.446
383.15*	0.608	0.587	0.551	0.517	0.487	0.451
393.15*	0.615	0.595	0.558	0.523	0.492	0.456

*Slightly above atmospheric pressure (0.3 MPa)

References

[1] Moresi, M.; Spinosi, M. Engineering factors in the production of concentrated fruit juices. 1. Fluid physical properties of orange juices. *J. Food. Technol.* 1980, *15*, 265-276.

[2] Crandall, P.G.; Chen, C.S.; Carter, R.D. Models for predicting viscosity of orange juice concentrate. *Food Technology*1982, *36*, 245-252.

[3] Famelart, M.-H.; Chapron, L.; Piot, M.; Brule, G.; Durier, C. High pressure-induced gel formation of milk and whey concentrates. *J. Food Eng.* 1998, *36*, 149-164.

[4] Farkas, D.F.; Hoover, D.G. High pressure processing. *J. Food Sci. Supplem.* 2000, *65*, 47-64.

[5] Farr, D. High pressure technology in the food industry. *Trends in Food Science & Technology* 1990, 14-16.

[6] Felipe, X.; Capellas, M.; Law, A.J.R. Comparison of the effect of high-pressure treatments and heat pasteurization on the whey proteins in goat's milk. *J. Agr. Food Chem.* 1997, *45*, 627-631.

[7] Wakeham, W.A.; Nagashima, A.; Sengers, J.V. (Editors), *Experimental Thermodynamics. Vol. III. Measurements of the Transport Properties of Fluids.* Blackwell Scientific Publications, Oxford, 1991.

[8] Choi, I.; Okos, M.R. Thermal properties of liquid foods-Review. In: *Physical and Chemical Properties of Food*, Editor M.R. Okos; ASAE: New York, NY, 1986; pp 35-77.

[9] Reidy, G.A.; Rippen, A.L. Methods for determining thermal conductivity in foods. *ASAE Trans.*, 1971, *14*, 248-254.

[10] [10] Reidy, G.A. Methods for determining thermal conductivity and thermal diffusivity of foods. II. Values for thermal properties of foods gathered from the literature. *MS Thesis*. Michigan State University, 1968.

[11] Tabil, L.G., Jr. Thermal conductivity and thermal diffusivity of agricultural and food materials, Ph.D., University of Saskatchewan,

[12] Jowitt, R.; Escher, F.; Hallstrom, B.; Meffert, H.F.Th.; Spiess, M.E.L.; Vos, G. (Editors). Thermal Properties of Foods. Part III. In: *Physical Properties of Foods*. Applied Sciences Publishers, London, 1983.

[13] Saravacos, G.D.; Maroulis, Z.B. *Transport Properties of Foods*; Marcel Dekker, Inc.: New York, NY, 2002.

[14] Mohsenin, N.N. Thermal Properties of Foods and Agricultural Materials. Gordon and Breach Science Publishers. New York, 1980.

[15] Kestin, J.; Wakeham, W.A. *Transport Properties of Fluids. Thermal Conductivity, Viscosity and Diffusion Coefficient*, Ed. by C.Y. Ho, Hemisphere Publ. Corp., New York, Vol. I-1, 1987.

[16] Assael, M.J.; Dix, M.; Lucas, A.B.; Wakeham, W.A. Absolute determination of the thermal conductivity of the noble gases and two of their binary mixtures as a function of density. *J. Chem. Soc. Faraday Trans.* 1981, *77*, 439-464.

[17] Assael, M.J.; Charitidou, E.; Georgiadis, G.P.; Wakeham, W.A. Absolute measurement of the thermal conductivity of electrically conducting liquids. *Ber. Bunsenges. Phys. Chem.* 1988, *92*, 627-631.

[18] Assael, M.J.; Charitidou, E.; Nieto de Castro, C.A. Absolute measurements of the thermal conductivity of alcohols by the transient hot-wire technique. *Int. J. Thermophys.* 1988, *9*, 813-824.

[19] Assael, M.J.; Charitidou, E.; Stassis, J.Ch.; Wakeham, W.A. Absolute measurement of the thermal conductivity of some aqueous chloride solutions. *Ber. Bunsenges. Phys. Chem.* 1989, *93*, 887-892.

[20] Assael, M.J.; Nieto de Castro, C.A.; Roder, H.M.; Wakeham, W.A. In: *Experimental Thermodynamics. III. Measurements of the Transport Properties of Fluids*. W.A. Wakeham, A. Nagashima, and J.V. Sengers, (Eds.), Blackwell Scientific Publications, Oxford, 1991, pp.161-195.

[21] Assael, M.J.; Karagiannidis, L.; Wakeham, W.A. Measurements of the thermal conductivity of R11 and R12 in the temperature range 250–340 K at pressures up to 30 MPa. *Int. J. Thermophys*. 1992, *13*, 735-751.

[22] Assael, M.J.; Karagiannidis, L.; Malamataris, N.; Wakeham, W.A. The transient hot-wire technique: A Numerical approach. *Int. J. Thermophys*. 1998, *19*, 379-389.

[23] Nagasaka, Y.; Nagashima, A. Absolute measurements of the thermal conductivity of electrically conducting liquids by the transient hot-wire method. *J. Phys. E.: Sci. Instrum.* 1981, *14*, 1435-1440.

[24] Nagasaka, Y.; Suziki, J.; Wada, Y.; Nagashima, A. A high-temperature, high-pressure transient hot-wire apparatus for aqueous electrolyte solutions. In: *Proc. 5th Jap. Symp. Thermophys. Prop.*, 1984, 175-178.

[25] Nagasaka, Y.; Hiraiwa H.; Nagashima A. Measurement of the thermal conductivity of liquid D_2O by the transient hot-wire method. In: "*Properties of Water and Steam*", Proc. of the 11th Intern. Conference on the Properties of Steam; eds. M. Pitchel. and O. Sifner; Hemis. Publ. Corp., 1989, pp 125-131.

[26] Mardolcar, U.V.; Fareleira, J.M.N.A.; Nieto de Castro, C.A. *High Temp.- High Press.* 1985, *17*, 469-488.

[27] Palavra, A.M.F.; Wakeham, W. A.; Zalaf, M. Thermal conductivity of n-pentane in the temperature range 306-360 K and at pressures up to 0.5 GPa. *Intern. J. Thermophys.* 1987, *8*, 305-315.

[28] Perkins, R. A.; Laesecke, A.; Nieto de Castro, C.A. Polarized transient hot-wire thermal conductivity measurements. *Fluid Phase Equilib.* 1992, *80*, 275-285.

[29] Perkins, R.A.; Roder, H.M.; Nieto de Castro, C.A. A high-temperature transient hot-wire thermal conductivity apparatus for fluids. *J. Res. Nat. Inst. Stand. Technol.* 1991, *96*, 247-269.

[30] Roder, H.M.; Perkins, R.A. Relation between wire resistance and fluid pressure in the transient hot-wire method. *J. Res. Nat. Inst. Stand. Technol.* 1989, *94*, 113-116.

[31] Roder, H.M.; Perkins, R.A.; Laesecke, A. Absolute steady-state thermal conductivity measurements by use of a transient hot-wire system. *J. Res. Nat. Inst. Stand. Technol.* 2000, *105*, 221-253.

[32] Wakeham, W.A.; Assael, M.J. *Chapter 5. Thermal Conductivity*, in *Handbook of Experimental Fluid Mechanics*, C. Tropea, J. Foss, A. Yarin (eds), Springer–Verlag, 2008, pp. 1-13.

[33] Abdulagatov, I.M.; Assael, M. In: *Hydrothermal Experimental Data. II. Thermodynamic and Transport Properties of Solutions. Thermal Conductity, Chapter 6*, Waley, 2009, in press.

[34] Todd, Q.W. *Proc. Roy. Soc.* A 1909, *83*, 19-39.

[35] Moster, R.; van der Berg, H.R.; van der Gulik, P.S. A guarded parallel-plate instrument for measuring the thermal conductivity of fluids in the critical region. *Rev. Sci. Instr.* 1989, *60*, 3466-3474.

[36] Amirkhanov, Kh.I.; Adamov, A.P. Heat transfer of steam in near critical and subcritical states. *Teploenergetika* 1963, *10*, 69-72.

[37] Amirkhanov, Kh.I.; Adamov, A.P.; Magomedov, U.B. experimental study of the thermal conductivity of heavy water at temperatures 25-350 °C and pressures 0.1-245.3 MN/m^2. *Teplofiz. Visok. Temp.* 1974, *13*, 75-78.

[38] Abdulagatov, I.M.; Magomedov, U.B. Thermal conductivity of aqueous solutions of NaCl and KCl at high pressures. *Intern. J. Thermophys.* 1994, *15*, 401-414.

[39] Abdulagatov, I.M.; Magomedov, U.B. In: "*Physical Chemistry of Aqueous Systems: Meeting the Needs of Industry,* ed. by H.J. White, J.V. Sengers, D.B.Neumann, and J.C.Bellows, Begell Hose, NY, 1995, pp.549-557.

[40] Abdulagatov, I.M.; Magomedov, U.B. Thermal conductivity of aqueous solutions of K_2CO_3 and NaI in the temperature range 298-473 K at pressures up to 100 MPa. In:

Proc. of the 4th Asian Thermophysical Properties Conference. Tokyo, 1995, pp. 499-502.

[41] Abdulagatov, I.M.; Magomedov, U.B. Thermal conductivity of aqueous $CdCl_2$ and $CdBr_2$ solutions from 293 K to 473 K at high pressures up to 100 MPa. *J. Chem. Eng. Data* 1997, *42*, 1165-1169.

[42] Abdulagatov, I.M.; Magomedov, U.B. Measurements of thermal conductivity of aqueous LiCl and LiBr solutions from 293 to 473 pressures up to 100 MPa. *Ber. Bunsenges. Phys. Chem.* 1997, *101*, 708-711.

[43] Abdulagatov, I.M.; Magomedov, U.B. Thermal conductivity of aqueous $ZnCl_2$ solutions at high temperatures and high pressures. *Ind. Eng. Chem. Res.* 1998, *37*, 4883-4888.

[44] Abdulagatov, I.M.; Magomedov, U.B. Thermal conductivity measurements of aqueous $SrCl_2$ and $Sr(NO_3)_2$ solutions in the temperature range between 293 and 473 K at pressures up to 100 MPa. *Int. J. Thermophys.* 1999, *20*, 187-196.

[45] Abdulagatov, I.M.; Magomedov, U.B. Measurements of the thermal conductivity of aqueous $CoCl_2$ solutions at pressures up to 100 MPa by parallel-plate apparatus. *J. Chem. Eng. Japan* 1999, *32*, 465-471.

[46] Abdulagatov, I.M.; Magomedov, U.B. Effect of temperature and pressure on the thermal conductivity of aqueous CaI_2 solutions. *High Temp. – High Press.* 2000, *32*, 599-611.

[47] Abdulagatov, I.M.; Magomedov, U.B. Thermal conductivity of aqueous BaI_2 solutions in the temperature range 293-473 and the pressure range 0.1-100 MPa. *Fluid Phase Equilib.* 2000, *171*, 243-252.

[48] Abdulagatov, I.M.; Magomedov, U.B. Thermal conductivity of aqueous KI and KBr solutions at high temperatures and high pressures. *J. Sol. Chem.* 2001, *30*, 223 -235.

[49] Abdulagatov, I.M.; Magomedov, U.B. Thermal conductivity of pure water and aqueous $SrBr_2$ solutions at high temperatures and high pressures. *High Temp. – High Press.* 2003/2004, *35/36*, 149-168.

[50] Sirota, A.M.; Latunin, V.I.; Belyaeva, G.M. An experimental investigation of the thermal conductivity maximu of water in the critical region. *Teploenergetika* 1974, *10*, 52-58.

[51] Sengers, J.V. Thermal conductivity measurements at elevated gas densities including the critical region. *Dissertation*, University Amsterdam, Amsterdam, 1962.

[52] [52] Michels, A.; Sengers, J.V.; van der Gulik, P.S. The thermal conductivity of carbon dioxide in the critical region. Part II-Measurements and conclusion. *Physica* 1962, *28*, 1201-1215.

[53] Michels, A.; Sengers, J.V.; van de Klundert, L.J.M. The thermal conductivity of argon at elevated gas densities. *Physica* 1963, *29*, 149-160.

[54] Guseynov, G.G. In: *Thermophysical Properties of Substances and Aqueous Electrolyte Solutions*, Institute of Physics of the DSC of the Russian Academy of Sciences, Makhachkala, 1987, pp.51-56.

[55] Guseynov, G.G. In: *Thermophysical Properties of Substances and Solutions*, Inst. Fiziki, Dag. FAN SSSR, Makhachkala, 1989, pp.67-74.

[56] Gitterman, M. *Hydrodynamics of fluids near a critical point.* Rev. Mod. Phys. *1978,* 50, *85-106.*

[57] De Groot, S.R.; Mazur, P. *Nonequlibrium Thermodynamics*, North – Holland Publishing Co., Amsterdam, 1962.

[58] Dietz, F.J.; de Groot, J.J.; Franck, E. F. *Ber. Bunsenges. Phys. Chem.* 1981, *85*, 1005-1009.

[59] Sirota, A.M. In: *Experimental Thermodynamics. III. The Measurement of Transport Properties of Fluids*, W.A. Wakeham, A. Nagashima and J.V. Sengers, eds., Blackwell Scientific, Oxford, 1991, pp.142-160.

[60] Yusufova, V.D.; Pepinov, R.I.; Nikolaev, V.A.; Guseynov, G.M. Thermal conductivity of aqueous NaCl solutions. *Inzh.-Fizich. Zh.* 1975, *9*, 600-605.

[61] Yusufova, V.D.; Pepinov, R.I.; Nikolaev, V.A.; Guseynov, G.M. Thermal conductivity of aqueous Na_2SO_4 solutions. *Zh. Fizich. Khim.* 1975, *49*, 2677-2679.

[62] Pepinov, R.L.; Guseynov, G.M. Thermal conductivity of aqueous KCl solutions at temperatures 200-340 °C. *Inzhen.-Fizich. Zh.* 1991, *60*, 742-747.

[63] Pepinov, R.L.; Guseynov, G.M. Experimental study of the thermal conductivity of aqueous KCl solutions at high temperatures. *Teplofiz. Visok. Temp.* 1991, *29*, 605-607.

[64] Pepinov, R.I.; Guseynov, G.M. Thermal conductivity of aqueous LiCl, KCl, and $CaCl_2$ solutions at high temperatures and pressures. In: "*Geotermiya, Geologich. i Teplofizich. Zadachi*", Institute of Geothermal Problems, Dagestan Scientific Center of the Russian Academy of Sciences, Makhachkala, 1992, pp. 204-211.

[65] Pepinov, R.I.; Guseynov, G.M. Thermal conductivity of aqueous LiCl solutions at high temperatures. *Zh. Fizich. Khim.* 1993, *67*, 1101-1103.

[66] Gratão, A.C.A.; Júnior, V.S.; Polizelli, M.A.; Telis-Romero, J. Thermal properties of passion fruit juice as affected by temperature and water content. *J Food Process Eng.* 2005, *27*, 413-431.

[67] Riedel, L. Thermal conductivity measurement on sugar solutions, fruit juices and milk. *Chem-Ing-Technik*, 1949, *21*, 340-341.

[68] Minim, L.A.;, Coimbra, J.S.R.; Minim, V.P.R.; Telis-Romero, J. Influence of temperature and water and fat contents on the thermophysical properties of milk. *J. Chem. Eng. Data* 2002, *47*, 1488-1491.

[69] Fernández-Martine, F.; Montes, F. Influence of temperature and composition on some physical properties of milk and milk concentrates. III. Thermal conductivity. *Milchwissenschaft* 1972, *27*, 772-776.

[70] Tadini, C.C.; Telis, V.R.N.; Telis-Romero, J. Influence of temperature and concentration on thermophysical properties of Caja juice (Spondia mombin, L). *Eurotherm Seminar 77- Heat and Mass Transfer in Food Processing*, Parma, Italy, June 20-22, 2005.

[71] Pedro, M.A.M.; Telis, V.R.N.; Telis-Romero, J. Transport and thermodynamic properties of lemon juice as affected by temperature and water content. *J. Chem. Eng. Data* 2008 in press.

[72] Assis, M.M.; Lannes, S.C.S.; Tadini, C.C.; Telis, V.R.N.; Telis-Romero, J. Influenece of temperature and concentration on thermophysical properties of yellow mombin (*Spondias mombin*, L.). *European Food Res. Technol.* 2006, *223*, 585-593.

[73] Coimbra, J.S.R.; Gabas, A.L.; Minim, L.A.; Garcia Rojas, E.E.; Telis, V.R.N.; Telis-Romero, J. Density, heat capacity and thermal conductivity of liquid egg products. *J. Food Eng.* 2006, *74*, 186-190.

[74] Telis-Romero, J.; Telis, V.R.N.; Gabas, A.L.; Yamashita, F. Thermophysical properties of Brazilian orange juice as affected by temperature and water content. *J. Food. Eng.* 1998, *38*, 27-40.

[75] Xu, S.; Lin, Q.; Chen, X.D.; Chen, Z.D.; Bandopadhayay, P. Shear rate dependent thermal conductivity measurement of two fruit juice concentrates. *J. Food Eng.* 2003, *57*, 217-224

[76] Magerramov, M.A.; Abdulagatov, A.I.; Azizov, N.D.; Abdulagatov, I.M. Thermal conductivity of peach, raspberry, cherry, and plum juices as a function of temperature and concentration. *J. Food Process Engineering* 2006, *29*, 304-326.

[77] gerramov, M.A.; Abdulagatov, A.I.; Azizov, N.D.; Abdulagatov, I.M. Thermal conductivity of pear, sweet-cherry, apricot, and cherry-plum juices as a function of temperature and concentration. *J. Food Sci. E. -Food Engineering and Physical Properties* 2006, *71*, 238-244.

[78] Keller, G.J.; Ballard, J.H. Predicting temperature changes in frozen liquids. *Ind. Eng. Sci.* 1956, *48*, 188-196.

[79] Woolf, J.F.; Sibbitt, W.L. Thermal conductivity of liquids. *Ind. Eng. Chem.* 1954, *46*, 1947-1952.

[80] Telis-Romero, J.; Gabas, A.L.; Polizelli, M.A.; Telis, V.R.N. Temperature and water content influence on thermophysical properties of coffee extract. Int. J. Food Prop. 2000, *3*, 375-384.

[81] Fikkin, K.A.; Fikiin, A.G. Prediction equation for thermophysical properties and enthalpy during cooling and freezing of ffod materials. *J. Food Engineering* 1999, *40*, 1-6.

[82] Vargaftik, N. B.; Smirnova, Y. V. On the temperature dependency of water vapor heat conductivity. *Zh. Tekh. Fiz.* 1956, *26*, 1221-1231.

[83] Ziebland, H. The thermal conductivity of nitrogen and argon in the liquid and gaseous states. *Brit. J. Appl. Phys.* 1958, *9*, 52-59.

[84] Ziebland, H.; Burton, J.T.A. Thermal conductivity of heavy water between 75 °C and 260 °C at pressures up to 300 atm. *Int. J. Heat Mass Transfer* 1960, *1*, 242-254.

[85] Vines, R.G. Measurement of thermal conductivity of gases at high temperatures. *J. Heat Transfer C* 1960, *82*, 48-52.

[86] Bailey, B.J.; Kellner, K. The thermal conductivity of argon near the critical point. *Brit. J. Appl. Phys.* 1967, *18*, 1645-1647.

[87] Le Neindre, B. Contribution àl'étude expérimentale de la conductivité thermique de quelques fluids a haute température et à haute pression. *Ph. D. Thesis*, Paris University, Paris, 1969.

[88] Le Neindre, B.; Garrabos, Y.; Tufeu, R. *Ber. Bunsenges. Phys. Chem.* 1984, *88*, 916-920.

[89] Le Neindre, B.; Bury, P.; Tufeu, R.; Vodar, B. Thermal conductivity of water and heavy water in the liquid state up to 370 °C. *J. Chem. Eng. Data* 1976, *21*, 265-274.

[90] Johannin, P. J. *Rech. Centre Nat. Rech. Sci.* 1958, *43*, 116-155.

[91] Abdulagatov, I.M.; Akhmedova-Azizova, L.A.; Azizov, N.D. hermal conductivity of aqueous $Sr(NO_3)_2$ and $LiNO_3$ solutions at high temperatures and high pressures. *J. Chem. Eng. Data* 2004, *49*, 688-704.

[92] Abdulagatov, I.M.; Akhmedova-Azizova, L.A.; Azizov, N.D. Thermal conductivity of binary aqueous NaBr and KBr and ternary H_2O+NaBr+KBr solutions at temperatures from 294 to 577 K and pressures up to 40 MPa. *J. Chem. Eng. Data* 2004, *49*, 1727-1737.

[93] Abdulagatov, I.M.; Azizov, N.D. Thermal conductivity and viscosity of the aqueous K_2SO_4 solutions at temperatures from 298 to 573 K and at pressures up to 30 MPa. *Intern. J. Thermophys.* 2005, *26*, 593-635.

[94] Gershuni, G. Z. Thermal convection in the space between vertical coaxial cylinders. *Dokl. Akad. Nauk SSSR* 1952, *86*, 697-698.

[95] Kestin, J.; Sengers, J. V.; Kamgar-Parsi, B.; Levelt Sengers, J. M. H. Thermophysical Properties of Fluid H_2O. *J. Phys. Chem. Ref. Data* 1984, *13*, 175-189.

[96] El'darov, V.S. Thermal conductivity of aqueous salt solutions. *Zh. Fizich. Khimii* 1980, *54*, 606-609.

[97] Eldarov, V.S. *Ph.D. Thesis*, Azer. State Institute of Oil and Chemistry, Baku, 1982.

[98] Eldarov, V.S. Thermal conductivity of aqueous solutions of nitrate salts. *Zh. Fizich. Khimii* 1986, *60*, 603-605.

[99] Eldarov, V.S.; Vakhabov, I.I.; Akhmedova, R.E. Study of thermal conductivity in ternary aqueous salt ($MgCl_2$ and$MgSO_4$) solutions. *Izv. Vyssh. Ucheb. Zaved., ser. Neft i Gaz.* 1992, *3-4*, 65-68.

[100] Eldarov, V.S.; Vakhabov, I.I.; Babaeva, S.Sh.; Akhmedova, R.E.; Yakubova, I.N. Analysis of studies of thermal conductivity in multi-component aqueous salt solutions. *Izv. Vissh. Ucheb. Zaved., ser. Neft i Gaz.* 1992, *9/10*, 59-62.

[101] Eldarov, V.S.; Babaeva, S.Sh.; Vakhabov, I.I.; Mirzoev, Kh.M.; Akhmedova, R.E. Thermal conductivity of mixed aqueous electrolyte solutions. In: *Geotermiya, Geologich. i Teplofiz. Zadachi,* Geothermal Res. Institute, DSC RAN, Makhachkala, 1992, pp.188-193.

[102] Eldarov, V.S.; Abdullaeva, G.K.; Yakubova, I.N.; Vakhabov, I.I.; Gafarova, D.S. Thermal conductivity of aqueous solutions in the system NaCl-$CaCl_2$ at ratio NaCl/$CaCl_2$=1/2 at high temperatures and high pressures. *Izv. Vyssh. Ucheb. Zaved., ser. Neft i Gaz.* 1996, *3/4*, 41-44.

[103] Eldarov, V.S. Thermal conductivity of aqueous KCl-NaCl-$CaCl_2$ solutions at high temperatures and pressures. *Teplofiz. Visok. Temp.* 2003, *41*, 381-385.

[104] Abdullaev, K.M.; Eldarov, V.S.; Munafov, Sh.M. thermal conductivity of mixing aqueous NaCl and $CaCl_2$ solutions at high temperatures and pressures. *Izv. Vyssh. Ucheb. Zaved., ser. Energetika* 1981, *5*, 63-67.

[105] Abdullaev, K.M.; El'darov, V.S. Study of the thermal conductivity of aqueous $NaNO_3$, KNO_3, and $AgNO_3$, solutions. *Izv. Vyssh. Ucheb. Zaved., ser. Energetika*. 1988, *6*, 78-84.

[106] Abdullaev, K.M.; El'darov, V.S.; Vakhabov, I.I.; Zul'fikarov, D.Sh. thermal conductivity of multicomponent aqueous electrolyte solutions. *Izv. Vyssh. Ucheb. Zaved., ser. Neft i Gaz.* 1992, *3/4*, 61-63.

[107] Abdullaev, K.M.; El'darov, V.S.; Vakhabov, I.I.; Babaeva, S.Sh. Thermal conductivity of aqueous solutions in the system with NaCl-Na_2SO_4-$MgCl_2$. *Izv. Vyssh. Ucheb. Zaved., ser. Neft i Gaz*. 1992, *8*, 45-48.

[108] Abdullaev, K.M.; Eldarov, V.S.; Vakhabov, I.I.; Garadagi, E.M.; Akhmedova, R.E.; Yakubova, I.N. Thermal conductivity of solutions in the systems H_2O-$NaNO_3$-KNO_3 near the saturation curve. *Izv. Vyssh. Ucheb. Zaved., ser. Neft i Gaz*. 1994, *3*, 52-55.

[109] Abdullaev, K.M.; Eldarov, V.S. Babaeva, S.Sh.; Mamedov, R.K.; Akhmedova, R.E.; Vakhabov, I.I. The thermal conductivity of mixing aqueous solutions of NaCl and $MgCl_2$ solutions. *Khimiya i Tekhnolog. Vodi* 1994, *16*, 271-276.

[110] Abdullaev, K.M.; Eldarov, V.S.; Vakhabov, I.I.; Gafarova, D.S. Study of the thermal conductivity of aqueous NaCl-$CaCl_2$ solutions at high temperatures. *Izv. Vyssh. Ucheb. Zaved., ser. Neft i Gaz*. 1995, *2*, 46-49.

[111] Abdullaev, K.M.; Eldarov, V.S.; Vakhabov, I.I.; Gafarov, D.S. Thermal conductivity of ternary aqueous NaCl and $CaCl_2$ solutions in the wide range of parameters. *Teploenergetika*. 1997, *5*, 61-64.

[112] Abdullaev, K.M.; Eldarov, V.S.; Mustafaev, A.M. Thermal conductivity of aqueous solutions of NaCl-$CaCl_2$ system. *Teplofiz. Visok. Temp.* 1998, *36*, 397-400.

[113] Abdullaev, K.M.; Eldarov, V.S.; Mustafaev, A.M. The thermal conductivity of mixing aqueous solutions of NaCl and $CaCl_2$ solutions at high temperatures and pressures. *Izv. Vyssh. Ucheb. Zaved., ser. Energetika* 1998, *1*, 63-67.

[114] Safronov, G.A.; Kosolap, Ya.G.; Rastorgnev, Yu.L. *Experimental studing of the thermal conductivity of binary solutions of electrolytes*. Dep. VINITI, No. 4262-B90, 1990.

[115] Grigor'ev, E.B. Thermal conductivity of aqueous binary and ternary solutions of lanthanides. *Ph.D.Thesis*, Geothermal Research Institute, DSC RAS, Makhachkala, Russia, 1995.

[116] Grigor'ev, E.B. Thermal conductivity of ternary aqueous solutions of lanthanides. *Teploenergetika* 2003, *6*, 64-66.

[117] Yata, J.M.; Minamiyama, T.; Tashiro, M.; Muragishi, H. Thermal conductivity of water and steam at high temperatures and pressures. I. Experimental apparatus and results with water up to 200 °C. *Bulleten of the JSME* 1979, *22*, 1220-1226.

[118] Yata, J.; Minamiyama, T.; Kadjimoto, K. Thermal conductivity of water and steam at high temperatures and pressures. II. Experimental results with water and steam up to 420 °C. *Jap. Soc. Mech. Eng.* 1979, *22*, 1227-1233.

[119] Yata, J.; Minamiyama, T.; Kataoka, H. In: "*Proc. 10th Int. Conf. Properties of Steam*", September 1984, Eds. V.V.Sytchev; A.A. Aleksandrov, Mir Publ., Moscow, USSR, 1986, V.2, pp. 348-357.

[120] Yata, J.; Hori, M.; Minamiyama, T.; Ohsako, K. In: "*Properties of Water and Steam. Proc. 11th Int. Conf. Properties of Steam*", September 1989, Prague, Eds. M.Pichal and O.Sifner, Hemisphere Publ. Corp., 1990, pp. 140-147.

[121] Healy, J.; de Groot, J.J.; Kestin, J. The theory of the transient hot-wires method for measuring thermal conductivity. *Physica C* 1976, *82*, 392-408.

[122] Stalhane, BB.; Pyk, S. *Technisk Tidskrift* 1931, *61*, 389-397.

[123] DiGuilio, R.M.; Lee, R.J.; Jeter, S.M.; Teja, A.S. Properties of lithium bromide – water solutions at high temperatures and concentrations I: Thermal conductivity. *ASHRAE Trans.* 1990, *96*, 702-708.

[124] DiGuilio, R.M.; Teja, A.S. Thermal conductivity of aqueous salt solutions at high temperatures and high concentrations. *Ind. Eng. Chem. Res.* 1992, *31*, 1081-1085.

[125] Bleazard, J.G.; DiGuilio, R.M.; Teja, A.S. Thermal conductivity of lithium bromide-water solutions. *AIChE Symp. Ser.* 1994, *298*, 23-28.

[126] Bleazard, J. G.; Teja, A. S. Thermal conductivity of electrically conducting liquids by the transient hot-wire method. *J. Chem. Eng. Data* 1995, *40*, 732-737.

[127] Kawamata, K.; Nagasaka, Y.; Nagashima, A. Measurements of the thermal conductivity of aqueous LiBr solutions at pressures up to 40 MPa. *Int. J. Thermophys.* 1988, *9*, 317-329.

[128] Quashou, M.S.; Vachon, R.I.; Touloukian, Y.W. Thermal conductivity of foods. Part 1; ASHRAE Semi-Annual Meeting. New Orleans, LA, 1972, *78*, 165-182.

[129] Muramatsu, Y.; Tagawa, A.; Kasai, T. Thermal conductivity of several liquid foods. *Food Science and Technology Research* 2005, *11*, 288-294.

[130] Frandas, A.; Bicanic, D. Thermal properties of fruit juices as a function of concentration and temperature determined using the photopyroelectric (PPE) method. *Journal of the Science of Food and Agriculture* 1999, *79*, 1361-1366.

[131] Ziegler, G.R.; Rizvi, S.S.H. Thermal conductivity of liquid foods by the thermal comparator method. *J. Food Sci.* 1985, *50*, 1458-1462.

[132] Morgan, D.A. Thermal conductivity in orange concentrate. *Florida State Horticultural Society* 1951, 192-198.

[133] Constenla, D.T.; Lozano, J.E.; Crapiste, G.H. Thermophysical properties of clarified apple juice as a function of concentration and temperature. *J Food Sci.* 1989, *54*, 663-668.

[134] Muramatsu, Y.; Tagawa, A.; Kasai, T.; Sakai, H.; Fukushima, M. Thermophysical properties of apple juice. *J. Jap. Soc. Food Sci. Technology* 2000, *47*, 548-550.

[135] Kolarov, K.M.; Gromov, M.A. A universal equation for computing the thermal conductivity of fruit and vegetable juices and syrups. *Khromitelna Promishlennost* 1973, *22*, 33-39.

[136] Dickerson, R.W. Thermal properties of foods. The freezing preservation of foods. Vol. 2, 4th edition. The AVI Publishing Co., Inc., Westport, Connecticut, 1968.

[137] Zainal, B.S.; Abdul Rahman, R.; Ariff, A.B.; Saari, B.N.; Asbi, B.A. Effect of temperature on the physical properties of pink guava juice at two different concentrations. *J. Food Engineering* 2000, *43*, 55-59.

[138] Voitko, A.M., Kovaleva, R.I., Tsaplin, V.A. The study of physical characteristics of concentrated grape juice. *Proc. of the Moldova NIIPP*, 1967, *7*, 61-74.

[139] Choi, I.; Okos, M.R. The thermal properties of tomato juice concentrates. *Transactions ASME* 1983, *26*, 305-311.

[140] Filkova, I.; Lawal, A.; Koziskova, B.; Mujumdar, A.S. Heat transfer to a power-law fluid in tube flow: Numerical and experimental study. *J. Food Engineering* 1987, *6*, 143-151.

[141] Maslikov, V.A.; Medvedev, O.K. Some thermophysical constants for tomato products. *Izv. Vuzov, ser. Pishevaya Tekhnologiya* 1969, *6*, 69-70.

[142] Shamsudin, R.; Mohamed, I.O.; Mohd Yaman, N. Kh. Thermophysical properties of Thai seedless guava juice as affected by temperature and concentration. *J. Food Engineering* 2005, *66*, 395-399.

[143] Lau, A.K.; March, A.C.; Lo, K.V.; Cumming, D.B. Physical properties of celery juice. *Can. Agric. Eng.* 1992, *34*, 105-110.

[144] Khelemskii, M. Z.; Zhadan,V. Z. , Thermal conductivity of normal Beet juice, A , Proc. All-Union Scientific Res. Inst. Of the Sugar Ind., Moscow, 1972, pp.11-13.

[145] Khelemshi, M.Z.; Zhadan, V.Z. The effect of dry solids concentration in beet juice on its thermphysical properties. *Russian J. Sugar Industry* 1963, *37*, 23-27.

[146] Kessler, H.G. Lebensmittel- und Bioverfahrenstechnik Molkereitechnologie: Verlag A. Kessler: Munchen, 1996.

[147] Konrad, H.; Rambke, K. Physical properties of liquid milk products. 4. Heat conductivity of milk, cream and milk concentrates. *Nahrung* 1971, *15*, 269-277.

[148] Muramatsu, *Y.*; Tagawa, *A.*; Kasai, T.; Takeya, K. Measurement of thermal conductivity and selection of heat conduction model for milk and whey. *J. Jap. Soc. Food Sci. Technology* 2003, *50*, 399-403.

[149] Spells, K.E. The thermal conductivities of some biological fluids. *J. Phys. In Medicine and Biology* 1960, *5*, 139-153.

[150] Reddy, Ch.S.; Datta, A.K. Thermophysical properties of concentrated reconstituted milk during processing. *J. Food Eng.* 1994, *21*, 31-40.

[151] Poppendiek, H.F.; Randall, R.; Breeden, J.A.; Chambers, J.E.; Murphy, J.R.; Thermal conductivity measurements and predictions for biological fluids and tissues. *Cryobiology* 1966, *3*, 318-327.

[152] Nowrey, J.E.; Woodams, E.E. Thermal conductivity of a vegetable oil-in-water emulsion. *J. Chem. Eng. Data* 1968, *13*, 297-301.

[153] Cuevas, R.; Cheryan, M. Thermal conductivity of liquid foods-Review. *J. Food Proc. Eng.* 1978, *2*, 283-306.

[154] Sweat, V.E. Thermal Properties of Foods. In: *Engineering Properties of Foods*, Second edition, Editors M.A. Rao, S.S.H. Rizvi; Marcel Dekker, Inc., New York, 1995; pp.99-138.

[155] Singh, R.P. Thermal diffusivity in food processing. *Food Technology*, 1982, *36*, 87-91.

[156] Woodams, E.E. Thermal conductivity of fluid foods. *Ms.D. Thesis*, Cornell University, 1965.

[157] Sweat, V.E.; Haugh, C.G. A thermal conductivity probe for small food samples. *Transections ASAE.* 1974, *17*, 56-58.

[158] De Moura, S.C.S.R.; Germer, S.P.M.; Jardim, D.C.P.; Sadahira, M.S. Thermophysical properties of tropical fruit juices. *Brazilian J. Food Technol.* 1998, *1*, 70-76.

[159] Leidenfrost, W. Measurements of the thermal conductivity of milk. *ASME Symp. Therm. Prop.*, Purdue University, Lafayette, Ind., 1959, pp.291-294.

[160] Sweat, V.E. Thermal properties of foods. In *Engineering Properties of Foods*, (M.A. Rao and S.S.H. Rizvi, Eds.), Marcel Dekker, Inc., New York, Chap. 1, 1986, pp.49-87.

[161] Becker, B.R.; Fricke, B.A. Food Thermophysical Properties Models, *Int. Communications in Heat and Mass Transfer* 1999, *26*, 627-636.

[162] Peacock, S., Predicting physical properties of factory juices and syrups. *Int. Sugar J.* 1995, *97*, 571-577.

[163] Bhumbla, V.K.; Singh, A.K.; Singh, Y.G.H. Prediction of thermal conductivity of fruit juices by thermal resistance model. *J Food Sci.* 1989, *54*, 1007-1012.

[164] Choi, I.; Okos, M.R. Effect of temperature and composition on thermal properties of foods. In *Food Engineering and process Applications* (M. Maguer and P. Jelen, Eds.), Elsevier Applied Science Publishers, London, 1986, pp. 93-101.

[165] Heldman, D.R.; Singh, R.P. *Food Process Engineering*, second edition, AVI Publishing Company, Inc., Westport, Connecticut (second edition), 1981.

[166] Miles, C.A.; Van Beek, G.; Veerkamp, C.H. Calculation of thermophysical properties of foods. In: Jowitt R, editor. Physical Properties of Foods. London and New York: Applied Science Publishers, 1983, pp.269-312

[167] Millat, J; Dymond, J.H., Nieto de Castro, C.A., Editors, *Transport properties of fluids. Their Correlation, Prediction and Estimation*. New York: IUPAC, Cambridge University Press, 1996.

[168] Aseyev, G. G. *Electrolytes. Properties of Solutions. Methods for Calculation of Multicomponent Systems and Experimental Data on Thermal Conductivity and Surface Tension.* Begell-House Inc., New York, 1998.

[169] Horvath, A.L. (1985) *Handbook of Aqueous Electrolyte Solutions: Physical Properties, Estimation Methods and Correlation Methods*. Ellis Horwood, West Sussex, England.

[170] Reid, R.C.; Prausnitz, J.M.; Poling, B.E. *The Properties of Gases and Liquids*. 4th ed., New York: McGaw-Hill, 1987.

[171] Ramires, M.L.V.; Nieto de Castro, C.A. Thermal conductivity of aqueous sodium chloride solutions. J. Chem. Eng. Data *1994, 39, 186-190.*

[172] Ramires, M.L.V.; Nieto de Castro, C.A. Thermal conductivity of aqueous potassium chloride solutions. *Int. J. Thermophys.* 2000, *21*, 671-679.

[173] Vargaftik, N.B.; Osminin, Y. P. Thermal conductivity of aqueous salt, acid, and alkali solutions. *Teploenergetika* 1956, *7*, 15-16.

[174] Hermans, F. Thermal diffusivity of foods. Ph.D. Thesis, University of Levan, The Nitherland, 1979.

[175] Alloush, A.; Gosney, W.B.; Wakeham, W.A. Transient hot-wire instrument for thermal conductivity measurements in electrically conducting liquids at elevated temperatures. *Intern. J. Thermophys.* 1982, *3*, 225-235.

[176] Chiquillo, A. *Measurements of the relative thermal conductivity of aqueous salt solutions with a transient hot-wire method*. Juris Druck+Verlag Zurich, 1967.

[177] Losenicky, Z. Thermal conductivity of aqueous solutions of alkali hydroxides. *J. Phys. Chem.* 1969, 73, 451-452.

[178] White, W.R.; Brunson, R.J.; Bearman, R.J.; Lindenbaum, S. Thermal conductivity of aqueous solutions of alkali hydroxides. *J. Sol. Chem.* 1975, 4, 557-570.

[179] Riedel, L. The heat conductivity of aqueous solutions of strong electrolytes. Chem-Ing-Techn 1951, *23*, 59-64.

[180] Dominguez, M.; De Elvira, C.; Fuster, C. Influence of air velocity and temperature on the two-stage cooling of perishable large-sized products. Annexe Bressanone, *Bull. IT Refrig.*, Annexe 1974, *3*, 83-90.

[181] Venart, J. E. S.; Prasad, R.C. Thermal conductivity of water and oleum. *J. Chem. Eng. Data* 1980, *25*, 196-198.

[182] Abdulagatov, I.M.; Abdulagatov, A.I.; Kamalov, A.N. *Thermophysical Properties of Pure Fluids and Aqueous Systems at High Temperatures and Pressures*. New York: Begell House, Inc, 2005.

[183] Klaas, D.M.; Viswanath, D.S. A correlation for the prediction of thermal conductivity of liquids. *Ind. Eng. Chem. Res.* 1998, *37*, 2064-2068.

[184] Rahman, R. A general form of thermal conductivity equation for an apple sample during drying. *Drying Technology*, 1995, *13*, 2153-2165.

[185] Watt, B.K.; Merrill, A.L., *Composition of Foods. Agriculture Handbook*, No. 8, U.S. Department of Agriculture, 1975.

[186] Maxwell, C.J. *A Treatise on Electrical and Magnetism*. Clarenton Press, Oxford, England, 3rd edition, 1904, pp. 440-445.

[187] Eucken, A. *Forsch. Gehiete Ingenieurue B3, Forschnung* 1932, *353*, 16-28.

[188] Waff, H.S. Theoretical considerations of electrical conductivity in partially molten mantle and implications for geothermometry. *J. Geophys. Res.* 1974, *79*, 4003-4010.

[189] Fricke, H. A mathematical treatment of the electric conductivity and capacity of disperse systems. *Phys. Rev.* 1924. *24*, 575-587.

[190] Dul'nev, G.N. *Thermal Conductivity of Mixtures and Composite Materials*. Leningrad, Energiya, 1974.

[191] Kunii, D.; Smith, J.M. Heat transfer characteristics of porous rocks. *J AIChE* 1960, *6*, 71-78.

[192] Odelevskii, V.I. Calculation of the generalized conductivity of heterogeneous systems. *Russ. J. Tech. Physics* 1951, *21*, 667-678.

[193] Özbek, H. Thermal conductivity of multi-fluid saturated porous media. *Ph.D. Thesis* Berkeley, University of California, 1976.

[194] Keller, Th.; Motschmann, U.; Engelhard, L. Modelling the poroelasticity of rocks and ice. *Geophys. Prospect* 1999, *47*, 509-526.

[195] Sugawara, A.; Yoshizawa, Y. An experimental investigation on the thermal conductivity of consolidated porous materials. *J. Appl. Phys.* 1962, *33*, 3135-3138.

[196] Zarichnyak, Yu.P.; Novikov, V.V. Effective conductivity of heterogenic system with chaotic structure. *Inzh. Fiz. Zhurnal* 1978, *34*, 412.

[197] Zehner, P.; Schlünder, E.U. Thermal conductivity of granular materials at moderate temperatures. *Chem. Ingr.-Tech.* 1970, *42*, 933-941.

[198] [Zimmerman, R.W. Thermal conductivity of fluid saturated rocks. *J. Pet. Sci. and Eng.* 1989, *3*: 219-227.

[199] Ghaffari, A. Model for predicting thermal conductivity of rock/fluid systems. *Ph.D. Thesis,* Berkeley, University of California, 1980.

[200] Gomaa, E.E. Thermal behavior of partially liquid saturated porous media, *Ph.D. Dissertation*, University of California, Berkeley, 1973.

[201] Chan, C. K.; Tien, C. L. Conductance of packed spheres in vacuum. *Trans. ASME,* 1973, *95*, 302-308.

[202] Cheng, H.; Torquato, S. Effective conductivity of periodic arrays of spheres with interfacial resistance. *Proc. R. Soc. London A* 1997, *453*, 145-161.

[203] Hsu, C.T.; Cheng, P.; Wong, K.W. Modified Zehner-Schlunder models for stagnant thermal conductivity of porous media. *Int. J. Heat Mass Transfer* 1994, *37*, 2751-2759.

[204] Hsu, C.T.; Cheng, P.; Wong, K.W. A Lumped –parameter model for stagnant thermal conductivity of spatially periodic porous media. *Transaction ASME*, 1995, *117*, 264-269.

[205] Kaviany, M. *Principles of heat transfer in porous media*. Second edition, New York, Springer, 1991.

[206] Mendel, A.M. Relation between thermal conductivity of rocks and structure of the pores. *Russ. J. Geol. Procpect.* 1997, *1*, 112-119.

[207] Miloh, T.; Benveniste, Y. On the effective conductivity of composites with ellipsoidal inhomogeneities and high highly conducting interfaces. *Proc. R. Soc., London A* 1996, *455*, 2687-2706.

[208] Nozad, S.; Carbonell, R.G.; Whitaker, S. Heat conduction in multiphase systems. I. Theory and Experiments for two-phase systems. *Chem. Eng. Sci.* 1985, *40*, 843-855.

[209] Yu, F.; Wei, G.; Zhang, X.; Chen, K. Two effective thermal conductivity models for porous media with hollow spherical agglomerates. *Int. J. Thermophys.* 2006, *27*, 293-303.

[210] Orr, C.; Dallavalle, J.M. Heat-transfer properties of liquid-solid suspensions. *Chem. Eng. Prog. Sym. Ser*. 1954, *50*, 29-45.

[211] Skelland, A.H.P. *Non – Newtonian Flow and Heat Transfer*, New York, John Wiley & Sons, 1967.

[212] Metzner, A.B. *Non – Newtonian technology: fluid mechanics, mixing, and heat transfer. In: Advances in Chemical Engineering,* T.B. Drew and J.W. Hoopes, Jr., eds. New York, Academic Press, 1956, Vol. 1, pp.77-153.

[213] Buntebarth, G.; Schopper, J. R. Experimental and theoretical investigations on the influence of fluids, solids and interactions between them on thermal properties of porous rocks. *J. Phys. Chem. Earth* 1997, *23*, 1141-1146.

[214] Aichlmayr, H.T.; Kulacki, F.A. The effective thermal conductivity of saturated porous media. *Advances in Heat Transfer*, (eds. G. Greene et al., New York: AP), 2006, vol. 39, 377-460.

[215] Hashin, Z.; Shtrikman, S.A. A variational approach to the theory of the effective magnetic permeability of multiphase materials. *J. Appl. Phys.* 1962, *33*, 3125-3131.

[216] Lichtencker, K.; Rother, K. Die Herleitung des logarithmischen Mischungs-gesetzes aus allegemeinen Prinzipien der stationaren Stromung. *Phys. Z.* 1931, *32*, 255-260.

[217] Brown, W.F. Solid mixture permitivities. *J. Chem. Phys.* 1955, *23*, 1514-1517.

[218] Ziman, J.M. *Electrons and phonons. The theory of transport phenomena in solids.* Clarendon Press: Oxford, 1962.

[219] Rzhevskii, V.; Novik, G. *The Physics of Rocks*, Moscow: Mir, 1971.

[220] Nieto de Castro, C.A.; Li, S. F.; Nagashima, A.; Trengove, R.D.; Wakeham, W.A. *J. Phys. Chem. Ref. Data* 1986, *15,* 1073-1086.

[221] Bálint, À. Prediction of physical properties of foods fro unit operations. *Periodica Polytechnica ser. Chem. Eng.* 2001, *45*, 35-40.

[222] Walsh, J.B.; Decker, E.R. Effect of pressure and saturating fluid on the thermal conductivity of compact rock. *J. Geophys. Res.* 1966, *71*, 3053-3061.

[223] More, G.R.; Prasad, S. Thermal conductivity of concentrated whole milk. *J. Food Proc. Eng.* 2007, *40*, 1105-1120.

[224] Mattar, H.L.; Minim, L.A.; Coimbra, S.R.; Minim, V.P.R.; Saraiva, S.H.; Telis-Romera, J. Modeling of thermal conductivity, specific heat, and density of milk. A neural network approach. *Int. J. Food Properties* 2004, *7*, 531-539.

In: Fruit Juices: Properties, Consumption and Nutrition ISBN: 978-1-60741-505-3
Editor: Pauline G. Scardina

Chapter 2

Cactus Pear Juice: A Source of Multiple Nutraceutical and Functional Components

Dedicated to the memory of my dear father

Hasna El Gharras [*]

Laboratoire de Chimie Organique et Analytique. Unité de Chimie Agroalimentaire, Université Sultan Moulay Slimane. Faculté des Sciences et Techniques BP523, Béni-Mellal. MAROC

Abstract

Recently, functional foods present in natural resources, such as fruits, vegetables, oilseeds, and herbs, have received a great attention both by health professionals and the common population for improving overall well-being, as well as in the prevention of diseases. In fact, regular consumption of fruits and vegetables is associated with reduced risks of chronic diseases such as cancer, cardiovascular disease, stroke, Alzheimer's disease, cataract and age-related functional decline.

The recent scientific investigations on cactus reported high content of some chemical constituents, which can give added value to cactus products in terms of functionality. The cactus pear (*Opuntia ficus-indica*) appears to be an excellent candidate for the inclusion in food. According to several studies, the great number of potentially active nutrients and their multifunctional properties make cactus pear perfect candidates for the production of health-promoting food and food supplements. Traditionally, it's appreciated for its pharmacological properties by the Native Americans. However, recent studies on

[*] E-mail: elgharrashasna@yahoo.fr

Opuntia have demonstrated cactus pear fruit and vegetative cladodes to be excellent candidates for the development of healthy food.

The objective of this chapter is to present a review in terms of cactus pear juice including its nutraceutical and functional properties.

Keywords: cactus pear, juice, nutraceutical, functional, betalains, antioxidants.

Introduction

The *Opuntia ficus-indica* plant, probably originated from Central Mexico, is a member of the Cactaceae family. It's widely distributed in Mexico and all American hemispheres and grows in many other parts of the world, such as Africa, Australia and the Mediterranean basin. As a xerophytic plant, cactus has developed phenological, physiological and a structural adaptation favourable to their development in arid environments, in which water is the main factor limiting the development of most plant species. Among these adaptations stand out its asynchronous reproduction, and its CAM metabolism, which combined with structural adaptations such as succulence allow this plant to continue the assimilation of carbon dioxide during long periods of drought and in this way reach acceptable productivity levels even in years of severe drought. Through succulence, the ability to store considerable quantities of water, the plant may survive despite harsh environmental conditions [1]. Furthermore, the same authors reported that *Opuntia* exhibits the highest production rate of aboveground-growing plants. Interestingly, the biomass production was even found to increase upon otherwise deleterious rise of atmospheric CO_2 concentrations [2], thus counteracting the greenhouse effect.

Cactus (*Opuntia*) has been used for many years as a common vegetable and as medicine by the Native Americans and Mexicans [3-6]. Cactus cladodes, fruits, and flowers were traditionally used as medicines in several countries, and particularly in Latin America. Recent scientific investigations showed that cactus products may be efficiently used as a source of food additives, mainly fibre, red dye and mucilages. The use of cactus products as cosmetics is even more developed than medicinal applications.

Cactus was largely ignored by the scientific world until the beginning of 1980, when there was a multiplication of research and symposia, resulting in a large number of publications. This renewed interest is to be ascribed in part to the multi-functionality of cactus fruits, pads and flowers. Recent data have, in fact, revealed the high content of some chemical constituents, which can give added value to cactus products. Additionally, some of the constituents show promising characteristics in terms of functionality. In recent years there has been a global trend toward the use of natural phytochemicals present in natural resources, such as fruit, vegetables, oilseeds, and herbs, as antioxidants and functional foods. Natural antioxidant can be used in the food industry, and there is evidence that these substances may exert their antioxidant effects within human body. Cactus has a global distribution and is an important nutrient and food source. The growing demand for neutraceuticals is paralleled by an increased effort in developing natural products for the prevention or treatment of human diseases. According to several studies demonstrating both cactus fruit and cladode yielding high values of important nutrients, such as betalains, amino compounds including taurine, minerals, vitamins, as well as further antioxidants, the cactus pear (*Opuntia* spp.) appears to be an excellent candidate for the inclusion in food. Even though Native Americans and ancient medicine have realized its antidiabetic and anti-inflammatory function, *Opuntia* spp. have hardly been considered in the development of health-promoting food, most probably due to the scattered information available.

The objective of this chapter is to present a review in terms of cactus pear juice including its nutraceutical and functional properties.

Physical Composition Of Cactus Pear Fruits

The fruits are unilocular, polyspermic, egg-shaped fleshy berries and highly appealing because of their attractive colours. However, the spines and glochids are embarrassing morphological features when peeling the fruit. The pericarp of fruits of *Opuntia ficus-indica* and the edible pulp may have soft-green, greenish-white, canary-yellow, lemon-yellow, red, cherry-red or purple hues [7]. Weight of fruit may range from 67 g to 216 g at the best stage of ripening. In our study, published in 2006, we have revealed a great variation in the weights of Moroccan yellow fruits of *Opuntia ficus-indica* at different stages of ripeness [8]. Also, the weight of the fruits varied as a function as the cultivar. The weight of green fruits was found to be significantly different than those of half-ripe and ripe fruits. On average, the weight of fruit varied from 62.27 to 91.23 g for first stage, from 77.68 to 110.13 g for second stage, and from 88.70 to 130.87g for the latest stage (**Table 1**) [8].

As reported by some authors, the fruit is composed of peel (33 % to 55 %), pulp (45 % to 67 %), and seeds (2 % to 10 %) [9-16]. As a function of maturity, we have observed in our study that the pulp increased, it varied from 51.93 to 54.73 % for green fruits, from 52.80 to 55.97 % for half ripe fruits, and from 53.99 to 56.36 % for ripe fruits (**Table 1**) [8].

Table 1. Weight of fruit and pulp of Moroccan yellow cactus pear [8].

Parameter Cultivar	Weight of fruit (g) Apparent maturity			Weight of pulp (g) Apparent maturity		
	Green	Half-ripe	Ripe	Green	Half-ripe	Ripe
ElKelaâ	62.2 ±6.90	77.68±2.76	88.70± 2.26	32.34±1.09	41.02±1.28	47.89±0.85
Skhour Rehamna	71.90±2.15	82.13± 2.06	113.93±5.33	37.81±1.40	44.95±0.62	63.46±1.25
AitBaâmrane	91.23±5.54	110.13±1.88	130.87±5.86	49.93±1.75	61.64±1.96	73.76±2.92
Average	75.13±14.75	89.98±17.59	111.17±21.22	40.03±9.00	49.20±10.95	61.70±13.02
CV %	19.63	19.55	19.09	22.48	22.26	21.10

However with advance in maturity, both the percent of weight of skin and seeds decreased. On average, the weight of skin varied from 41.20 to 39.45 % for the green stage to the latest and the percent of weight of seeds varied from 5.20 to 5.72 % from the first stage to the latest (**Table 2**) [8].

The large variability in percentages depends on cultivar, cultural practices, fecundated- and aborted-seed number, fruit load, lighting period, climate, and harvesting season [9-16].

Table 2. Weight of skin and seeds of Moroccan yellow cactus pear fruits [8].

Parameter Cultivar	Weight of skin (g)			Weight of seeds (g)		
	Apparent maturity			Apparent maturity		
	Green	Half-ripe	Ripe	Green	Half-ripe	Ripe
ElKelaâ	26.05±0.83	32.18±1.17	35.82±0.90	3.89±0.50	4.47±0.50	4.98±0.57
Skhour Rehamna	29.92±1.12	32.56±0.57	44.61±1.34	4.17±0.38	4.61±0.36	5.86±0.57
AitBaâmrane	36.64±1.61	43.01±2.48	50.79±3.21	4.66±0.36	5.48±0.88	6.32±0.60
Average	30.87±5.36	35.92±6.15	43.74±7.52	4.24±0.39	4.85±0.55	5.72±0.68
CV %	17.36	17.12	17.19	9.20	11.34	11.89

Chemical Characteristics of Cactus Pear Fruits Juices

Humidity

The pulp is the edible part of the fruit and is composed of water with a rate varying from 84 % to 90 % [15-20]. In Moroccan cactus pears, we have revealed an amounts varying from 878.00 to 902.70 (g/Kg of juice) for green fruits, from 857.80 to 899.60 (g/Kg of juice) for half ripe fruits, and from 839.20 to 888.80 (g/Kg of juice) for ripe fruits (**Table 3**) [8]. It decreased slightly with advances in maturity. On average, the humidity of Moroccan cactus pears varied from 855.10 to 881.33 (g/Kg of juice) [8].

Ash

As reported by Piga (2004), the ash varied from 3-10 (g/Kg) [15-20]. In Moroccan yellow cactus pears, the amount of ash varied from 1.98 to 3.41 (g/Kg of juice) (**Table 3**) [8].

Table 3. Chemical composition of Moroccan yellow cactus pear fruits per 1 Kg of juice [8].

Parameter Cultivar	Dry matter (g)			Ash (g)		
	Apparent maturity			Apparent maturity		
	Green	Half-ripe	Ripe	Green	Half-ripe	Ripe
ElKelaâ	97.30±8.30	100.40±8.90	111.20±5.40	3.15±0.16	2.80±0.25	3.15±0.16
Skhour Rehamna	136.70±8.00	151.40±5.00	162.70±7.80	1.98±0.64	2.85±0.33	2.03±0.92
AitBaâmrane	122.00±9.40	142.20±4.60	160.80±8.20	2.77±0.25	2.98±0.56	3.41±0.13
Average	118.67±19.91	131.33±27.18	144.90±29.20	2.63±0.60	2.88±0.09	2.86±0.73
CV %	16.78	20.70	20.15	22.81	3.13	25.52

Brix

Saenz-Hernandez (1995), reported that the total soluble solids varied from 12 to 17 % for Mexican cultivars [21]. In Moroccan yellow cactus pear juices, we have observed that the average soluble solid (°Brix) content was lowest (12.56 %) in green fruits, increased to (13.67 %) in half-ripe fruits and reached the maximum (14.89 %) in ripe fruits (**Table 4**) [8]. On average, total soluble solids for Moroccan yellow cactus pear juices range between 10.16 and 16.61 % [8].

Table 4. Physico-chemical parameters of juices of Moroccan yellow cactus pear fruits [8].

Parameter	Degree Brix (%)			pH			Titrable acidity (g of monohydrate citric acid per 1Kg of juice)		
Cultivar	Apparent maturity			Apparent maturity			Apparent maturity		
	Green	Half-ripe	Ripe	Green	Half-ripe	Ripe	Green	Half-ripe	Ripe
ElKelaâ	10.16±0.81	10.32±0.88	11.53±0.49	6.01±0.07	6.01±0.07	6.16±0.05	0.60±0.02	0.60±0.02	0.57±0.02
Skhour Rehamna	14.24±0.70	15.68±0.43	16.54±0.68	6.07±0.07	6.19±0.10	6.34±0.12	0.59±0.02	0.57±0.02	0.55±0.02
AitBaâmrane	13.27±0.99	15.00±0.31	16.61±0.57	5.95±0.08	6.05±0.08	6.15±0.07	0.59±0.02	0.58±0.02	0.55±0.02
Average	12.56±2.13	13.67±2.92	14.89±2.91	6.01±0.06	6.08±0.09	6.22±0.11	0.59±0.01	0.58±0.02	0.56±0.01
CV %	16.96	21.36	19.54	1.00	1.48	1.77	1.69	3.45	1.79

Organic acids

Several studies reported values of pH of the pulp ranging from 5.5 to 6.4 [15-19], which characterizes cactus pears as low acid food (pH>4.5), because of the extremely low content of organic acids. This makes them rather liable to pathogen growth if not acidified. Hence, acidification prior to thermal treatment is a prerequisite to allow pasteurization instead of more rigid sterilization, thereby retaining nutritionally important components such as betalains [20,22-25]. Citric acid is the main organic acid (62 mg/100g) of cactus pears followed by malic acid (23.3 mg/100g). Quinic (19.1 mg/100g) and shikimic acids (2.8 mg/100g) are also important, iso-citric, fumaric, glycolic, and succinic acids could only be detected in traces [17,25]. In Australian fruits oxalic acid was found at amounts of 40 mg/100g [26] whereas in Italian fruits oxalic acid amounted to 50 % of the total acids [27].

The pH measured for Moroccan yellow cactus pear juices turns out to be very high, with values of the order of 6.1 commonly measured (**Table 4**) [8]. The pH of the fruits increased with the advance in maturity, being 6.0 for green mature, 6.1 for half-ripe and 6.2 for ripe fruits [8]. Accompanying the pH value, the titrable acidity decreased slightly with advances in maturity (**Table 4**) [8]. On average, the total acid content in the cactus pear fruits varied from 0.55 to 0.60 (g/Kg) and it did not differ significantly among the cultivars with regard to the stage of ripeness [8].

The total acid content in cactus pear juice is very low in comparison with the acidity of other fruit juices, expressed according to monohydrate citric acid, such as pear (3 g/Kg), orange (8 g/Kg), apple (9 g/Kg), peach (9 g/Kg), strawberry (9 g/Kg), pineapple (11 g/Kg), raspberry (18 g/Kg), plum (22 g/Kg), and apricot (24 g/Kg) [28,29].

Functional Compounds Of Fruits

Hydrocolloids

The mucilaginous components in leaves and fruit from *Opuntia* are related to pectic substances. Investigations on the fruit revealed average pectin levels of the pulp of 0.18 g/100g on a fresh weight basis [15,16,30]. The polysaccharide fraction of cactus pear pulp was only recently reported to be composed of a complex mixture of polysaccharides of which less than 50 % corresponded to a pectin-like polymer. The hydrocolloid fraction from the fruit pulp of *Opuntia ficus-indica* fruits obtained by ethanol precipitation yielded 3.8 % and contained 93.5 % sugars. Whereas, after saponification, uronic acid content of 42.3 % was determined; neither proteins nor nitrogen were detected. After total hydrolysis, the presence of arabinose, rhamnose, xylose, and galactose in the molar ratio of 1.0:1.7:2.5:4.1 was found. However, further studies are required to completely characterize the hydrocolloid fraction of cactus pear fruit pulp [31].

In a more detailed investigation pectin was found to be 70.3 % of the pulp fiber substances. Hemicellulose, cellulose and lignin were 15.5, 14.2 and 0.01 %, respectively, in peel and seeds [32]. In cactus pear peel pectin was characterized by a galacturonic acid content of 64 %, a low degree of methoxylation (10 %) and a high degree of acetylation (10 %) and neutral sugar content (51 %) of which 34.5 % was galactose and rhamnose [33].

The high fiber content, which gives cactus pear juice a pleasant mouthfeel, might be advantageous for the design of new soft drinks, dairy or cereal products. Furthermore, these mucilaginous substances are associated with blood sugar regulation in humans suffering from diabetes mellitus type II, the non-insulin dependent diabetes mellitus [7,34-36]. A potential for lowering plasma cholesterol levels has also been discussed [37,38]. Cactus pear pectin consumption modified low density lipoprotein (LDL) composition.

Sugars

In cactus pear juices total soluble solids range between 12 and 17 °Bx [21] with glucose and fructose being the predominant carbohydrates. Because of high invertase activity, sucrose is mostly converted to absorbable sugars and therefore little represented in the pulp [32,39,40]. Some authors additionally reported the occurrence of galactose [41] and maltose [42]. Depending on invertase activity, colour of fruit and fruit origin, different ratios of glucose and fructose were found. Kuti and Galloway (1994) reported varying enzyme activity in differently coloured fruits without giving information about their botanical origin [39]. Differences in the relative enzyme activity are reflected by the ratio of sucrose, glucose and fructose in peel and pulp. The question as to whether a correlation between skin colour and invertase activity exists remains still to be confirmed. Relative amounts of glucose and fructose of about 1:1 have been reported in two studies [15,39], whereas another investigation found glucose and fructose at a ratio of 11:1 [17]. These conflicting results may also be due to different analytical methods applied. The degree of ripeness of the fruit material investigated should be considered during invertase activity measurement as well as sugar analysis.

In Moroccan yellow cactus pear juices, the sugar contents were significantly different during different stages of maturity and as function as the cultivar [8]. They increased with maturity and reached the higher values especially in completely ripe cactus pear fruits. On average, reducing sugars increased from (117.24 g/Kg) for the green mature to (152.26 g/Kg) for the ripe stage of maturity (**Table 5**) [8]. Consequently, the °Brix/acid ratio increased from 211.36 for green mature to 268.92 for ripe fruits, being significantly different among all stages of maturity [8]. The reducing sugars content in cactus pear fruits, cited in bibliography, is higher when compared with that of other common fruit juices such as pineapple (123 g/Kg), apple (111 g/Kg), pear (98 g/Kg), peach (85 g/Kg), plum (78 g/Kg), orange (70 g/Kg), apricot (61 g/Kg), strawberry (57 g/Kg), and raspberry (45 g/Kg) [8,29,43,44].

Table 5. Chemical composition of Moroccan yellow cactus pear fruits per 1 Kg of juice [8].

Parameter Cultivar	Reduced sugars (g)			Protein (g) Conversion factor (=6.25)		
	Apparent maturity			Apparent maturity		
	Green	Half-ripe	Ripe	Green	Half-ripe	Ripe
ElKelaâ	97.93±2.14	99.91±4.27	111.22±1.57	1.35±0.28	1.62±0.24	2.43±0.39
Skhour Rehamna	131.56±8.23	153.67±7.81	170.44±12.16	1.91±0.80	2.03±0.70	2.09±0.76
AitBaâmrane	122.22±8.74	143.78±5.87	175.11±12.81	2.11±0.42	3.31±0.47	3.77±0.55
Average	117.24±17.36	132.45±28.61	152.26±35.62	1.79±0.39	2.32±0.88	2.76±0.89
CV %	14.81	21.60	23.39	21.79	37.93	32.25

With respect to bioavailability, cactus pear containing mainly fructose and glucose is an ideal energy source for brain and central nervous system.

The high sugar content of the pulp results in sugar:acid ratios within the range of 90:1 up to 490:1, which is responsible for the bland taste and, therefore, far from a sensory pleasant ratio of 10 to 18 [18,45-47].

Proteins

For Chilean cultivars, Saenz *et al.* 2001 have reported amounts of proteins ranging from (2.1 g/Kg) to (16 g/Kg) [48]. We revealed for Moroccan yellow cactus pear, that the amounts of proteins in juices increased during the stages of maturity [8]. On average the amount of proteins varied from (1.79 g/Kg) to (2.79 g/Kg) (**Table 5**). The differences between results may be attributed to the conditions in which cactus pears were grown in those studies.

Finally, the amount of protein present in cactus pear are comparables to those found in other common fruits such as apple (2 g/Kg), pear (3 g/Kg), apricot (4 g/Kg), pineapple (5 g/Kg), plum (5 g/100 g), orange (7 g/Kg), peach (8 g/Kg), and strawberry (9 g/Kg) [29,44].

Amino acids

Stintzing *et al.* 1999 have reported that free amino acids comprised all essential amino acids found in *Opuntia ficus-indica* [19]. Proline was found to be the predominant amino acid in the pulp of six different cultivars ('Apastillada', 'Bianca', 'Gialla', 'Gymno carpo', 'Morado', and 'Rossa') from *Opuntia ficus-indica* fruits amounting to (883.4 mg/L) and even (1929.1 mg/L) followed by the nutraceutical taurine (323.6 to 407.3 mg/L), glutamine (98.3 mg/L to 574.6 mg/L), and serine (130.6 mg/L to 392.6 mg/L) [19,49,50].

Vitamins

Significant amounts of ascorbic acid are generally found in fruits of different *Opuntia* spp. ranging from (10 mg/kg) to (410 mg/kg). The most common *Opuntia ficus-indica* (L.) Mill. shows ascorbic acid contents from (180 mg/kg) to (300 mg/kg) [20,47]. So, cactus pear is higher in ascorbic acid than other common fruits, such as apple, pear, grape, and banana.

Though it is a good source of vitamin C with levels ranging from 18 to 23 mg per 100 g fresh fruit, the vitamin spectrum in cactus pear is not very spectacular. Carotenoids, thiamin, riboflavin and niacin were only found in trace amounts [15,16,26,51,52].

Minerals

Cactus pear is rich in magnesium and calcium, whereas sodium, potassium, iron and phosphorus content are in the typical range of other fruits [17,26,53]. High calcium (up to 59 mg/100g) and magnesium (up to 98.4 mg/100g) contents make cactus pear juices useful in the prevention of osteoporosis and cramps, respectively. Suited for energy and sports drinks in upholding the mineral pool during periods of physical exhaustion, low levels of sodium and chloride are preferred in the diet for curing high blood pressure [54,55].

In Moroccan fruits, the content of sodium varied from 96.49 to 144.43 (mg/Kg) (**Table 6a**) [8]. These values are comparables to those reported for Mexican cultivars (120-160 mg/Kg) [56].

The potassium content varied from 1666.91 to 1897.41 (mg/Kg) (**Table 6a**) [8]. These data are higher than those reported for Mexican cultivars (610 to 720 mg/Kg) [56], and significantly very higher than those reported for Chilean cultivars (12.8 to 27.6 mg/Kg) [15,16].

Table 6a. Mineral content (mg/Kg of juice) of juices of Moroccan yellow cactus pear fruits [8].

Parameter Cultivar	Sodium			Potassium		
	Apparent maturity			Apparent maturity		
	Green	Half-ripe	Ripe	Green	Half-ripe	Ripe
ElKelaâ	236.78±0.74	115.60±0.59	136.48±0.87	963.90±0.60	2025.40±0.57	1649.97±1.17
Skhour	145.74±0.59	110.72±0.58	90.82±0.68	2338.00±1.15	1348.62±0.39	1957.76±1.25
Rehamna	50.78±0.38	63.15±0.40	166.70±0.59	1698.84±1.54	2318.20±1.50	1909.50±3.64
AitBaâmrane	144.43±93.01	96.49±28.98	131.33±38.2	1666.91±687.61	1897.41±497.30	1839.08±165.54
Average CV %	64.40	30.03	29.09	41.25	26.21	9.00

In Moroccan fruits, the amount of calcium increased during the stages of maturity (**Table 6b**) [8]. It increased from (161.47 mg/Kg) for the green mature to (214.60 mg/Kg) for the ripe stage of maturity (**Table 6b**) [8]. These results were higher than those reported for Mexican cultivars [56] (110 to 170 mg/Kg) and relatively lower than those reported for Chilean cultivars (154 to 328 mg/Kg) [15,16].

The amount of copper varied during the stage of maturity, but the variation was not very significant (**Table 6b**) [8]. The content varied from (0.18 mg/Kg) for the green fruits to (0.19 mg/Kg) for the half-ripe and ripe fruits (**Table 6b**) [8]. These results were very lower than those reported in the literature for Mexican cultivars (5 mg/Kg) [56].

On average, the amount of zinc decreased as function as the stages of maturity (**Table 6b**) [8]. It decreased from (0.62 mg/Kg) for the green fruits, to (0.37 mg/Kg) for the half-ripe and for the ripe to (0.29 mg/Kg) (**Table 6b**) [8]. The content of zinc in Moroccan cultivars is in good agreement with those reported for Italian cultivars (0.3 to 0.4 mg/Kg) [43] but very lower than those reported for Mexican cultivars (12 to 16 mg/Kg) [56].

Table 6b. Mineral content (mg/Kg of juice) of juices of Moroccan yellow cactus pear fruits [8].

Parameter Cultivar	Calcium			Copper			Zinc		
	Apparent maturity			Apparent maturity			Apparent maturity		
	Green	Half-ripe	Ripe	Green	Half-ripe	Ripe	Green	Half-ripe	Ripe
ElKelaâ	188..60±1.54	228.30±1.49	263.00±1.18	0.21±0.02	0.20±0.02	0.19±0.02	1.18±0.02	0.48±0.02	0.38±0.02
Skhour	111.11±0.61	125.90±0.36	129.60±0.48	0.16±0.01	0.15±0.01	0.16±0.01	0.31±0.02	0.18±0.01	0.08±0.01
Rehamna	184.70±1.16	239.39±1.18	251.20±1.46	0.17±0.01	0.22±0.01	0.21±0.01	0.37±0.02	0.45±0.01	0.41±0.02
AitBaâmrane	161.47±43.66	197.86±62.57	214.60±73.85	0.18±0.03	0.19±0.04	0.19±0.03	0.62±0.49	0.37±0.17	0.29±0.18
Average CV %	27.04	31.62	34.41	16.67	21.05	15.79	79.03	45.95	62.07

Authors reported a large variation in the mineral composition of the fruits of different regions [15,16,43,56]. The mineral pattern is dependent on fruit origin, the edaphic factors at the site of the cultivation, thus explaining conflicting literature data.

Pigments

Because the appearance of food is as important as its taste, modern food manufacturers have become greatly concerned with conserving the aspect of foods that have lost their natural colours during processing. Adding colorants preserves the aspect of foods while also reducing batch-to-batch colour variations and enhancing the natural colour [22]. Nevertheless, synthetic colorants have increasingly been perceived as undesirable or harmful by consumers. At the same time, the European Union and the United States have restricted the use of synthetic colorants as food additives. These restrictions on the use of artificial colorants have increased the need to study the use of natural pigments in the food industry [22,23].

Cactus fruits contain betalains [57], which can be used in agri-food. Cactus pear pulps offer different colours based on betalains covering a wide spectrum from white to purple with pigment contents of (66 mg/Kg) to (1140 mg/kg) fruit pulp [58,59]. Cactus betalains contains two types of pigments: betacyanins (red) and betaxanthins (yellow) (**Figure 1**) in betaxanthin:betacyanin ratios varying between 0 to 11.7 resulting in different colour shades [46,59,60]. These betalain pigments were used for yaourts [61] and orange juice [62] preparations.

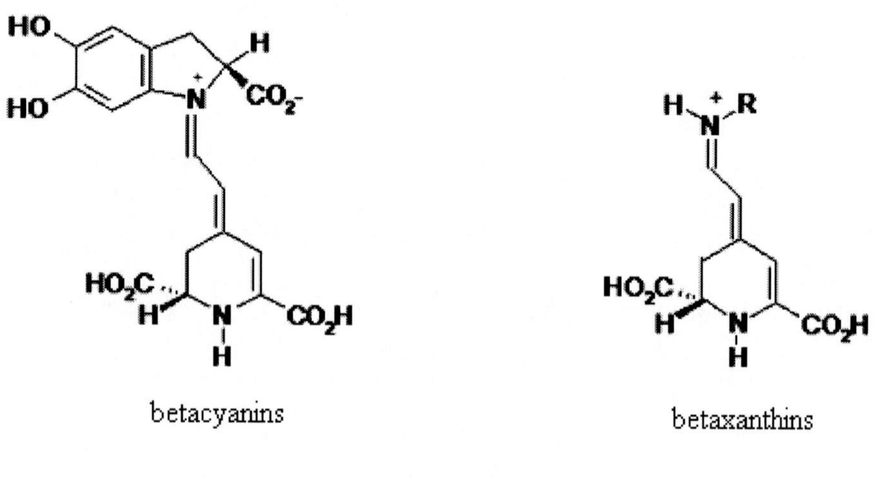

Figure 1. Chemical structure of betacyanins and betaxanthins.

The water-soluble pigments of cactus pear are localized in the plant vacuole. Unlike the widely distributed anthocyanins, betalains are nitrogenous chromoalkaloids characteristic of the ten families of the order Caryophyllales, except the Caryophyllaceae and the Molluginaceae, which accumulate anthocyanins instead.

Little has been published with respect to the physiological role of betalains in mammals. In earlier reports, it was found that red beet neither exerted hepatotoxic nor mutagenic action [63, 64]. Kapadia *et al.* (1996) showed a significant inhibitory effect of beetroot towards skin and lung cancer in mice [65]. In other animal feeding trials, purple cactus pear [66] and garambullo (myrtillocactus geometrizans [67] proved to be devoid of toxicity and their pigments did not provoke any allergic reactions [68,69]. The excretion of red urine after ingestion of beetred in 10-14 % of the population, the so-called beeturia, was classified as an idiosyncratic reaction being dependent on individual's physiology constitutions rather than representing a pathological event or a genetic defect [70].

Recent findings rank beet among the 10 most potent vegetables with respect to their antioxidant capacities [71,76]. Betalains from beet [77,80] but also from cactus pears [60] were at least in part responsible for these benefical properties. A very recent study investigated structure-activity relationships of various betaxanthins and betacyanins from members of the amaranthaceae with respect to free radical scavenging capacities [81]. The antioxidant potential was found to be related to structural features of the respective betalains. In betaxanthins, an increasing number of hydroxyl and imino residues improved free radical scavenging. In betacyanins, glycosylation reduced activity while acylation generally raised the antioxidant potential. Furthermore, 5-*O*-glycosylated structures produced lower antioxidant values than 6-*O*-glycosylated betacyanins. Future studies will have to ascertain the alleged promising physiological and pharmacological effects of betalains on humans published only very recently [80,82].

Polyphenols

Phenolics are an important constituent of fruit quality because of their contribution to the taste, colour and nutritional properties of fruit. Phenolic compounds have long been regarded as the UV-B screen for plants [83]. Their significance as dietary antioxidants has also been highlighted in recent years and thought to account for the cholesterol lowering, anticancer, antinflamintory or other physiological activity [84,85]. Environmental and developmental factors have been reported to affect the accumulation of polyphenols.

Flavonoids have a wide range of biological effects, such as inhibition of key enzymes in mitochondrial respiration, protection against coronary heart disease and anti-inflammatory, antitumour, and antimicrobial activities [86]. Hydroxycinnamic acid compounds inhibit the oxidation of low-density lipoprotein [87] and have anticancer [88] and antimicrobial activities [89].

Based on investigations of flowers and stems, *Cactaceae* were found to be low in polyphenols [90-92]. The presence of polyphenols in the juice at a level of (393 mg/kg), without differentiating between individual substances, has been reported [93]. Recently fruits of *Opuntia ficus-indica* cv. Saboten were subjected to polyphenol analysis, which indicated higher levels in the fruit than in the stem and seed [94]. Several author have recently reported the presence of polyphenols in the pulp [60,95-97]. Quercetin, kaempferol, and isorhamnetin derivatives were found to be the major flavonoids in cactus pear pulp [95]. However, more in-depth studies should be envisaged to fully assess the phenolic composition of cactus pear fruits neglected so far.

Regarding their antioxidative properties, polyphenols in fruit tissue are an attractive target. Whereas inter-and intramolecular stacking of polyphenols and anthocyanins has been intensively studied [98,101], similar stabilization principles have only been reported for acylated betacyanins [102,103]. With respect to betalain stability and colour shifts, analogous investigations appear to be of interest.

Flavour compounds

The high ratio of sugar and organic acids (exceeding 16:1) gives cactus pear a mildly sweet taste with little acid character. Cactus pear flavour is similar to honeydew melon or cucumber. The pulp flavour is characterized by a faint melon or cucumber-like aroma determined by alcohols and esters with 2-(E/Z)-2,6-nonadien-1-ol and 2-methylbutanoic acid methyl ester being the key aroma substances [104-108]. The flavour intensity was found to be strongest for yellow, followed by red, and, finally, white cactus pear fruits [104].

Alcohols, especially unsaturated, aldehydes, ketones, esters, ethers and hydrocarbons contribute to the spectrum of volatiles. Differences in the pattern of volatiles are attributed to climate, ripeness degree, postharvest conditions as well as to the species investigated [106,107]. The rather modest melon or cucumber-like flavour does not interact with stronger flavour impacts from other fruit or vegetable preparations which destine cactus pear as food colouring stuff not requiring declaration.

Sixty one aromas have been found in cactus fruit flesh of *Opuntia ficus-indica* [107], most of them are alcohols.

Lipids, sterols and fat-soluble vitamins

Lipids are present at very low levels ranging from 0.1 to 1.0 % in mesocarp or pulp of fruits [109]. In cactus pear pulp oils, linoleic acid was reported the dominating fatty acid, followed by palmitic and oleic acids. Also, the polyunsaturated fatty acids γ-linolenic and α-linolenic acids were detected in higher amounts [110,111]. The major sterol in pulp oils was β-sitosterol followed by campesterol, together constituting about 90 % of the total sterol portion. Interestingly, δ-tocopherol was the predominant vitamin E homologue, followed by α-, β-, and γ-tocopherols in far less amounts [110,111].

Medicinal Uses Of Cactus Pear

Antioxidant capacity

The antioxidative action is one of many mechanisms by which fruit and vegetable substances might exert their beneficial health effects [112]. The presence of several antioxidants (ascorbic acid, carotenoids, reduced glutathione, cysteine, taurine and flavonoids such as quercetin, kaempferol and isorhamnetin) has been detected in the fruits and vegetables of different varieties of cactus pear [96,97,112-114]. More recently, the antioxidant properties of the most frequent cactus pear betalains (betanin and indicaxanthin) have been revealed [6,59,96,97,115,116].

Lee *et al.* (2002) investigated *Opuntia ficus-indica* var Saboten (OFS), widely spread cactus in Southwestern Korea, and where is used as a functional food [117]. Antioxidant activity of OFS is reported to correspond to well-known antioxidants, such as catalase, -tocopherol, and ascorbic acid in a cell-free reactive oxygen species (ROS) generating system. It well established that oxidative stress may play a role in several diseases, such as heart disease, degenerative neuronal disease, and cancers. Many biochemical and clinical studies suggest that natural and synthetic antioxidant compounds are helpful in treating diseases mediated by oxidative stresses.

On the other hand, numerous *in vitro* studies have demonstrated the beneficial effect of colourless phenolics and betalains [59,118]. These are generally attributed to the ability of antioxidants to neutralize reactive oxygen species such as singlet oxygen, hydrogen peroxide or H_2O_2, or suppression of the xanthine/xanthineoxidase system, all of which may induce oxidative injury, i.e. lipid peroxidation.

Polyphenolics are antioxidants with well-known cardioprotective, anticancer, antiviral and antiallergenic properties [119,120].

Lee *et al.* (2002) demonstrated that antioxidative flavonoids, quercetin, (+) -dihydroquercetin and quercetin 3-methyl ether, isolated from *Opuntia ficus-indica* var. Saboten have neuroprotective effects [117]. They evaluated their protective effects against oxidative neuronal injuries induced in primary cultured rat cortical cells and their antioxidant activities. They found that quercetin inhibits H_2O_2- or xanthine (X)/xanthine oxidase (XO)-induced oxidative neuronal cell injury. Moreover, quercetin 3-methyl ether potently and dramatically inhibited H_2O_2 and X/XO-induced neuronal injuries. All above mentioned three principles markedly inhibited lipid peroxidation and scavenged 1,1-diphenyl-2-picrylhydrazyl free radicals. These results indicate that quercetin, (+)-dihydroquercetin, and quercetin 3-methyl ether are the active antioxidant principles in the fruits and cladodes of *Opuntia ficus-indica* var. Saboten. Furthermore, quercetin 3-methyl ether appears to be the most potent neuroprotectant of the three flavonoids isolated from this plant.

The betalain distribution in the three Sicilian cultivars of cactus pear (*Opuntia ficus-indica*) of yellow, red, and white fruits and the antioxidant activities of methanolic extracts from edible pulp were investigated by Buetra *et al.* (2002) [60]. The yellow cultivar exhibited the highest amount of betalains, followed by the red and white ones. Indicaxanthin accounted for about 99 % of betalains in the white fruit, while the ratio of betanin to indicaxanthin varied from 1:8 (w:w) in the yellow fruit to 2:1 (w:w) in the red one. Polyphenol pigments were negligible components only in the red fruit. When measured as 6-hydroxy-2,5,7,8-tetramethylchroman-2-carboxylic acid (Trolox) equivalents per gram of pulp, the methanolic fruit extracts showed a marked antioxidant activity. Vitamin C did not account for more than 40 % of the measured activity. In addition, the extracts dose-dependently inhibited the organic hydroperoxide-stimulated red cell membrane lipid oxidation, as well as the metaldependent and -independent low-density lipoprotein oxidation. The extract from the white fruit showed the highest protection in all models of lipid oxidation. These findings suggest that the above betalains contribute to the antioxidant activity of cactus pear fruits.

It is appears that supplementation with cactus pear (*Opuntia ficus-indica*) fruit decreases oxidative stress in healthy humans. Short-term supplementation with cactus pear fruit compared with vitamin C alone on total-body oxidative status in healthy humans was investigated by Butera *et al.* (2002) [60]. After supplementation with cactus pear fruit, malondialdehyde decreased by approximately 75 %; GSH:GSSG shifted toward a higher value; and LDL hydroperoxides were reduced by almost one-half. Supplementation with vitamin C did not significantly affect any marker of oxidative stress. Authors concluded that consumption of cactus fruit positively affects the body's redox balance, decreases oxidative damage to lipids, and improves antioxidant status in healthy humans. Supplementation with vitamin C at a comparable dosage enhances overall antioxidant defense but does not significantly affect body oxidative stress.

Galati and collaborators (2005) investigated the protective effects of cactus fruit (*Opuntia ficus-indica*) juice against carbon tetrachloride (CCl4)-induced hepatotoxicity in rats [121]. The animals were treated orally with the juice (3 mL/rat) 2 h after administration of the hepatotoxic agent. Preventive effects were studied by giving the juice (3 mL/rat) for 9 consecutive days. On day 9 the rats received the hepatotoxic agent. Morphological and biochemical evaluations were carried out 24, 48 and 72 h after induction of the hepatic damage. Data show that *Opuntia ficus-indica* fruit juice administration exerts protective and curative effects against the CCl_4-induced degenerative process in rat liver. Histology evaluation revealed a normal hepatic parenchyma at 48 h; the injury was fully restored after 72 h. Moreover, a significant reduction in CCl_4-induced increase of GOT and GPT plasma levels is evident; these data are in agreement with the functional improvement of hepatocytes. Authors assumed that cactus fruit juice contains many phenol compounds, ascorbic acid, betalains, betacyanins, and a flavonoid fraction, which consists mainly of rutin and isorhamnetin derivatives. Hepatoprotection may be related to the flavonoid fraction of the juice, but other compounds, such as vitamin C and betalains could, synergistically, counteract many degenerative processes by means of their antioxidant activity.

Cactus fruits have high antioxidant activity conferred by the presence of vitamin C, betacarotens, flavonoids, and betalains [95,122]. Fruits extract have an antioxidant activity of 4.2 to 5.3 mol Trolox f-1 for white and yellow variety, respectively.

The antioxidant activity of fruit extract is twice higher than pears, apples, tomato, bananas, white grapes, and similar to red grapes and grape fruit [60].

Significant amounts of ascorbic acid are present in *Opuntia ficus-indica* ranging from 180 to 300 mg/Kg. Cactus fruit is higher in vitamin C than other common fruits. The identification of vacuolar pigments contained in cactus pear fruit has been of renewed interest recently [22,23,49]. In addition to colour, the same pigments have shown antioxidant properties being higher than for ascorbic acid [96,97].

The presence of phenolics has been detected in cactus pulp fruit [60,95,97]. Kuti (1992) has reported an antioxidative effect due to the major flavonoids encountered in cactus fruits (quercetin, kaempferol and isorhamnetin) [113]. There is clear evidence that these compounds are more efficient antioxidants than vitamins, since phenolic compounds are able to delay prooxidative effects on proteins, DNA and lipids by the generation of stable radicals [123]. *Opuntia ficus-indica* polyphenolic compounds have been shown to induce a hyperpolarization of the plasma membrane and to raise the intracellular pool of calcium in human Jurkat T-cell lines [124]. Flavonol derivatives detected in *Opuntia* ssp. have been recently compiled [59]. When fruits are investigated, it must be taken into account that higher phenolic contents are expected in the peel, rather than the pulp. Consequently, from a nutritional point of view processing both peel and pulp appears to be advantageous.

The fat soluble vitamin E or tocopherols, and beta-carotene are found in the lipid fraction of both the cactus fruit seed and pulp. The vitamin E homologues isoforms gamma- and delta-tocopherol are the main components in seed and pulp oils, respectively, amounting to about 80 % of the total vitamin E content. Similar to beta-carotene, it is predominant in pulp lipids [110,111].

Anti-inflammatory and analgesic properties

Numerous studies have evocated the analgesic and anti-inflammatory actions of the genus *Opuntia* by using either the fruit extract from *Opuntia dillenii*, the lyophilized cladodes [125], or the phytosterols from fruit and stem extracts [114]. Park *et al.* (2001) identified beta-sitosterol as the active anti-inflammatory principle from the stem extract [126]. Gastric lesions in rat animal studies were reduced both by stem and fruit powders [117,127].

The ethanol extracts of *Opuntia ficus-indica* fruits inhibited the writhing syndrome induced by acetic acid, indicating that they contain analgesic effect [114]. The oral administrations of these extracts suppressed carrageenan-induced rat paw edema and also showed potent inhibition in the leukocyte migration of CMC-pouch model in rats. Moreover, the extracts suppressed the release of beta-glucuronidase, a lysosomal enzyme in rat neutrophils. It was also noted that the extracts showed the protective effect on gastric mucosal layers. From these results it is suggested that the cactus extracts contain anti-inflammatory action having protective effect against gastric lesions.

Antiulcerogenic effect and healing properties

In a work published in (2003), Galati *et al.* investigated the cactus fruit juice contents of ascorbic acid, total polyphenols, and flavonoids [122]. In the juice, ferulic acid was the chief derivative of hydroxycinnamic acid and the mean concentration of total phenolic compounds was 746 μg/mL. The flavonoid fraction, analyzed by high-performance liquid chromatography-diode array detection, consisted of rutin and isorhamnetin derivatives. The juice showed antioxidant activity, probably due to the phenolic compounds that are effective radical scavengers. The preventive administration of the juice inhibited the ulcerogenic activity of ethanol in rat. Light microscopy observations showed an increase in mucus production and the restoration of the normal mucosal architecture.

Additionally, Lee *et al.* (2001,2002) postulated an antiulcerogenic effect of the cladode or fruit powder from *Opuntia ficus-indica* var. saboten Makino [117,127]. Stomach lesions triggered by hydrochloric acid/ethanol or hydrochloric acid/acetylsalicylic acid were reduced, but no anti-inflammatory effect could be proven. The secretion rate of both gastric juice as well as the pH value remained constant, which has been confirmed by Galati *et al.* (2001) [125].

Anti-hyperlipidemic and cholesterol lowering effect

In a recent study it was shown that a daily consumption of 250 g of cactus pear pulp reduced the risk of thrombosis in patients suffering from hyperlipidemia and diabetes [128]. Wolfram *et al.* (2002) reported a reduction of total cholesterol, LDL, apolipoprotein levels, triglycerides, fibrinogen, blood glucose, insulin and urate, while body weight, high-density lipoprotein (HDL)-cholesterol, apolipoprotein A-1 and lipoprotein A levels were found to remain unchanged [129]. The anti-hyperlipidemic effects were ascribed to the pulp pectin, which both reduced lipid absorption and increased fecal sterol excretion, thus disrupting the enterohepatic circle.

Anti-cancer effect

It has been noted that Native Americans have a lower cancer rate when compared to white and African Americans [130]. Both cactus fruits and cladodes which contain multiple antioxidants have been used as a dietary supplement for centuries by Native Americans.

The goal of cancer prevention is to delay or block the processes of initiation and progression from pre-cancerous cells into cancer. Cancer chemoprevention, which targets normal and high risk populations, involves the use of drugs or other chemical agents to inhibit, delay, or reverse cancer development [131]. Medical benefits from plant forms have been recognized for centuries. Herbs have been used in Chinese medicine for thousands of years to cure diseases and heal wounds.

Recently, it has been found that Grape seed extracts have anti-cancer activities and protect chromosome [132]. Researchers at University of Alabama at Birmingham found that grape seed extract was chemo-preventive from their studies using animal model of breast cancer. However, diet had a strong impact to the grape seed extract's chemopreventive activity. Also, as a rule, herbs and natural products lack much of the toxicity that is present in synthetic chemicals, thus, enhancing their appeal for long term preventive strategies. Although hundreds of agents have been developed in the United States during the past decade, only a few new drugs have actually been approved [133]. The development of chemopreventive agents is slow and inefficient. More effective and less toxic agents, including natural products, are needed if we are to reach the goal of cancer prevention, both primary and secondary.

The development of effective and safe agents for prevention and treatment of cancer remains slow, inefficient, and costly. The key to effective chemoprevention is the identification of a chemopreventive agent(s) that can effectively inhibit cancer development without toxic side effects. Therefore, chemopreventive agents may need to be used for a long period of time to be effective. As a result, identification of agents with little or no toxicity becomes important.

Recent studies suggests that the cactus fruit extract (i) inhibits the proliferation of cervical, ovarian and bladder cancer cell lines *in vitro,* and (ii) suppresses tumor growth in the nude mice ovarian cancer model *in vivo* [134]. The intra-peritoneal administration of cactus extract solution into mice did not affect the animal body weight, which indicated that cactus did not have a significant toxic effect in animals.

Zou *et al.* (2005) showed that growth inhibition of cultured-cancer cells was associated with an increase in apoptotic cells and the cell cycle arrest at the G1-phase [134]. The same authors confirm that cactus fruit extract inhibited growth of different cancer cells *in vitro* and *in vivo*. Cactus products inhibited cancer cell growth with concentrations as low as 5 %; cell cycle was also affected at this concentration with an increase in G1 phase.

However, apoptosis was observed at a higher concentration of 10 % and 25 %. They have also compared cactus with the chemopreventive agent 4-HPR in nude mice. Both cactus and 4-HPR inhibited ovarian cancer growth. The anti-carcinogenic properties of natural and synthetic retinoids have been suggested to be due, in part, to the antioxidant effect, increased consumption of fruit and vegetables is associated with prevention of various human diseases, and the oxidative damage is an important etiologic risk factor for many diseases, including cancer and heart disease.

Carcinogenesis may be viewed as a process of progressive disorganization. This process is characterized by the accumulation of genotypic changes and corresponding tissue and cellular abnormalities including loss of proliferation and apoptosis controls. A dietary agent that can increase anti-proliferation pathways and change cell cycle in cancer cells without toxicity would be a potential agent for chemoprevention. Although the mechanism for cactus pear extract in cancer prevention is unclear, the study conducted by Zou *et al.* (2005) shows that cactus fruit extracts alter the expression of certain genes related to cell growth and apoptosis [134]. Quercetin is one of the components of cactus pear extracts. Results of Zou *et al.* (2005) and Hansen *et al.* (1997) suggest quercetin might be one of the active compounds responsible for the anticarcinogenetic and apoptosis-induction effects of cactus pear extracts [134,135]. Cactus pear extracts might have inhibitory effects on angiogenesis, an important factor contributing to tumor growth and metastasis.

It can be concluded that cactus pear extracts could be a candidate in cancer prevention for both normal and high-risk populations and prevention of recurrence in patients with previous cancers [134]. This product holds promise for long-term use because of the safety of food-derived products and the fact that they are not perceived as a "chemical", and that mechanisms involved need to be further investigated.

Conclusions

Both cactus pear (*Opuntia ficus-indica*) and red beet (*Beta vulgaris*) are rich on betalain pigments and particularly suitable for application in low acid food. The high nitrate levels [136] and the earthy smell by geosmin and pyrazine derivatives [137,138] restrict the application for red beet. While the use of cactus pear as a betalain source is an interesting possibility because they are highly flavored and show better nutritional properties than red beet [8,20,25,137]. In addition, *Opuntia* species have minimal soil and water requirements and may be regarded as an alternative for the agricultural economy of arid and semiarid regions. Cactus pear concentrates may be suitable for colouring yoghurts, ice creams, and fruit preparations. While the market potential of plain *Opuntia* juices is considered fair due to their faint flavour and high sugar:acid ratio, their utilization as a functional additive or for food colouring appears to be more promising. Cactus pear juices are considered a valuable ingredient for sports and energy drinks due to the high contents of amino acids, particularly proline and taurine, and minerals such as calcium and magnesium [139,140]. Moreover, cactus pear juice is considered a valuable source for enhancing colour of fruit-juice blends, such as orange-apple juice blends [141]. In addition to their use as colorants, the recently reported effects of betalains on human health [6,24,60,115] may open broader applications. Furthermore, the untapped potential of the hydrocolloid fraction and polyphenolics of both cactus pear fruit pulp and peel remains to be evaluated both from a nutritional and a technological point of view. Moreover, because of its high glucose and fructose contents, cactus pear is considered a potential raw material for the manufacture of high fructose glucose syrup [142]. Finally, for complete exploitation of the fruit, seeds may be used for oil extraction [110,137]. Hitherto, the main limitation of broader commercialization of cactus pear derivatives is the current market prices and the lack of know-how in cactus pear fruit processing.

In conclusion, cactus pear is a promising plant with a big potential for breeders, agriculturists and food technologists alike.

References

[1] Nobel, P.S; De la Barrera, E. (2003). Tolerances and acclimation to low and high temperatures for cladodes, fruits and roots of a widely cultivated cactus, Opuntia ficus indica. New Phytologist, 157, 271–279.

[2] Nobel, P. S; Pimienta-Barrios, E; Zaeudo Hernandez, J; Ramirez-Hernandez, B. (2002). Historical aspects and net CO_2 uptake for cultivated Crassulacean acid metabolism plants in Mexico. Annals of Applied Biology, 140, 133–142.

[3] Cornett, J. (2000). Nature trails Press: How Indians used desert plants.

[4] Kay, M.A. (1996). Healing with plants in the America, and Mexican west. The University of Arizona Press.

[5] Knishinsky, R. (1971). Prickly pear cactus medicine. Healing Arts Press. Rochester, Vermont.

[6] Tesoriere, L.D; Butera, A.M; Pintaudi, M.Allegra & Livrea, M.A. (2004). Supplementation with cactus pear (Opuntia ficus-indica) fruit decreases oxidative stress in healthy humans: a comparative study with vitamin C. American Journal of Clinical Nutrition, 80, 391-395.

[7] Munoz-de-Chavez, M.A; Chavez. V.Valles and Roldan, J.A. (1995). The nopal: a plant of manifold qualities. World Review of Nutrition and Dietetics, 77, 109-134.

[8] El Gharras, H; Hasib, A; Jaouad, A; El-bouadili, A. (2006). Chemical and physical characterisation of three Moroccan yellow prickly pears (*Opuntia ficus-indica*) at three different stages of maturity. Ciencia y Tecnologia Alimentaria, 5(2), 93-99.

[9] Barbera, G; Inglese, P. and La Mantia.T. (1994). Seed content and fruit characteristics in cactus pear (Opuntia ficus- indica Mill.). Scientia Horticulturae, 58, 161-165.

[10] Inglese, P; Barbera, G; La Mantia, T. and Portolano, S. (1995). Crop production and ultimate size of cactus pear fruit following fruit thinning. Horticultural Science, 30, 227-230.

[11] Lakshminarayana, S; Alvarado, L. and Perez, F. (1979). The development and postharvest physiology of the fruit of prickly pear (Opuntia amyclaea Tenore). Tropical Foods, 1, 69-93.

[12] Mondragon-Jacobo, C. and Perez-Gonzalez, S. (1996). Native cultivars of cactus pear in Mexico. In Progress in new crops, J. Janick (ed.), ASHS Press, Arlington, Va, pp. 446-450.

[13] Nerd, A; Karadi, A. and Mizrahi, Y. (1991). Out of season prickly pear: fruit characteristics and effect of fertilization and short droughts on productivity. Horticultural Science, 26, 527-529.

[14] Nieddu, G., De Pau, L ; Schirra, M. and D'hallewin, G. (1997). Chemical composition of fruit and seeds of cactus pears during early and late-induced crop ripening. Acta Horticulturae, 438, 105-111.

[15] Sawaya, W. N; Khatchadourian, H. A; Safi, W. M. and Al-Muhammad, H. M. (1983). Chemical Characterization of Prickly Pear Pulp, Opuntia Ficus Indica, and the Manufacturing of Prickly Pear Jam. Journal of Food Technology, 18, 183-193.

[16] Sepulveda, E; Saenz, C. (1990). Caracteristicas Quimicas y Fisicas de Pulpa de Tuna (Opuntia Ficus Indica). Revista de Agroquimica y Tecnologia de Alimentos, 30, 51-555.

[17] Askar, A; El-Samahy, S. K. (1981). Chemical composition of prickly pear fruits. Deutsche Lebensmittel-Rundschau, 77, 279-281.

[18] Joubert, E. (1993). Processing of the Fruit y Pear Cultivars Grown in South Africa. International Journal of Food Science and Technology, 28, 377-387.

[19] Stintzing, F.C; Schieber, A. and Carle, R. (1999). Amino acid composition and betaxanthin formation in fruits from Opuntia ficus-indica". Planta Medica, 65(7), 632-635.

[20] Piga, A. (2004). Cactus pear: A fruit of nutraceutical and functional importance. Journal of the Professional Association for Cactus Development, 6, 9-22.

[21] Saenz-Hernandez, C. (1995). Food manufacture and by-products. In: Barbera, G.; Inglese, P.; Pimienta-Barrios, E. (eds.). Agro-ecology, cultivation and uses of cactus pear. FAO Plant Production and Protection Paper, 132, 137-143.

[22] El Gharras, H; Hasib, A; Jaouad, A; El-bouadili, A. and Schoefs, B. (2008). Stability of vacuolar betaxanthin pigments in juices from Moroccan yellow *Opuntia ficus indica* fruits. International Journal of Food Science and Technology, 43, 351–356.

[23] EL Gharras, H. Betalains: Vacuolar pigments. Plant Cell Compartments - Selected Topics, (2008). ISBN: 978-81-308-0104-9. Research Signpost. India. Editor: Benoît SCHOEFS. Chapter 11, 309-334.

[24] Feugang, J.M; Konarski, P; Zou, D; Stintzing, F.C. and Zou, C. (2006). Nutritional and medicinical use of cactus pear (Opuntia spp.) cladodes and fruits. Frontiers in Bioscience, 11, 2574-2589.

[25] Stintzing, F. C; Schieber, A; Carle, R. (2001). Phytochemical and nutritional significance of cactus pear. International Food Research Technology, 212, 396-407.

[26] Wills, R. B. H; Lim, J. S. K; Greenfield, H. (1986). Composition of Australian foods. 31. Tropical and sub-tropical fruit. Food Technology in Australia, 38, 118-123.

[27] Barbera, G; Carimi, F; Inglese, P. and Panno, M. (1992). Physical, morphological and chemical changes during fruit development and ripening in three cultivars of prickly-pear (Opuntia ficus-indica (L.) Miller). Journal of Horticultural Science, 67, 307-312.

[28] Tateo, F. (1978). Analisi dei Prodotti Alimentari; Chiriotti Editori: Pinerolo (TO), Italy.

[29] Belitz, H. D; Grosch, W. (1999). Food Chemistry, Springer-Verlag: Berlin, Germany.

[30] Villareal, F; De Alva, B.E; Romero, G. (1964). Estudio quimico sobre jugos de tunas enlatadas. Ciencia (Méx.), 23, 75-82.

[31] Matsuhiro, B; Lillo, L.E; Sáenz, C; Urzúa, C. C. and Zárate, O. (2006). Chemical characterization of the mucilage from fruits of Opuntia ficus indica. Carbohydrate Polymers, 63, 263-267.

[32] El Kossori, R. L ; Villaume, C; El Boustani, E ; Sauvaire, Y. and Méjean, L. (1998). Composition of pulp, skin and seeds of prickly pears fruits (Opuntia ficus indica sp.). Plant Foods for Human Nutrition, 52, 263-270.

[33] Forni, E; Penci, M. and Polesello, A. (1994). A preliminary characterization of some pectins from quince fruit (Cydonia oblonga Mill.) and prickly pear (Opuntia ficus-indica) peel. Carbohydrate Polymers, 23, 231-234.

[34] Cruse, R. R. (1973). Desert Plant Chemurgy: a current review. Economic Botany, 27, 210-230.

[35] Felker, P; Singh, G; Pareek, O. P. (1997). Opportunities for development of cactus (Opuntia spp.) in arid and semi-arid regions. Annals of Arid Zone, 36, 267-278.

[36] Trejo-Gonzalez, A; Gabriel-Ortiz, G; Puebla-Perez, A. M; Hulzar-Contreras, M. D; Mungula-Mazariegos, M. R; Mejia-Arreguln, S; Calva, E. (1996). A purified extract from prickly pear cactus (Opuntia fuliginosa) controls experimentally induced diabetes in rats. Journal of Ethnopharmacology, 55, 27-33.

[37] Luz-Fernandez, M ; Trejo, A ; McNamara, D. J. (1990). Pectin isolated from prickly pear (Opuntia sp.) modifies low density lipoprotein metabolism in cholesterol-fed guinea pigs. Journal of Nutrition, 120, 1283-1290.

[38] Luz-Fernandez, M; Lin, E. C. K; Trejo, A; McNamara, D. J. (1992). Prickly pear (Opuntia sp.) pectin reverses low density lipoprotein receptor suppression induced by a hypercholesterolemic diet in guinea pigs. Journal of Nutrition, 122, 2330-2340.

[39] Kuti, J.O. and Galloway C-M. (1994). Sugar composition and invertase activity in prickly pear fruit. Journal of Food Science, 59, 387-393.

[40] Ouelhazi, N.K; Ghrir, R; Diêp Le, K. H; Lederer, F. (1992). Invertase from Opuntia ficus-indica fruits. Phytochemisry, 31, 59-61.

[41] Espinosa, J; Borrocal, R; Jara, M; Zorilla, C; Zanabria, C; Medina, J. (1973). Quelques propriétés et essais préliminaires de conservation des fruits et du jus de figue de Barbarie (Opuntia ficus-indica). Fruits, 28, 285-289.

[42] Lakshminarayana, S. (1980). Sapodilla and prickly pear. In: NAGY, S.; SHAW, P.E., 1980. Tropical and subtropical fruits. Composition, properties and uses. AVI Publishing, Inc., Westport, Connecticut. Chapter 12, 415-441.

[43] Gurrieri, S; Miceli, L; Lanza, C. M; Tomaselli, F; Bonomo, R. P; Rizzarelli, E. (2000). Chemical Characterization of Sicilian Prickly Pear (Opuntia ficus indica) and Perspectives for the Storage of Its Juice. Journal of Agricultural and Food Chemistry, 48, 5424-5431.

[44] Cappelli, P. and Vannucchi, V. Chimica degli Alimenti-Conservazione e Trasformazioni; Zanichelli: Bologna, Italy, (1990).

[45] Felker, P; Del C, Rodriguez, S; Casoliba, R. M; Filippini, R; Medina, D. and Zapata, R. (2005). Comparison of Opuntia ficus-indica varieties of Mexican and Argentine origin for fruit yield and quality in Argentina. Journal of Arid Environments, 60, 405-422.

[46] Odoux, E. and Domínguez-López, A. (1996). Le figuier de Barbarie: une source industrielle de bétalaines? Fruits, 51, 61-78.

[47] Moßhammer, Markus. R; Stintzing, Florian. C. and Carle, Reinhold. (2006). Cactus Pear Fruits (Opuntia spp.): A Review of Processing Technologies and Current Uses. Journal of the Professional Association for Cactus Development, 1-25.

[48] Sáenz, C; Berger, H; Galletti, L. and Coronado, F. (2001). Sensory and microbiological changes in minimally processed cactus pear (Opuntia ficus-indica). Acta Horticulturae, 553, 709-710.

[49] Stintzing, F. C; Schieber, A. and Carle, R.C. (2003). Evaluation of colour properties and chemical quality parameters of cactus juices. European Food Research Technology, 216, 303-311.

[50] Kugler, F; Graneis, S; Schreiter, P; Stintzing, F. C. and Carle, R. (2006). Determination of free amino compounds in betalainic fruits and vegetables by gas chromatography with flame ionization and mass spectrometric detection. Journal of Agricultural and Food Chemistry, 54, 4311-4318.

[51] Herrmann, K. (1998). Uber die Inhaltsstoffe und die Verwendung wichtiger exotischer Obstarten. XIII. Kaktusfeigen. Industrielle Obst- und Gemüseverwertung 11/12, 335-337.

[52] Teles, F. F. F; Stull, J. W; Brown, W. H; Whiting, F. M. (1984). Amino and organic acids of the prickly pear cactus (Opuntia ficus-indica L.). Journal of the Science of Food and Agriculture, 35, 421-425.

[53] Dominguez-Lopez, A. (1995). Review: use of the fruits and stems of the prickly pear cactus (Opuntia spp.) into human food. Food Science and Technology International, 1, 65-74.

[54] Blenford, D. E. (1996). Winner Drinks. The use of amino acids and peptides in sports nutrition. International Food Ingredients, 3, 20-23.

[55] Pszczola, D. E. (1998). Natural colors: Pigments of imagination. Food Technology, 52, 70-82.

[56] Silos-Espino, H; Fabian-Morales, L; Osuna-Castro, J. A; Valverde, M. E; Guevara-Lara, F; Paredes Lopez, O. (2003). Chemical and Biochemical changes in prickly pears with different ripening behaviour. Nahrung Food, 47(5), 334-338.

[57] Sepúlveda Jiménez, G; Rueda Benítez, P; Porta, H; Rocha Sosa, M. (2003) Wounding and infiltration with Pseudomonas syringae pv. tabaci of Agrobacterium tumefaciens induced the synthesis of betacyanins in red beet (Beta vulgaris vad. CrosbyEgyptian)

leaves. Participation of oxygen reactive species. In 7th International Congress of Plant Molecular Biology, Barcelona.

[58] Castellar, M. R; Obón, J. M; Alacid, M. and Fernández-López, J. A. (2003). Color properties and stability of betacyanins from Opuntia fruits. Journal of Agricultural and Food Chemistry, 51, 2772-2776.

[59] Stintzing, F. C; Herbach, K. M; Moßhammer, M. R; Carle, R; Yi, W. E; Sellappan, S; Akoh, C. C; Bunch, R. and Felker, P. (2005). Color, betalain pattern and antioxidant properties of cactus pear (Opuntia sp.) clones. Journal of Agricultural and Food Chemistry, 53, 442-451.

[60] Butera, D; Tesoriere, L; Di Gaudio, F; Bongiorno, A; Allegra, M; Pintaudi, A. M; Kohen, R. & Livrea, M. A. (2002). Antioxidant activities of Sicilian prickly pear (Opuntia ficus-indica) fruit extracts and reducing properties of its betalains: betanin and indicaxanthin. Journal of Agricultural and Food Chemistry, 50, 6895–6901.

[61] Nefzaoui, A; Nazareno, M; El Mourid, M. (2008). Review of Medicinal Uses of cactus. CactusNet, Issue 11, 3-17.

[62] Moreno Alvarez, M. J; Medina,C; Antón, L; García, D; Belén Camacho, D. R. (2003). Uso de pulpa de tuna (Opuntia boldinghii) en la elaboración de bebidas cítricas pigmentadas. Interciencia, 28, 539-543.

[63] Schwartz, S. J; Von Elbe, J. H; Pariza, M. W; Goldsworthy, T. & Pitot, H. C. (1983). Inability of red beet betalain pigments to initiate or promote hepatocarcinogenesis. Food and Chemical Toxicology, 21, 531–535.

[64] Von Elbe, J. H. & Schwartz, S. J. (1981). Absence of mutagenic activity and short-term toxicity study of beet pigments as food colorants. Archives of Toxicology, 49, 93–98.

[65] Kapadia, G. J; Tokuda, H; Konoshima, T. & Nishino, H. (1996). Chemoprevention of lung and skin cancer by Beta vulgaris (beet) root extract. Cancer Letters, 100, 211–214.

[66] Krifa, F; Villet, A; Roussel, A.-M. & Alary, J. (1987). Pourpre de Barbarie, nouveau colorant naturel extrait d'Opuntia stricta. Annales des Falsifications de l'Expertise Chimique et Toxicologique, 928, 183–191.

[67] Reynoso, R. C; Giner, T. V. & Gonzalez de Mejia, E. (1999). Safety of a filtrate of fermented garambullo fruit: biotransformation and toxicity studies. Food and Chemical Toxicology, 37, 825–830.

[68] Kuramoto, Y; Yamada, K; Tsuruta, O. & Sugano, M. (1996). Effect of natural food colorings on immunoglobulin production in vitro by rat spleen lymphocytes. Bioscience, Biotechnology and Biochemistry, 60, 1712–1713.

[69] Pourrat, A; Lejeune, B; Grand, A; Bastide, P. & Bastide, J. (1987). Propriétés du jus et des colorants de la betterave rouge. Médecin et Nutrition, 23, 166–172.

[70] Mitchell, S. C. (2001). Food idiosyncrasies: beetroot and asparagus. Drug Metabolism and Disposition, 29, 539–543.

[71] Cao, G; Sofic, E. & Prior, R. L. (1996). Antioxidant capacity of tea and common vegetables. Journal of Agricultural and Food Chemistry, 44, 3426–3431.

[72] Halvorsen, B. L; Holte, K; Myhrstad, M. C. W; Barikmo, I; Hvattum, E; Remberg, S. F; Wold, A.-B; Haffner, K; Baugerod, H; Andersen, L. F; Moskaug, J. O; Jacobs jr, D.

R., & Blomhoff, R. (2002). A systematic screening of total antioxidants in dietary plants. Journal of Nutrition, 132, 461–471.

[73] Kähkönen, M. P; Hopia, A. I; Vuorela, H. J; Rauha, J.-P; Pihlaja, K; Kujala, T. S. & Heinonen, M. (1999). Antioxidant activity of plant extracts containing phenolic compounds. Journal of Agricultural and Food Chemistry, 47, 3954–3962.

[74] Ou, B; Huang, D; Hampsch-Woodill, M; Flanagan, J. A. & Dee-mer, E. K. (2002). Analysis of antioxidant activities of common vegetables employing oxygen radical absorbance capacity (ORAC) and ferric reducing antioxidant power (FRAP) assays: a comparative study. Journal of Agricultural and Food Chemistry, 50, 3122–3128.

[75] Vinson, J. A; Hao, Y; Su, X. & Zubik, L. (1998). Phenol antioxidant quantity and quality in foods: vegetables. Journal of Agricultural and Food Chemistry, 46, 3630–3634.

[76] Wettasinghe, M; Bolling, B; Plhak, L. & Parkin, K. (2002). Screening for phase II enzyme-inducing and antioxidant activities of common vegetables. Journal of Food Science, 67, 2583–2588.

[77] Escribano, J; Pedreňo, M. A; Garcĭa-Carmona, F. & Muňoz, R. (1998). Characterization of the antiradical activity of betalains from Beta vulgaris L. roots. Phytochemical Analysis, 9, 124–127.

[78] Pavlov, A; Kovatcheva, P; Georgiev, V; Koleva, I. & Ilieva, M. (2002). Biosynthesis and radical scavenging activity of betalains during the cultivation of red beet (Beta vulgaris) hairy root cultures. Zeitschrift für Naturforschung C, 57, 640–644.

[79] [79] Pedreňo, M. A. & Escribano, J. (2001). Correlation between antiradical activity and stability of betanine from Beta vulgaris L roots under different pH, temperature and light conditions. Journal of the Science of Food and Agriculture, 81, 627–631.

[80] [80] Wettasinghe, M; Bolling, B; Plhak, L; Xiao, H. & Parkin, K. (2002). Phase II enzyme-inducing and antioxidant activities of beetroot (Beta vulgaris L.) extracts from phenotypes of different pigmentation. Journal of Agricultural and Food Chemistry, 50, 6704–6707.

[81] [81] Cai, Y; Sun, M. & Corke, H. (2003). Antioxidant activity of betalains from plants of the Amaranthaceae. Journal of Agricultural and Food Chemistry, 51, 2288–2294.

[82] [82] Kanner, J. & Lapidot, T. (2001). The stomach as a bioreactor: dietary lipid peroxidation in the gastric fluid and the effects of plant-derived antioxidants. Free Radical Biology & Medicine, 31, 1388–1395.

[83] [83] Schmitz-Hoerner, R. &Weissenböck, G. (2003). Contribution of phenolic compounds to the UV-B screening capacity of developing barley primary leaves in relation to DNA damage and repair under elevated UV-B levels. Phytochemistry, 34, 243–255.

[84] Prior, R. L; Cao, G; Martin, A; Sofic, E; McEven, J; O'Brien, C. (1998). Antioxidant capacity as influenced by total phenolics and anthocyanin content, maturity and variety of vaccinum species. Journal of Agricultural and Food Chemistry, 26, 2686–2693.

[85] Velioglu, Y. S; Mazza, G; Gao, L. & Oomah, B. D. (1998). Antioxidant activity and total phenolics in selected fruits, vegetables, and grain products. Journal of Agricultural and Food Chemistry, 46, 4113–4117.

[86] Harborne, J. B. & Williams, C. A. (2000). Advances in flavonoid research since 1992. Phytochemistry, 55, 481–504.

[87] Meyer, A. S; Donovan, J. L; Pearson, D. A; Waterhouse, A. L. & Frankel, E. N. (1998). Fruit hydroxycinnamic acids inhibit human low-density lipoprotein oxidation in vitro. Journal of Agricultural and Food Chemistry, 46, 1783–1787.

[88] Kual, A. & Khanduja, K. L. (1998). Polyphenols inhibit promotional phase of tumorigenesis: relevance of superoxide radicals. Nutrition Cancer, 32, 81–85.

[89] Kernan, M. R; Amarquay, A; Chen, J. L; Chan, J; Sesin, D. F; Parkinson, N. (1998). Antiviral phenlypropanoid glycosides from the medicinal plant Markhamia lutea. Journal of Natural Product, 61, 564–570.

[90] Reznik, H. (1957). Die Pigmente des Centrospermen als systhematisches Element. II. Untersuchungen über das Ionophoretische Verhalten. Planta, 49, 406-434.

[91] Hegnauer, R. (1964). Chemotaxonomie der pflanzen. Dicotyledoneae: acanthaceae-cyrillaceae, vol 3. birkhauser, basel, pp 324-336.

[92] Hegnauer, R. (1989). Chemotaxonomie der pflanzen. Bd. 8: Nachträge zu Band 3 und Band 4 (Acanthaceae-Lythraceae). Birkhauser-Verlag Basel, pp 176-183, 648, 670.

[93] Lercker, G; Lerici, C. R; Capella, P. (1976). Caratteri chimici del fico d'India (Cactus opuntia). 1: Carboidrati e lipidi del frutto. La Rivista Italiana delle Sostanze Grasse, 53, 250-254.

[94] Lee, Y. L; Hwang, K. H; Han, D. H; Kim, S. D. (1997). Compositions of Opuntia ficus-indica. Korean Journal of Food Science and Technology, 29, 847-853.

[95] Kuti, J. O. (2004). Antioxidant compounds from four Opuntia cactus pear fruit varieties. Food Chemistry, 85, 527-533.

[96] Tesoriere, L; Fazzari, M; Allegra, M. & Livrea, M. A. (2005). Biothiols, taurine, and lipid-soluble antioxidants in the edible pulp of Sicilian cactus pear (Opuntia ficus-indica) fruits and changes of bioactive juice components upon industrial processing. Journal of Agricultural and Food Chemistry, 53, 7851-7855.

[97] Tesoriere, L; Butera, D; Allegra, M; Fazzari, M. & Livrea, M. A. (2005). Distribution of betalain pigments in red blood cells after consumption of cactus pear fruits and increased resistance of the cells to ex vivo induced oxidative hemolysis in humans. Journal of Agricultural and Food Chemistry, 53, 1266-1270.

[98] Bloor, S. J. (1997). Blue flower colour derived from flavonol—anthocyanin co-pigmentation in Ceanothus papillosus. Phytochemistry, 45(7), 1399-1405.

[99] Brouillard, R; Figueiredo, P; Elhabiri, M; Dangles, O. (1997). Vegetables. In: tomas-barberan fa, robins rj (eds) phytochemistry of fruit and vegetables, clarendon press, oxford, pp 29-49.

[100] Davies, A. J; Mazza, G. (1993). Copigmentation of simple and acylated anthocyanins with colorless phenolic compounds. Journal of Agricultural and Food Chemistry, 41(5), 716-720.

[101] Goto, T. (1987). Structure, stability and color variation of natural anthocyanins - Prog. Chem. Org. Nat. Prod. 52, 113-158.

[102] Heuer, S; Wray, V; Metzger, J. W; Strack, D. (1992). Betacyanins from flowers of Gomphrena globosa. Phytochemistry, 31(5), 1801-1807.

[103] Schliemann, W. and Strack, D. (1998). Intramolecular stabilization of acylated betacyanins. Phytochemistry, 49(2), 585-588.

[104] Agozzino, P; Avellone, G; Ceraulo, L; Ferrugia, M. and Filizzola, F. (2005). Volatile profiles of Sicilian prickly pear (Opuntia ficus-indica) by SPME-GC/MS analysis. Italian Journal of Food Science, 17, 341-348.

[105] Arena, E; Campisi, S; Fallico, B; Lanza, M. C. and Maccarone, E. (2001). Aroma value of volatile compounds of prickly pear (Opuntia ficus-indica (L.) Mill, Cactaceae). Italian Journal of Food Science, 13, 311-319.

[106] Di Cesare, L. F. and Nani, R. (1992). Analyse der flüchtigen Inhaltsstoffe in Kaktusfeigensaft (Opuntia ficus-indica var. Fructa sanguineo). Flüssiges Obst, 59: 12-14.

[107] Flath, R. A. and Takahashi, J. M. (1978). Volatile constituents of prickly pear (Opuntia ficus indica Mill.), de Castilla variety. Journal of Agriculture and Food Chemistry, 26, 835-837.

[108] Weckerle, B; Bastl-Bormann, R; Richling, E; Hör, K; Ruff, C. and Schreier, P. (2001). Cactus pear (Opuntia ficus indica) flavour constituents – chiral evaluation (MDGC-MS) and isotope ratio (HRGC-IRMS) analysis. Flavour and Fragrance Journal, 16, 360-363.

[109] Kamel, B. S. and Kakuda, Y. (2000). Fatty acids in fruits and fruit products. In C.K. Chow (Ed.), Fatty acids in foods and their health implications (2nd ed.) (pp. 239-270). New York: Marcel Dekker.

[110] Ramadan, M. F. & Mörsel, J.-T. (2003). Oil cactus pear (Opuntia ficus-indica L.). Food Chemistry, 82, 339–345.

[111] Ramadan, M. F. and Mörsel, J.-T. (2003). Lipid profile of prickly pear pulp fractions. Food, Agriculture & Environment, 1, 66-70.

[112] Lee, Y. C; Hwang, K. H; Han, D. H; Kim, S. D. (1999). Compositions of Opuntia ficus-indica. Korean Journal of Food Science and Technology, 29, 847–853.

[113] Kuti, J. O. (1992). Growth and compositional changes during the development of prickly pear fruit. Journal of Horticultural Science, 67, 861-868.

[114] Park, E.-H; Kahng, J.H. & Paek, E.-A. (1998). Studies on the pharmacological actions of cactus: identification of its anti-inflammatory effect. Archives of Pharmacal Research, 21, 30–34.

[115] Gentile C; Tesoriere,L; Allegra, M; Livrea, M. A. & D'Alessio, P. (2004). Antioxidant betalains from cactus pear (Opuntia ficus-indica) inhibit endothelial ICAM-1 expression. Annals of the New York Academy of Sciences, 1028, 481–486.

[116] Tesoriere, L; Butera, D; D'Arpa,D; Di Gaudio,F; Allegra, M; Gentile, C. & Livrea, M. A. (2003). Increased resistance to oxidation of betalainenriched human low density lipoproteins. Free Radical Research, 37, 689–696.

[117] Lee, J-C; Kim, H. R; Kim, J; Jang, Y.-S. (2002). Antioxidant property of an ethanol extract of the stem of Opuntia ficus indica var. saboten. Journal of Agricultural and Food Chemistry, 50, 6490– 6496.

[118] Dok-Go, H; Lee, K. H; Kim, H. J; Lee, E. H; Lee, J; Song, Y. S; Lee, Y.-H; Jin, C; Lee, Y.S. & Cho, J. (2003). Neuroprotective effects of antioxidative flavonoids,

quercetin, (+)- dihydroquercetin and quercetin 3-methyl ether, isolated from Opuntia ficus-indica var. saboten. Brain Research, 965, 130-136.

[119] Carbo, N; Costelli, P; Baccino, F. M; Lopez-Soriano, F. J. & Argiles, J. M. (1999). Resveratrol, a natural product present in wine, decreases tumour growth in a rat tumour model. Biochemical and Biophysical Research Communications, 254, 739-743.

[120] Tapiero, H; Tew, K. D; Ba, G.N. & Mathe, G. (2002). Polyphenols: Do they play a role in the prevention of human pathologies? Biomedicine & Pharmacotherapy, 56, 200–207.

[121] Galati, E. M; Mondello, M. R; Lauriano, E. R; Taviano, M. F; Galluzzo, M. & Miceli, N. (2005). Opuntia ficus indica (L.) Mill. Fruit Juice Protects Liver from Carbon Tetrachlorideinduced Injury. Phytotherapy Research, 19, 796–800.

[122] Galati, E. M; Tripodo, M. M; Trovato, A; d'Aquino, A. & Monforte, M. T. (2003). Biological activity of Opuntia ficus indica cladodes II: Effect on experimental hypercholesterolemia in rats. Pharmaceutical Biology, 41, 3, 175-179.

[123] Shahidi, F; Janitha, P. K. & Wanasundara, P. D. (1992). Phenolic antioxidanta, Critical previous term Reviews next term. Journal of Food Science and Nutrition, 32, 67–103.

[124] Aires, V; Adote, S; Hichami, A; Moutairou, K. E. S; Boustani, E. & Khan, N. A. (2004). Modulation of intracellular calcium concentrations and T cell activation by prickly pear polyphenols. Molecular and Cellular Biochemistry, 260, 103-110.

[125] Galati, E. M; Monforte, M. T; Tripodo, M. M; d'Aquino A. & Mondello, M. R. (2001). Antiulcer activity of Opuntia ficus-indica (L.) Mill. (Cactaeceae): ultrastructural study. Journal of Ethnopharmacology, 76, 1-9.

[126] Park, E. H; Kahng J. H; Lee, S. H. & Shin, K. H. (2001). An anti-inflammatory principle from cactus. Fitoterapia, 72, 288-290.

[127] Lee, E. B; Hyun, J. E; Li, D. W. & Moon, Y. I. (2001). The effect of Opuntia ficus-indica var. saboten fruit on gastric lesion and ulcer in rats. Natural Product Science, 7, 90-93.

[128] Wolfram, R. M; Budinsky, A; Efthimiou, Y; Stomatopoulos, J; Oguogho, A; Sinzinger, H. (2003). Daily prickly pear consumption improves platelet function. Prostagland. Leukotr. Ess. Fatty Acids, 69, 61–66.

[129] Wolfram, R. M; Kritz, H; Efthimiou, Y; Stomatopoulos, J; Sinzinger, H. (2002). Effect of prickly pear (Opuntia robusta) on glucose- and lipid-metabolism in nondiabetics with hyperlipidemia – a pilot study. Wiener Klin. Wochenschr., 114, 840–846.

[130] Cancer statistics, (2004). American cancer society.

[131] Kelloff, G. J; Sigman, C. C; Greenwald, P. (1999). Cancer chemoprevention: progress and promise. European Journal of Cancer, 35, 2031-2038.

[132] Kim, H; Hall, P; Smith, M; Kirk, M; Prasain, J. K; Barnes, S; Grubbs, C. (2004). Chemoprevention by grape seed extract and genistein in carcinogen-induced mammary cancer in rats is diet dependent. Journal of Nutrition, 134(12 Suppl), 3445S-3452S.

[133] Kelloff, G. J; Crowell, J. A; Vernon, E; Steele, R. A; Lubet, W. A; Malone, C. W; Boone, L. K. E. T; Hawk, R; Lerman, J. A; Lawrence, I. A, Jaye, L. V. and Sigman, C. C. (2000). Progress in Cancer Chemoprevention: Development of Diet-Derived Chemopreventive Agents. Journal of Nutrition, 130, 467S-471S.

[134] Zou, D. M; Brewer, M; Garcia, F; Feugang, J. M; Wang, J; Zang, R; Liu, H. & Zou, C.P. (2005). Cactus Pear - a Natural Product in Cancer Chemoprevention. Nutrition Journal, 4:25.

[135] Hansen, R. K; Oesterreich, S; Lemieux, P; Sarge, D.K; Fuqua, S. A. W. (1997). Quercetin inhibits heat shock protein induction but not heat shock factor DNA-binding in human breast carcinoma celles. Biochemical and Biophysical Research Communications, 239, 851-856.

[136] Bednar, C. M; Kies, C; Carlson, M. (1991). Nitrate-nitrite levels in commercially processed and home-processed beets and spinach. Plant Foods for Human Nutrition, 41, 261-8.

[137] Stintzing, F. C; Schieber, A; Carle, R. (2000). Cactus pear-a promising component to functional food. Forschung, 2000, 40-47.

[138] Lu, G; Edwards, C. G; Fellman, J. K; Mattinson, D. S. and Navazio, J. (2003). Quantitative determination of geosmin in red beets (Beta vulgaris L.) using headspace solid-phase microextraction. Journal of Agricultural and Food Chemistry, 51, 1026-1029.

[139] Reyner, L. A. and Horne, J. A. (2002). Efficacy of a 'functional energy drink' in counteracting driver sleepness. Physiology & Behavior, 75, 331-335.

[140] Seidl, R; Peyrl, A; Nicham, R. and Hauser, E. (2000). A taurine and caffeine-containing drink stimulates cognitive performance and well-being. Amino Acids, 19, 635-642.

[141] Moreno-Alvarez, M. J; Medina, C; Antón, L; García, D. and Belén-Camacho, D. R. (2003). Uso de pulpa de tuna (Opuntia boldinghii) en la elaboración de bebidas cítricas pigmentadas. Interciencia, 28, 539-543.

[142] Hamdi, M. (1997). Prickly pear cladodes and fruits as a potential raw material for the bioindustries. Bioprocess Engineering, 17, 387-391.

In: Fruit Juices: Properties, Consumption and Nutrition
Editor: Pauline G. Scardina
ISBN: 978-1-60741-505-3

Chapter 3

Preservation of Fruit Juices by Pulsed Electric Fields

Pedro Elez-Martínez, Robert Soliva-Fortuny and Olga Martín-Belloso*

Department of Food Technology. University of Lleida
Av. Alcalde Rovira Roure, 191. 25198 Lleida, Spain

Abstract

Pulsed electric fields (PEF) is a nonthermal processing technology that could be used to pasteurize fluid foods avoiding the negative effects of heat. The application of PEF to preserve fruit juices has been extensively studied in the last years. Both microbiological safety and spoilage delay can be achieved when juices are treated with PEF. Furthermore, PEF treatments have also been shown to inactivate varying amounts of several deleterious enzymes. Because of the inactivation of microorganisms and enzymes with a minimal impact on quality and nutritional properties, it is suggested that PEF is a technology of choice to obtain safe and high-quality fruit juices with a shelf-life similar to the attained with mild heat pasteurization treatments. Moreover, the combination of PEF with other food preservation techniques is currently being studied in order to further extend the shelf-life of juices. Future efforts will be devoted to successfully implement PEF processing at an industrial scale as an alternative to traditional heat processing or even as a way of improving quality of the final product by reducing heat treatment intensities.

* e-mail: omartin@tecal.udl.es

Introduction

Pulsed electric fields (PEF) is a non-thermal food processing technology that has been studied in recent years as an alternative or complement to heat treatments. This technique involves applying electrical pulses of high intensity (kV/cm) during a very short period of time (μs) at moderate or low temperatures. Inactivation of pathogenic and spoilage microorganisms can be attained together with a minimal impact on food quality and nutritional properties, which suggests that it is possible to obtain safe PEF-treated foods of high quality with an acceptable shelf life.

The use of electricity to stabilize food is very old. It was initially applied as a thermal treatment by increasing the product temperature to treat grape juice (Tracy, 1932) and milk (Moses, 1938). However, it felt almost into oblivion during the mid-40's (Palaniappan and Sastry, 1991; Martín et al., 1994).

In the 50's, a new kind of food processing, which consisted in the implementation of high-intensity discharges causing the formation of an electric arc, was called "electrohydraulic treatment". This treatment caused the destruction of microorganisms and enzymes but, at the same time, induced the formation of electrolysis products. In addition, this technique produces changes in the composition of the food and a large warming (Palaniappan and Sastry, 1991).

It was in 1967 when Sale and Hamilton applied the electricity in the form of pulses, thus allowing to process the food without heating, Hence, they could demonstrate that the effect on the microorganisms was due to electricity and not to heat or electrolysis. However, it has not been until the end of the twentieth century, when extensive studies have been conducted to improve this technique of food preservation, and several application systems of PEF have been patented (Bushnell et al., 1993; Zhang et al., 1996; Yin et al., 1997). As a result, not only promising results have been achieved regarding the inactivation of microorganisms and enzymes, but also an outstanding minimal modification of the nutritional and sensory properties of the treated products has been reported (Bendicho et al. 2002a; Espachs-Barroso et al., 2003; Martín-Belloso, et al., 2005; Martín-Belloso and Elez-Martínez, 2005ab). Because of these evidences, there has been an increasing interest by the fruit juice processing industry in the technology and its future industrial implementation (Espachs-Barroso et al., 2003). Currently, the most important juices in terms of economics are orange, apple and tomato, which are also the juices on which more studies regarding PEF processing have been carried out.

Different authors have evaluated the effect of PEF treatment on the microorganisms inoculated into juices and have come to the conclusion that the microbial inactivation depends on factors such as field strength, treatment time (number and pulse width), pulse shape, frequency and polarity of the treatments (Qin et al. 1995a; Qiu et al., 1998; Elez-Martínez et al., 2004, 2005). The destruction of microorganisms also depends on the type of microorganism, the concentration of initial inoculum, the stage of growth and the medium in which they are located (Pothakamury 1995; Zhang et al 1994). Therefore, an appropriate selection of treatment conditions is needed to achieve an effective application. Also the electrical properties of the food to be processed has to be considered. Resistivity may greatly vary upon the fruit from which a juice is obtained. In general, the resistivity is higher for juices than for the rest of liquids susceptible of being treated by PEF. In addition, resistivity decreases with increasing temperature (Arántegui et al., 1999).

On the other hand, inactivation of enzymes by PEF has been studied by several authors (Elez-Martínez et al., 2007). In some cases, reported inactivation levels are high, whereas in other cases there is virtually no inactivation, depending on the type of juice and processing conditions.

To a lesser degree, there are studies related to the impact of PEF on juice quality, sensory characteristics and bioactive compounds, issues which are being currently investigated.

This chapter presents the most outstanding results obtained so far concerning the implementation of PEF for orange, apple and tomato juice processing. The effects of PEF on those juices in relation to microorganisms, enzymes, quality and bioactive components are described hereby.

Effects Of Pulsed Electric Fields On Juices

Orange juice

The effects of PEF on both pathogenic and spoilage microorganisms inoculated in orange juice have been extensively studied. McDonald et al. (2000) achieved 5-6 log reductions of *Listeria innocua* and *Escherichia coli*, while *Leuconostoc mesenteroides* was destroyed by about 3.5 log reductions after processing orange juice with up to 6 pulses of 2 μs at 30 kV/cm. They also found that microbial inactivation was not always increased when pulses of 50 kV/cm were applied. Furthermore, *Leuconostoc mesenteroides* (Gram negative) was shown to be the most resistant bacteria to treatments of short duration (< 8 μs) whereas *Listeria innocua* (Gram positive) was the most sensitive. In a later study, about 3 logarithmic reductions in the counts of *Escherichia coli* were achieved by processing an inoculated orange juice at 30 kV/cm for 200 μs (Rodrigo et al., 2003a). Liang et al. (2002) reported roughly 6 decimal reductions after treating an orange juice inoculated with *Salmonella typhimurium* with pulses of 90 kV/cm for 100 μs at 55 °C. Other authors have observed more than 5 logarithmic reductions in the counts of *Salmonella enteritidis* and *E. coli* O157: H7 in an inoculated orange juice processed at 35 kV/cm for 2000 μs without heating the product above 40 °C during the process (Mosqueda-Melgar et al., 2008).

Grahl and Märkl (1996) reported an elimination of an initial *Saccharomyces cerevisiae* inoculum of 10^6 cfu/ml by applying 5 pulses of 7 kV/cm to an inoculated orange juice. Furthermore, a reduction of 5.1 logs has been observed after processing orange juice at 35 kV/cm for 1000 μs without exceeding 40 °C (Elez-Martínez et al., 2004). The effect of PEF on the growth of other spoilage microorganisms such as *Lactobacillus* has also been studied. Elez-Martínez et al. (2005) attained nearly 6 logarithmic reductions when treating orange juice inoculated with *L. brevis* during 1000 μs at 35 kV/cm below 40 °C (Figure 1). Gómez et al. (2005a) processed orange juice inoculated with *L. plantarum* at 25 kV/cm for 1000 μs and reduced the initial load by at least 3 log cycles.

(a)

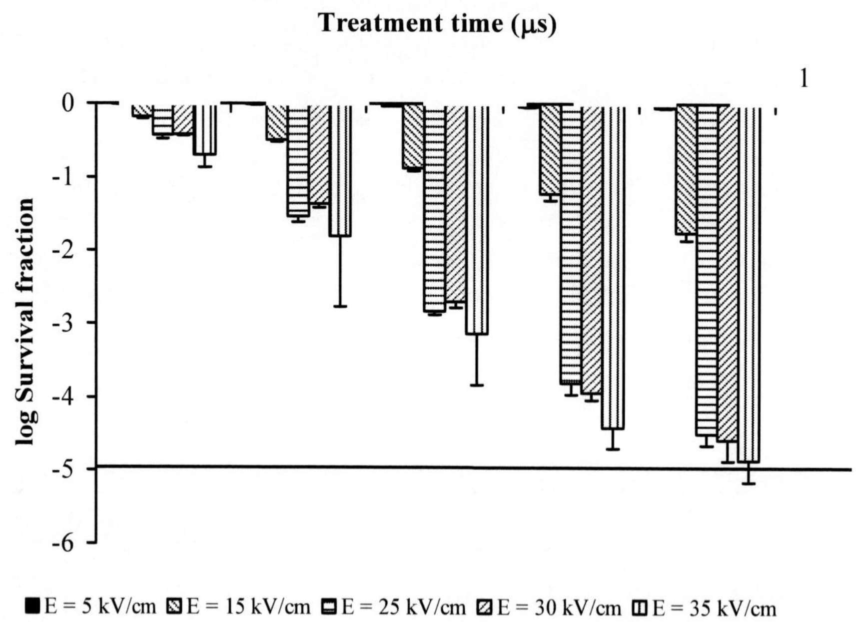

(b)

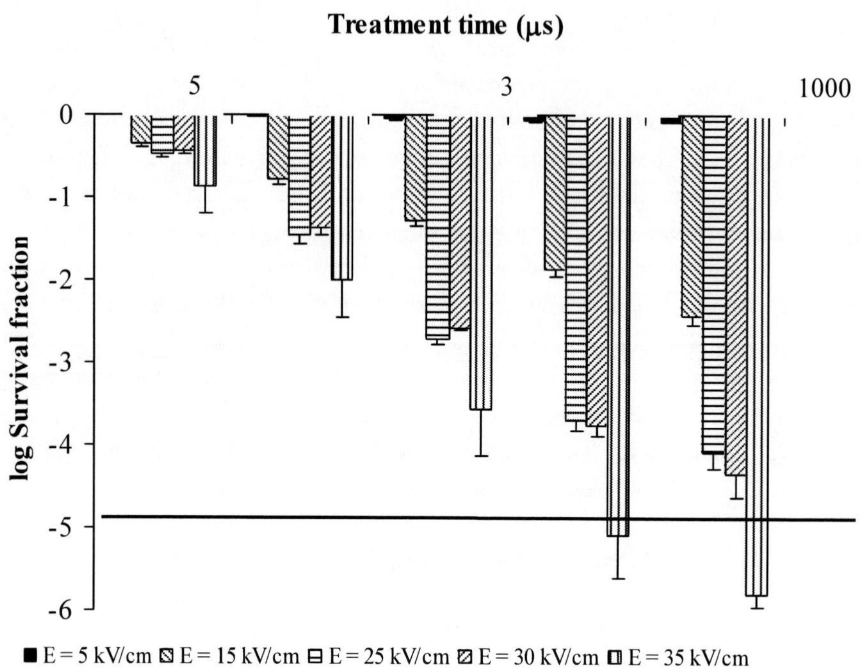

Figure 1.- Inactivation of *Lactobacillus brevis* in orange juice exposed to mono- (a) and bipolar (b) PEF. Pulse frequency = 200 Hz; pulse width = 4 μs. Square pulses. E, electric field strength. Thermal treatment = 90 °C / 1 minute (horizontal line) (from Elez-Martínez et al., 2005).

Moreover, studies on the effect of PEF-treatments in ascospores of *S. cerevisiae* in freshly squeezed orange juice have been conducted. When treatments of 30 kV/cm for 14 μs or 50 kV/cm for 6 μs with 2-μs pulses were applied, less than 1 log reduction at temperatures below 60 ° C was achieved (McDonald et al., 2000). Raso et al. (1998a) applied treatments from 32.3 to 36.5 kV/cm to inactivate ascospores of *Zygosaccharomyces bailii* in orange juice at low temperature (<22 ° C). After 2 pulses, they observed 4.7 log reductions in the counts of vegetative cells and 3.8 log reductions in their ascospores. Raso et al. (1998b) also studied the effects of PEF on the inactivation of various moulds, thus finding that ascospores of *Byssochlamys nivea* and *Neosartorya fischeri* were resistant to a treatment of 40 pulses at 51 kV/cm. On the other hand, 4.5 log reductions were achieved in the counts of conidiospores of *Byssochlamys fulva* in an orange juice treated with 12 pulses at 30 kV/cm.

With regard to enzymes, pectin methyl esterase (PME) and peroxidase (POD) have been the most studied in orange juice. A continuous PEF treatment of 35 kV/cm over 59 μs and 60.1 °C was reported to inactivate up to a 90% of the native PME in orange orange (Yeom et al., 2002). Elez-Martínez et al. (2007) inactivated a 80% of PME when processing orange juice at 35 kV/cm for 1500 μs applying bipolar pulses of 4 μs without exceeding 37.5 ° C. In the same study, higher levels of inactivation were observed when treatment frequency and pulse width were increased from 50 to 450 Hz and from 1 to 10 μs, respectively. Furthermore, some authors have found synergistic effects between PEF and heat treatments when aiming at inactivating PME in fruit juices (Yeom et al, 2002; Rodrigo et al., 2003b).

Almost total inactivation of POD was attained when processing orange juice at 35 kV/cm for 1500 μs with bipolar pulses of 4 μs at 200 Hz and a treatment temperature always below 35 °C (Elez-Martínez et al., 2006a). The applied energy density to achieve complete inactivation of POD in orange juice was 8067 MJ/m^3.

Another aspect evaluated when treating orange juice by PEF is the influence of the process on the bioactive potencial of the juices. A treatment of 35 kV/cm for 1000 μs with bipolar pulses of 4 μs at 200 Hz resulted in a 8% decrease of the vitamin C content of orange juice, which contrasts with the 17% loss achieved with a heat treatment (90 °C, 1 min) (Elez-Martínez and Martín-Belloso, 2007). Cortés et al. (2006a) observed that thermal pasteurization had a greater impact on the total carotenoids in orange juice (12% decrease) than PEF treatments applied at 25, 30 and 40 kV/cm, which depleted carotenoids by 9.6%, 6.4% and 7.8%, respectively. Likewise, Sanchez-Moreno et al. (2005) concluded that PEF did not change the flavanones content, namely naringenine and hesperitine, in orange juice. The antioxidant capacity of the PEF-processed juice has not been reported to undergo substantial modifications and, in any case, it is lower than that which takes place after heat-treating the juice (Sanchez-Moreno et al., 2005; Elez-Martínez and Martín-Belloso, 2007).

Some physicochemical and sensory properties of orange juice processed by PEF have been studied by Cserhalmi et al. (2006). The pH, soluble solids, electrical conductivity, viscosity, color, non-enzymatic browning index and hydroximethyl furfural unchanged with respect to the untreated controls after processing orange juice at 28 kV/cm for 100 μs at temperatures not exceeding 34 °C. There were no changes reported in the contents of organic acids and volatile compounds when processing orange juice by PEF (Cserhalmi et al., 2006). For instance, the amount of aroma compounds accounting for the juice flavor was reduced to

22-25% after a thermal pasteurization treatment, whereas, in contrast, only a 3-9% was lost when PEF-treating at 30 kV/cm for 240-480 μs (Qiu et al., 1998; Jia et al., 1999).

Apple juice

Several studies have been conducted to determine the effect of PEF on the pathogenic and deletereous microbiota of apple juice. *E. coli* has been the most studied pathogenic microorganism in this juice. Evrendilek et al. (1999) compared the effect of PEF on 2 strains of *E. coli* (O157: H7 and 8739) in apple juice. The samples were exposed to pulses of 18-30 kV/cm with a treatment duration ranging from 86 to 172 μs at temperatures below 35 °C. No difference was observed in the destruction of both strains, with a maximum inactivation of 5 logarithmic reductions. In addition, the number of viable microorganisms decreased when increasing the treatment time at a constant field intensity of 29 kV/cm. On the other hand, Gupta et al. (2003) reported 5 logarithmic reductions when applying 100 pulses of 40 kV/cm at 20°C to an apple juice inoculated with *E. coli* K12, whereas Heinz et al. (2003) managed to achieve a 6.2 log decrease in the counts when delivering pulses of 34 kV/cm with an energy density of 40 kJ/kg at 55 °C In this same way, roughly 6 logarithmic reductions were attained in an apple juice inoculated with *Listeria monocytogenes* and processed at 28 kV/cm for 400 μs (Gómez et al., 2005b).

The inactivation effect of PEF on Lactobacilli inoculated in apple juice has been also investigated. The initial population of *Lactobacillus plantarum* inoculated in apple juice was diminished by 4.5 logs after processing at 25 kV/cm for 1000 μs (Gómez et al., 2005a). In apple juice inoculated with *Saccharomyces cerevisiae*, Qin et al. (1995b) observed a virtual elimination of an initial inoculum of 10^6 cfu/ml by applying 10 pulses of 2.5 μs at 35 kV/cm.

Heinz et al. (2003) reported a reduction of 4.3 logs in *L. monocytogenes*, 4.9 logs in *Lactobacillus rhamnosus*, 4.3 logs in *Aspergillus niger* and 6.5 logs in *Rhizopus rubra* inoculated into an apple juice subjected to a PEF treatment at 55 °C with 34 kV/cm and an energy density of 40 kJ/kg. Raso et al. (1998a) applied PEF treatments from 32.3 to 36.5 kV/cm on ascospores of *Zygosaccharomyces bailii* in apple juice with a maximum treatment temperature of 22 °C. After delivering 2 pulses, 4.8 log units of the vegetative cells and 3.6 logs of their ascospores were inactivated. Raso et al. (1998b) also found that ascospores of *Byssochlamys nivea* and *Neosartorya fischeri* were resistant to a treatment of 40 pulses at 51 kV/cm. About 5 logarithmic reductions in the counts of conidiospores of *Byssochlamys fulva* were attained in a juice after treating with 15 pulses of 30 kV/cm.

Regarding enzymes inactivation, a treatment of 40 kV/cm for 100 μs at 35 °C led to a decrease of 50% of POD activity and 60% of PPO activity in the juice (Rien et al., 2008). Authors, highlighted that an increase in treatment time and electric field strength enhanced the degree of inactivation of the enzymes.

On the other hand, the effect of the PEF on some bioactive compounds of apple juice was studied by Aguilar-Rosas et al. (2007). These authors found that the total phenol content of apple juice decreased by 14% when processing the juice by PEF (35 kV/cm, bipolar pulses of 4 μs, 1200 Hz), whereas it dropped by 32% after a heat treatment (90 °C, 30 s). They also observed that losses in volatile components of apple juice processed by PEF were lower than those observed for a heat treatment. Zarate-Rodríguez et al. (2000) found that applying PEF, none of the attributes of apple juice (soluble solids, pH, acidity and color) varied apart from the color, since the juice developed certain browning. Aguilar-Rosas et al. (2007) did not observe changes in pH or acidity of the juice treated with PEF. Similarly, Qin et al. (1995a) did not find differences between treated and untreated juices when evaluating the sensory profile of a concentrated apple juice after applying 10 pulses of 50 kV/cm and that of a fresh apple juice subjected to 16 pulses of 50 kV/cm.

Tomato juice

The inoculated population of *Salmonella enterica* ser. Enteritidis in tomato juice was reduced by 4.2 logs after applying a bipolar treatment of 35 kV/cm for 1000 μs, rendering pulses of 4 μs at 100 Hz without exceeding 36 °C (Mosqueda-Melgar et al., 2008b). Roughly 4 logarithmic reductions were achieved in the counts of conidiospores of *Byssochlamys fulva* in tomato juice with a PEF treatment,of 15 pulses of 30 kV/cm (Raso et al., 1998b).

The enzymes studied in tomato juice have been pectin methyl esterase (PME), polygalacturonase (PG), lipoxygenase (LOX) and peroxidase (POD). PEF reduced the activity of PME by about a 55% when processing at 80 kV/cm for 40 μs at 5 °C, whereas PG activity was almost unaffected (Nguyen and Mittal, 2007). LOX was inhibited by 80% when processing tomato juice with 20 kV/cm for 60 μs at 30 °C (Min et al. 2003a). POD of tomato juice was completely inactivated when processing with bipolar 7-μs pulses of 35 kV/cm for 2000 μs at 200 Hz (Aguiló-Aguayo et al., 2008a). It was also noted that the higher the treatment time, the pulse width and the pulse frequency, the higher the level of POD inactivation. Aguiló-Aguayo et al. (2008b) observed a PME inactivation of 82%, a PG inactivation of 12% and a POD inactivation of 97% after processing tomato juice at 35 kV/cm fro 1500 μs using 4-μs bipolar pulses at 100 Hz. In addition, viscosity of tomato juice increased after PEF treatment, whereas color changed slightly (Aguiló-Aguayo et al., 2008b).

The maximum relative content of lycopene (131.8%) and vitamin C (90.2%), as well as the greatest antioxidant capacity retention (89.4%) of tomato juice was obtained when processing juice at 35 kV/cm for 1000 μs with bipolar pulses of 1 μs at 250 Hz (Odriozola-Serrano et al., 2007) (Table 1). Nguyen and Mittal (2007) also reported the maintenance of vitamin C in tomato juice processed by PEF. No significant differences were found in the phenolic content of PEF-processed (35 kV/cm for 1500 μs in bipolar 4-μs pulses at 100 Hz) and unprocessed tomato juices (Odriozola-Serrano et al., 2008). Furthermore, PEF processing (40 kV/cm, 59 μs) produced tomato juice with a greater retention of aromas, a smaller non-enzymatic browning and redder coloration than that obtained by thermal processing (92 ° C, 90 s) (Min and Zhang, 2003).

Table 1.- Effect of PEF on lycopene, vitamin C and antioxidant capacity of tomato juice[a] (adapted from Odriozola-Serrano et al., 2007)

Frecuency (Hz)	Pulse width (μs)	Relative content Lycopene (%)		Retention Vitamin C (%)		Retention Antioxidant Capacity (%)	
		Monopolar	Bipolar	Monopolar	Bipolar	Monopolar	Bipolar
50	1	101.0	103.2	99.0	98.3	50.7	66.5
50	7	112.3	114.2	84.4	82.1	81.8	86.1
250	1	113.4	129.1	93.8	86.1	77.5	90.4
250	7	135.1	146.2	66.0	60.6	67.8	75.9
50	4	110.2	101.1	92.2	88.4	62.3	74.6
150	1	107.0	118.7	98.6	89.2	60.4	80.1
150	7	118.9	128.1	80.2	58.2	78.3	81.3
250	4	127.0	142.7	82.6	78.8	72.6	81.0
150	4	109.6	119.4	76.6	74.8	81.3	92.3

[a] Electric field strength of 35 kV/cm, total treatment time of 1000 μs

Shelf Life Of Juices Processed By Pulsed Electric Fields

PEF treatment is as efficient as thermal pasteurization to stabilize juices microbiologically during storage in refrigeration. Irreversible inactivation of deleterious enzymes was observed during storage of juices processed by PEF. Moreover, health-promoting properties as well as sensory characteristics were better retained in PEF-treated juices than in those processed by traditional thermal treatments.

Orange juice is the most popular juice worldwide and therefore numerous studies have been published concerning the effects of PEF on the juice shelf life. A PEF treatment of 480 μs at 30 kV/cm has been reported to effectively reduce the total microbiological counts of an orange juice, thus extending its shelf life up to 42 days (Jia et al., 1999). Indeed, a treatment of 35 kV/cm and 59 μs was shown to be at least as effective as a thermal pasteurization treatment (94.6 °C for 30 s) in keeping below 1 log cfu/ml the number of viable microorganisms in orange juice stored at 4, 22 and 37 ° C during 112 days (Yeom et al., 2000ab; Ayhan et al., 2002). Consistently, Min et al. (2003b) observed that, after processing orange juice with a commercial-scale PEF system (40 kV/cm, 97 μs), the counts of both total aerobic microorganisms and molds and yeasts were always below 10 cfu/ml thoughout 112 days at 4 ° C. Elez-Martínez et al. (2006b) reported that a treatment of 35 kV/cm and 1000 μs combined with refrigerated storage (4 °C) ensured the microbial stability of orange juice for at least 56 days (Figure 2).

(a)

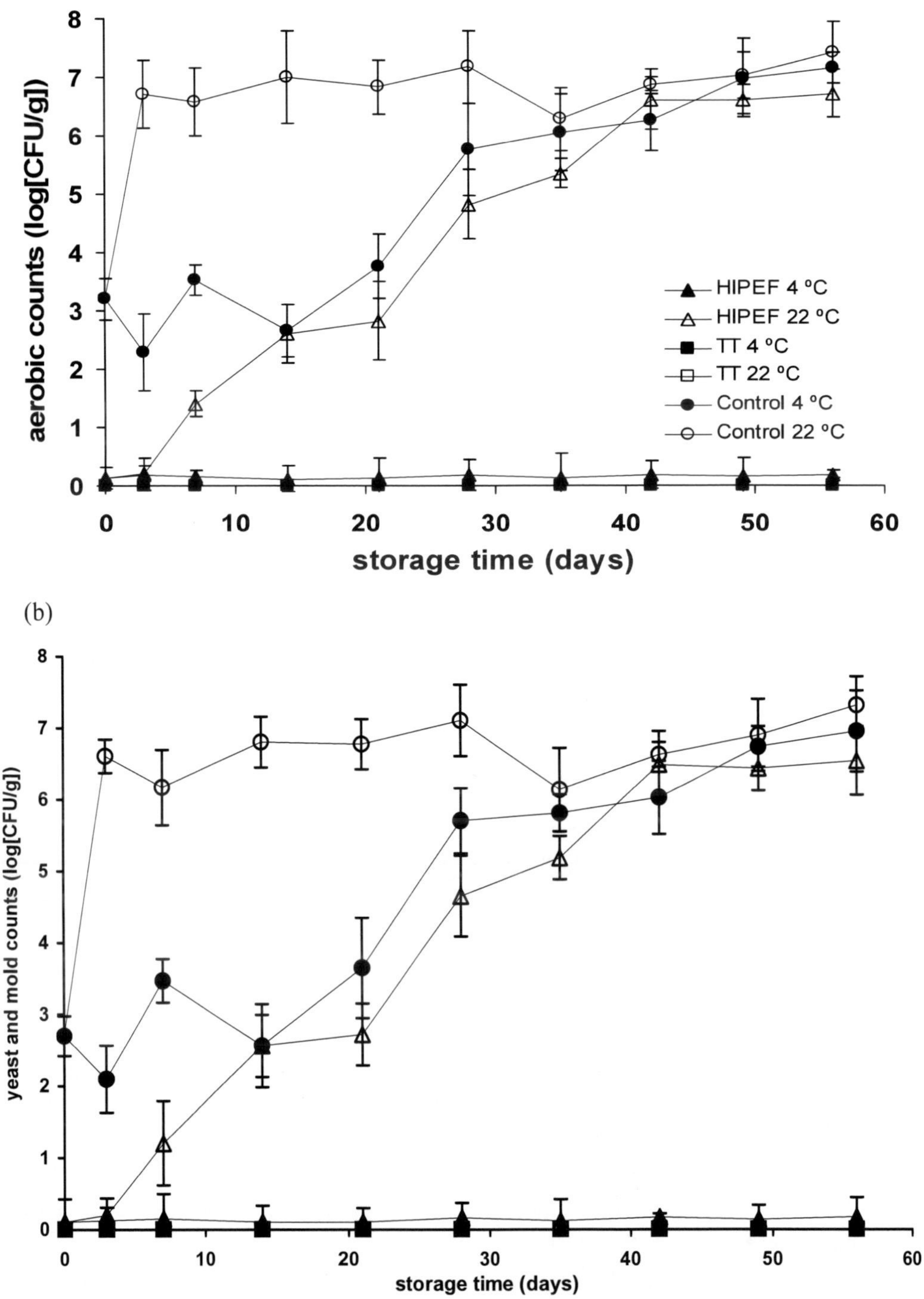

(b)

Figure 2.- Effects of PEF treatment and heat pasteurization (TT) on the microbial counts (total aerobic bacteria [A] and yeasts and molds [B]) of orange juice throughout storage at 4 and 22 °C (from Elez-Martínez et al., 2006b).

Yeom et al. (2000b) studied the effects of a PEF treatment on the PME activity of orange juice compared with the effects of traditional thermal pasteurization. The analysis after the treatments showed 88% and 98% reduction of enzyme activity, respectively. The juice treated and stored at 4 and 22 °C did not exhibit any increase in PME activity throughout 112 days. Elez-Martínez et al. (2006b) did not observe any activation of PME or POD enzymes in orange juice stored at 4 and 22 °C for 56 days after processing juice with PEF.

Changes on physico-chemical and sensory properties (color, pH, acidity, °Brix, viscosity, aromas) of orange juice processed by PEF occurred throughout storage, but these changes were smaller than those occurring in a heat-processed juice (Yeom et al., 2000b; Min et al., 2003b; Elez-Martínez et al., 2006b; Cortés et al., 2008). Orange juice processed by PEF exhibited a certain loss of vitamin C throughout storage under both refrigeration and room temperatures. However, the losses were smaller than those observed in a heat-treated juices or even in an untreated juice (Yeom et al. 2000b; Min et al. 2003b; Elez-Martínez et al., 2006b). Likewise, Cortés et al. (2006b) reported a decrease of 12.6% in the total carotenoids of a heat-treated juice (90 °C, 20 s), whereas a PEF treatment (30 kV/cm, 100 μs) depleted the carotenoids content of treated orange by 6.7% after 7 weeks of storage. On the other hand, antioxidant capacity was shown to decrease smoothly during storage of a PEF-processed orange juice but no further differences were observed with an untreated juice (Elez-Martínez et al., 2006b; Plaza et al., 2006).

Shelf life of PEF-treated apple juice has been also studied. A shelf life of at least 3 weeks at either 4 ° C or 25 ° C was achieved when the juice was treated with 250 μs at 36 kV/cm (Qin et al. 1995b). Indeed, when processing apple juice at 35 kV/cm for 94 μs, shelf-life was at least 67 days under refrigerated storage (Evrendilek et al., 2000). In this study, PEF-treated apple juices exhibited a slight browning, though these color changes were less noticeable than those occurring during the storage of a heat-processed juice. In addition, PEF treatments favoured retention of vitamin C in apple juice stored regardless of the storage temperature.

On the other hand, Min et al. (2003c) evaluated the refrigerated shelf life of a tomato juice processed by PEF (40 kV/cm for 57 μs) in comparison to that of a heat-tread juice (92 °C for 90 s). Both treatments provided a microbiological shelf life of at least 112 days. LOX activity during storage of a PEF-treated tomato juice was studied by Min et al. (2003c). Residual activity measured immediately after the treatment (46%) was not shown to increase throughout 112 days of storage at 4 °C. Aguiló-Aguayo et al. (2008b) observed that residual POD and PME activities remained around 5% during 56 days and around 14% during 77 days of storage, respectively. However, PG activity decreased during storage of PEF-processed and heat-treated tomato juice (Aguiló-Aguayo et al., 2008b) (Figure 3).

Furthermore, physico-chemical and sensory characteristics (color, pH, acidity, °Brix, viscosity, aromas) were maintained in a PEF-treated tomato juice much better than in a heat-treated juice (Min and Zhang, 2003; Min et al., 2003c; Aguiló-Aguayo et al., 2008b). Regarding the antioxidant potential, PEF-processed juices retained more vitamin C and lycopene than the heat-treated when stored under both cooling and room temperature (Min et al., 2003c). Consistently, a PEF treated tomato juice (35 kV/cm, 1500 μs) exhibited a higher content of vitamin C and lycopene during storage at 4 °C than heat-treated juices (90 °C-30 s and 90 °C-60 s). The total phenolic content remained unchanged during refrigerated storage regardless of the treatment applied to tomato juice, whereas the antioxidant capacity decreased without significant differences between PEF-treated and heat-treated juices (Odriozola-Serrano et al., 2008).

(a)

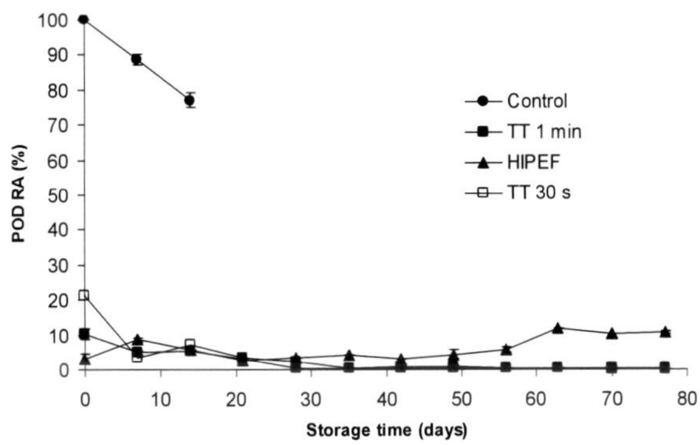

(b)

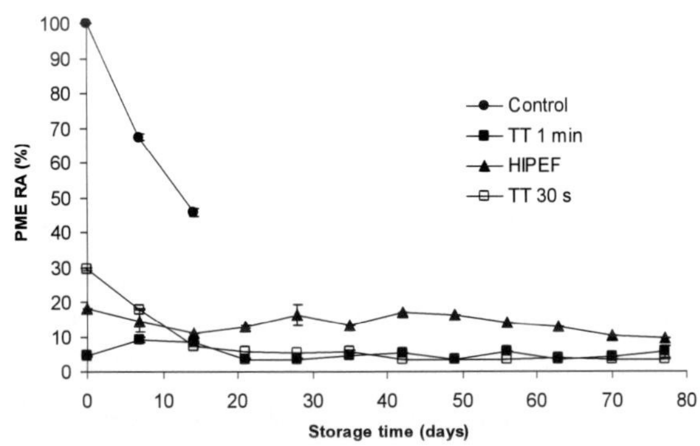

(c)

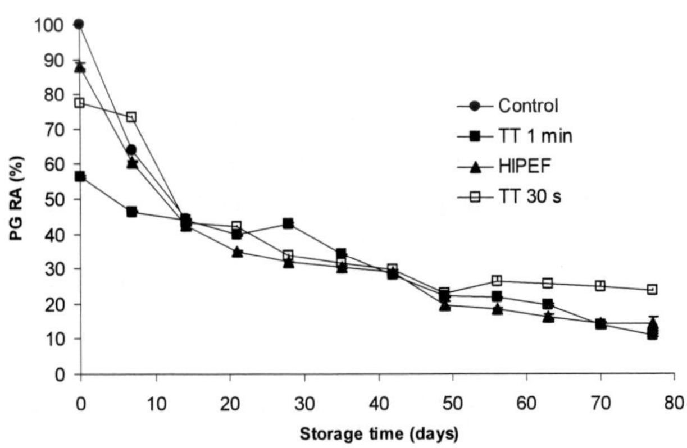

Figure 3.- Effects of PEF treatment and thermal treatments, 90°C for 1 min (TT 1 min) or for 30 s (TT 30 s) on residual POD (a), PME (b) and PG (c) activities of tomato juice throughout storage at 4°C (adapted from Aguiló-Aguayo et al., 2008b).

Preservation Of Juices By Combining Pulsed Electric Fields And Other Processing Technologies

The use of PEF combined with other processing technologies has been recently studied in order to find synergies to better maintain juice quality and safety. In this regard, the implementation of PEF in combination with moderate heat treatments can attain levels of microbial inactivation similar to those achieved with intense heat treatments and, at the same time, allows for better keeping the original physico-chemical and nutritional properties of juices. Heinz et al. (2003) reported more than 5.5 logarithmic reductions when applying pulses of 36 kV/cm at 60 ºC, whereas roughly 3 log reductions were achieved when treating at 35 ° C and 36 kV/cm. Furthermore, the treatment at 60 ºC reduced by more than 5-fold the specific energy input needed compared to the treatment at 35 ºC. Likewise, Liang et al. (2002) treated orange juice with 20 pulses of 90 kV/cm applied within the range of 30-50 ºC. They found that when treatments were applied below 45 ºC, inactivation of *Salmonella typhimurium* inoculated in the juice did not exceed 1.4 log cycles. In contrast, treatments performed at 50 ºC led to a destruction of 4.2 log units. The increase in microbial inactivation has been attributed to the reduction in the thickness of cell walls, which has been attributed to a change of state of the membrane phospholipids, from gel to liquid-crystalline phase, as temperature increases.

In general, the combination of heat and PEF allows a much greater inactivation of microorganisms and enzymes responsible for the reactions of deterioration of juice. Yeom et al. (2002) observed a decrease of 90% in the PME activity of an orange juice by applying a treatment of 25 kV/cm for 250 μs at 50 ºC. On the contrary, only a 35% of the native enzyme was inactivated when applying the same electrical treatment at 20 ºC.

Several authors have proposed the addition of antimicrobial compounds as a complementary technique to the application of PEF in fruit juices. The use of nisin (100 IU/ml) or lysozyme (2400 IU/ml) in orange juice treated with PEF (90 kV/cm, 30 pulses, 45° C) yielded 4.8 and 4.3 logarithmic reductions in *Salmonella typhimurium*, compared to 2.2 logarithmic reductions achieved without addition of antimicrobials (Liang et al., 2002). Moreover, a decrease of 6.5 log units was reported when combining a PEF treatment with a mixture of nisin (27.5 IU/ml) and lysozyme (690 IU/ml). Hodgins et al. (2002) obtained a maximum inactivation of 6 log units on the native mibrobiota of orange juice when combining a treatment of 20 pulses at 80 kV/cm and 44 ºC with nisin (100 IU/ml). With this treatment, a 97.5% of the initial vitamin C content was mantained, whereas a 92.7% of the orange juice native PME was inactivated. In tomato juice, 4.4 log reductions were attained through the application of 20 pulses (80 kV/cm, 50 ºC) in combination with nisin (100 IU/ml) (Nguyen and Mittal, 2007).

Mosqueda-Melgar et al. (2008a) studied the inactivation of *Salmonella enteritidis* in apple and orange juices processed by PEF with the addition of antimicrobials. Combining a treatment of 35 kV/cm for 1000 μs with 0.1% cinnamon oil resulted in 6 log decrease (Figure 4). Similarly, Mosqueda-Melgar et al. (2008b) reported more than 6 logarithmic reductions in the counts of *S. enteritidis* inoculated in tomato juice when applying similar treatment conditions.

(a)

(b)

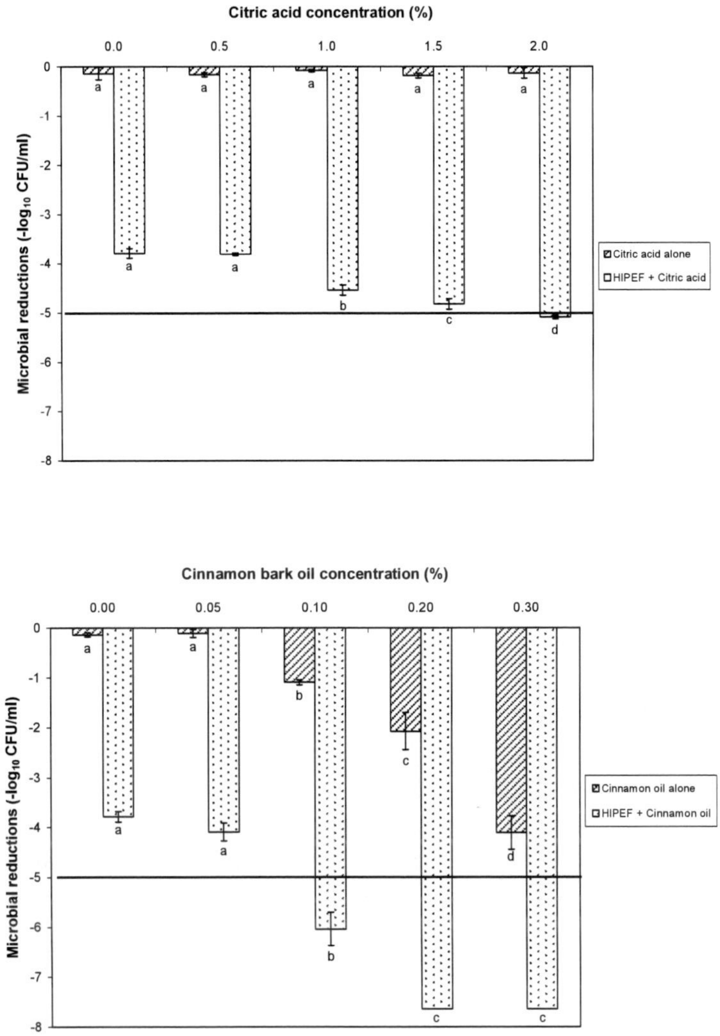

Figure 4.- Inactivation of *Salmonella enterica* ser. Enteritidis in tomato juice by combining PEF with citric acid (a) or cinnamon bark oil (b). Treatment conditions: 35 kV/cm for 1000 μs at 100 Hz, 4 μs pulse width and 38.8 ± 1.8 °C (adapted from Mosqueda-Melgar et al., 2008b).

The influence of pH on the bacterial inactivation by PEF has not been established clearly. Some studies in model solutions have led to inconclusive results. Álvarez et al. (2000) found that *Salmonella senftenberg* suspended in solutions of the same regulatory conductivity was more resistant to PEF at acid pH than at neutral pH. Regardless of the influence of pH on the bacterial inactivation by PEF, acid or acidified fruit juices are good candidates for processing using this technology because a low pH prevents the germination of bacterial spores.

Recently, Noci et al. (2008) have proposed the combined application of electrical pulses (40 kV/cm, 100 μs) and ultraviolet light (30 W, 30 min, d = 30 cm) to reduce the spoilage microbiota of an apple juice. These researchers found that ultraviolet treatments and PEF yielded 2.2 and 5.4 logarithmic reductions, respectively, if applied separately. The concatenation of the two treatments represented more than 6 logarithmic reductions if PEF was applied first and more than 7 reductions if the juice was treated first with ultraviolet light. In addition, the combination of treatments led to better preservation of the color and phenolic content of the juice.

Because of the rigidity of their structures, bacterial spores are highly resistant to PEF processing. The application of PEF combined with other emerging processing technologies, such as high hydrostatic pressure or ultrasound, can allow the inactivation of spores. Pagan et al. (1998) explored the possibility of germinating spores of *Bacillus* by applying high pressure treatments and then inactivating the germinated cells with a PEF treatment. High pressure processing (1500 atm, 30 min, 40 °C) induced the germination of more than 5 log of spores. Then, PEF treatment (60 kV/cm, 75 pulses) render satisfactory inactivation of germinated spores.

Conclusion

The application of pulsed electric fields (PEF) for processing juices looks promising. This treatment may be an alternative to heat-pasteurization, thus providing safe and stable juices and, at the same time, avoiding the negative effects of heat on their sensory and nutritional properties.

With the investigations carried out so far, it is expected that PEF technology could be incorporated into the juice processing industry as a unique form of preservation or as part of a combined system of preservation methods. However, further research should be conducted with the aim of designing equipment for processing that allows treating high juice productions. Finally, a reliable assessment of the economic costs of the implementation at an industrial scale is also necessary to facilitate the transference of the technology to the juice processing industry.

Acknowledgments

This work has been carried out with the financial support from the Commission of the European Communities, Framework 6, Priority 5 “Food Quality and Safety”, Integrated Project Novel Q (FP6-CT-2006-015710). This work was also supported by the Spanish Ministry of Education and Science through the Projects AGL2005-05768/ALI and AGL2006-12758-C02-02/ALI.

References

Aguilar-Rosas, S.F.; Ballinas Casarrubias, M.L.; Nevarez-Moorillon, G.V.; Martin-Belloso, O.; Ortega-Rivas, E. (2007). Thermal and pulsed electric fields pasteurization of apple juice: effects on physicochemical properties and flavour compounds. *Journal of Food Engineering*, 83, 41-46.

Aguiló-Aguayo, I.; Odriozola-Serrano, I.; Quintao-Teixeira, L.J.; Martín-Belloso, O. (2008a). Inactivation of tomato juice peroxidase by high-intensity pulsed electric fields as affected by process conditions. *Food Chemistry*, 107, 949-955.

Aguiló-Aguayo, I.; Soliva-Fortuny, R.; Martín-Belloso, O. (2008b). Comparative study on color, viscosity and related enzymes of tomato juice treated by high-intensity pulsed electric fields or heat. *European Food Research and Technology*, 227, 599-606.

Álvarez, I.; Raso, J.; Palop, A.; Sala, F. J. (2000). Influence of different factors on the inactivation of *Salmonella senftenberg* by pulsed electric fields. *International Journal of Food Microbiology*, 55, 143–146.

Arántegui, J.; Rosell, J.R.; Purroy, P.; Barbosa-Cánovas, G.V.; Martín, O. (1999). Electrical properties of peach juice and milk. *European Conference of Emerging Food Science and Technology*, Tampere, Finland.

Ayhan, Z.; Zhang, Q.H.; Min, D.B. (2002). Effects of pulsed electric field processing and storage on the quality and stability of single-strength orange juice. *Journal of Food Protection*, 65, 1623-1627.

Bendicho, S.; Barbosa-Cánovas, G.V.; Martín, O. (2002). Milk processing by high intensity pulsed electric fields. *Trends in Food Science and Technology*, 13, 195-204.

Bushnell, A.H.; Dunn, J.E.; Clark, R.W.; Pearlman, J.S. (1993). High pulsed voltage systems for extending the shelf life of pumpable food products. U.S. Patent n° 5,235,905.

Cortés, C.; Esteve, M.J.; Rodrigo, D.; Torregrosa, F.; Frígola, A. (2006a). Changes of colour and carotenoids contents during high intensity pulsed electric field treatment in orange juices. *Food and Chemical Toxicology*, 44,1932-1939.

Cortés, C.; Torregrosa, F.; Esteve, M.J.; Frígola, A. (2006b). Carotenoid profile modification during refrigerated storage in untreated and pasteurized orange juice and orange juice treated with high-intensity pulsed electric fields. *Journal of Agricultural and Food Chemistry*, 54, 6247-6254.

Cortés, C.; Esteve, M.J.; Frígola, A. (2008). Color of orange juice treated by high intensity pulsed electric fields during refrigerated storage and comparison with pasteurized juice. *Food Control*, 19, 151-158.

Cserhalmi, Zs.; Sass-Kiss, Á.; Tóth-Markus, M.; Lechner, N. (2006). Study of pulsed electric field treated citrus juices. *Innovative Food Science and Emerging Technologies*, 7, 49-54.

Dutreux, N.; Notremans, S.; Witjzes, T.; Góngora-Nieto, M.M.; Barbosa-Cánovas, G.V.; Swanson, B.G. (2000) Pulsed electric field inactivation of attached and free-living *Escherichia coli* and *Listeria innocua* under several conditions. *International Journal of Food Microbiology*, 54, 91–98.

Elez-Martínez, P.; Escolà-Hernández, J.; Soliva-Fortuny, R.C.; Martín-Belloso, O. (2004). Inactivation of *Saccharomyces cerevisiae* suspended in orange juice using high-intensity pulsed electric fields. *Journal of Food Protection*, 67, 2596-2602.

Elez-Martínez, P.; Escolà-Hernández, J.; Soliva-Fortuny, R.C.; Martín-Belloso, O. (2005). Inactivation of *Lactobacillus brevis* in orange juice by high-intensity pulsed electric fields. *Food Microbiology*, 22, 311-319.

Elez-Martínez, P.; Aguiló-Aguayo, I.; Martín-Belloso, O. (2006a). Inactivation of orange juice peroxidase by high-intensity pulsed electric fields as influenced by process parameters. *Journal of the Science of Food and Agriculture*, 86, 71-81.

Elez-Martínez, P.; Soliva-Fortuny, R.C.; Martín-Belloso, O. (2006b). Comparative study on shelf life of orange juice processed by high intensity pulsed electric fields or heat treatment. *European Food Research and Technology*, 222, 321-329.

Elez-Martínez, P.; Martín-Belloso, O. (2007). Effect of high intensity pulsed electric field processing conditions on vitamin C and antioxidant capacity of orange juice and gazpacho, a cold vegetable soup. Food Chemistry, 102, 201-209.

Elez-Martínez, P.; Rodrigo, D.; Sampedro, F.; Martín-Belloso O. (2007). Impact of pulsed electric fields on food enzymes and shelf life. In Lelieveld, H.L.M.; Notermans, S.; De Haan, S.W.H. (Eds.). *Food preservation by pulsed electric fields: from research to application*. Woodhead Publishing Limited, Cambridge, UK, pp. 212-246.

Elez-Martínez, P.; Suárez-Recio, M.; Martín-Belloso, O. (2007). Modeling the reduction of pectin methyl esterase activity in orange juice by high intensity pulsed electric fields. Journal of Food Engineering, 78, 184-193.

Espachs-Barroso, A.; Barbosa-Cánovas, G. V.; Martín-Belloso, O. (2003). Microbial and enzymatic changes in fruit juice induced by high-intensity pulsed electric fields. Food Reviews International, 19, 253-273.

Evrendilek, G.A.; Zhang, Q.H.; Richter, E.R. (1999). Inactivation of *Escherichia coli* O157:H7 and Escherichia coli 8739 in apple juice by pulsed electric fields. *Journal of Food Protection*, 62, 793-796.

Evrendilek, G.; Jin, Z. T.; Ruhlman, K. T.; Qiu, X.; Zhang, Q. H.; Richter, E. R. (2000). Microbial safety and shelf-life of apple juice and cider processed by bench and pilot scale PEF systems. *Innovative Food Science and Emerging Technologies*, 1, 77-86.

Gómez, N.; García D.; Álvarez, I.; Raso, J.; Condón, S. (2005a). A model describing the kinetics of inactivation of *Lactobacillus plantarum* in a buffer system of different pH and in orange and apple juice. *Journal of Food Engineering*, 70, 7-14.

Gómez, N.; García, D.; Álvarez, I.; Condón, S.; Raso, J. (2005b). Modelling inactivation of *Listeria monocytogenes* by pulsed electric fields in media of different pH. *International Journal of Food Microbiology*, 103, 199-206.

Grahl, T.; Märkl, H. (1996). Killing of microorganisms by pulsed electric fields. *Applied Microbiology and Biotecnology*, 45, 148-157.

Gupta, B.S.; Masterson, F.; Magee, T.R.A. (2003). Inactivation of *E. coli* K12 in apple juice by high voltage pulsed electric fields. *European Food Research and Technology*, 217, 434-437.

Heinz, V.; Toepfl, S.; Knorr, D. (2003). Impact of temperature on lethality and energy efficiency of apple juice pasteurization by pulsed electric fields treatment. *Innovative Food Science and Emerging Technologies*, 4, 167-175.

Hodgins, A.M.; Mittal, G.S.; Griffiths, M.W. (2002) Pasteurization of fresh orange juice using low-energy pulsed electrical field. *Journal of Food Science*, 67, 2294-2299.

Jia, M., Zhang, Q.H., Min, D.B. (1999). Pulsed electric field processing effects on flavor compounds and microorganisms of orange juice. *Food Chemistry*, 65, 445-451.

Liang, Z.; Mittal, G.S.; Griffiths, M.W. (2002). Inactivation of *Salmonella typhimurium* in orange juice containing antimicrobial agents by pulsed electric field. *Journal of Food Protection*, 65, 1081-1087.

Martín, O.; Zhang, Q.; Castro, A. J.; Barbosa-Canovas, G. V.; Swanson, B. G. 1994. Revisión: Empleo de pulsos eléctricos de alto voltaje para la conservación de alimentos. Microbiología e ingeniería del proceso. *Revista Española de Ciencia y Tecnología Alimentaria [Spanish Journal on Food Science and Technology]*, 1 (34): 1-34.

Martín-Belloso, O.; Bendicho, S.; Elez-Martínez, P.; Barbosa-Cánovas, G.V. (2005). Do high intensity pulsed electric fields induce changes in enzymatic activity, protein conformation and vitamin and flavor stability? In Barbosa-Cánovas, G.V.; Tapia, M.S.; Cano, M.P. (Eds.). *Novel Food Processing Technologies*. Marcel Dekker/CRC Press. New York, USA. pp. 87-104.

Martín-Belloso, O.; Elez-Martínez, P. (2005a). Enzymatic inactivation by pulsed electric fields. In Sun, D.W. (Ed.). *Emerging Technologies for Food Processing*. Elsevier. London, UK. pp. 155-181.

Martín-Belloso, O.; Elez-Martínez, P. (2005b). Food safety aspects of pulsed electric fields. In Sun, D.W. (Ed.). *Emerging Technologies for Food Processing*. Elsevier. London, UK. pp. 183-217.

McDonald, C.J.; Lloyd, S. W.; Vitale, M.A.; Petersson, K.; Innings, F. (2000). Effects of pulsed electric fields on microorganisms in orange juice using electric field strenghts of 30 and 50 kV/cm. *Journal of Food Science*, 65, 984- 989.

Min, S.; Min, S.K.; Zhang, Q.H. (2003a). Inactivation kinetics of tomato juice lipoxygenase by pulsed electric fields. *Journal of Food Science*, 68, 1995-2001.

Min, S.; Jin, Z. T.; Min, S. K.; Yeom, H.; Zhang, Q. H. (2003b). Commercial-scale pulsed electric field processing of orange juice. *Journal of Food Science*, 68, 1265-1271.

Min, S.; Jin, Z. T.; Zhang, Q. H. (2003c). Commercial scale pulsed electric field processing of tomato juice. *Journal of Agricultural and Food Chemistry*, 51, 3338-3344.

Min, S.; Zhang, Q.H. (2003). Effects of commercial-scale pulsed electric field processing on flavor and color of tomato juice. *Journal of Food Science*, 68, 1600-1606.

Moses, B. D. (1938). Electric pasteurization of milk. Agricultural Engineering, december 1938.

Mosqueda-Melgar, J.; Raubaudy-Massilia, R.M.; Martín-Belloso, O. (2008a). Non-thermal pasteurization of fruit juices by combining high-intensity pulsed electric fields with natural antimicrobial. *Innovative Food Science and Emerging Technologies*, 9, 328-340.

Mosqueda-Melgar, J.; Raubaudy-Massilia, R.M.; Martín-Belloso, O. (2008b). Inactivation of *Salmonella enterica* ser. Enteritidis in tomato juice by combining of high-intensity pulsed electric fields with natural antimicrobials. *Journal of Food Science*, 73, M47-M53.

Noci, F.; Riener, J.; Walkling-Ribeiro, M.; Cronin, D.A.; Morgan, D.J.; Lyng, J.G. (2008). Ultraviolet irradiation and pulsed electric fields (PEF) in a hurdle strategy for the preservation of fresh apple juice. *Journal of Food Engineering*, 85, 141-146.

Nguyen, P.; Mittal, G.S. (2007). Inactivation of naturally occurring microorganisms in tomato juice using pulsed electric field (PEF) with and without antimicrobials. *Chemical Engineering and Processing*, 46, 360-365.

Odriozola-Serrano, I.; Aguiló-Aguayo, I.; Soliva-Fortuny, R.; Gimeno-Añó, V.; Martín-Belloso, O. (2007). Lycopene, vitamin C, and antioxidant capacity of tomato juice as affected by high-intensity pulsed electric fields critical paramenters. *Journal of Agricultural and Food Chemistry*, 55, 9036-9042.

Odriozola-Serrano, I.; Soliva-Fortuny, R.; Martín-Belloso, O. (2008). Changes of health-related compounds throughout cold storage of tomato juice stabilized by thermal or high intensity pulsed electric field treatments. *Innovative Food Science and Emerging Technologies*, 9, 272-279.

Pagán, R.; Esplugas, S.; Góngora-Nieto, M.M.; Barbosa-Cánovas, G.V.; Swanson, B.G. (1998) Inactivation of *Bacillus subtilis* spores using high intensity pulsed electric fields in combination with other food conservation technologies. *Food Science and Technology International*, 4, 33–44.

Palaniappan, S.; Sastry, S. K. (1991). Electrical conductivity of selected juices: influences of temperature, solids content, applied voltage, and particle size. *Journal of Food Processing and Engineering*, 14: 247-260.

Plaza, L.; Sánchez-Moreno, C.; Elez-Martínez, P.; De Ancos, B.; Martín-Belloso, O.; Cano, M.P. (2005). Effect of refrigerated storage on vitamin C and antioxidant activity of orange juice processed by high-pressure or pulsed electric fields with regard to low pasteurization. *European Food Research and Technology*, 223, 487-493.

Pothakamury, U.R.; Monsalve-Gonzalez, A.; Barbosa-Cánovas, G.V.; Swanson, B.G. (1995). Inactivation of *Escherichia coli* and *Staphylococcus aureus* in model foods by pulsed electric field technology. *Food Research International*, 28, 167-171.

Qin, B.L.; Pothakamury, U.R.; Vega, H.; Martin, O.; Barbosa-Cánovas, G.V.; Swanson, B.G. (1995a). Food pasteurization using high-intensity pulsed electric fields. *Food Technology*, 49, 55-60.

Qin, B.L.; Chang, F.J.; Barbosa-Cánovas, G.V.; Swanson, B.G. (1995b). Non-thermal inactivation of *Saccharomyces cerevisiae* in apple juice using pulsed electric fields. *Food Science and Technology-LWT*, 28, 564-568.

Qiu, X.; Sharma, S.; Tuhela, L.; Jia, M.; Zhang, Q. (1998). An integrated PEIAC pilot plant for continuous nonthermal pasteurization of fresh orange juice. *Agricultural Engineering*, 41, 1069-1074.

Raso, J.; Calderón, M. L.; Góngora, M.; Barbosa-Cánovas, G. V.; Swanson, B.G. (1998a). Inactivation of *Zygosaccharomyces bailii* in fruit juices by heat, high hidrostatic presure and pulsed electric fields. *Journal of Food Science*, 63, 1042- 1044.

Raso, J.; Calderón, M. L.; Góngora, M.; Barbosa-Cánovas, G. V.; Swanson, B.G. (1998b). Inactivation of mold ascospores and conidospores suspended in fruit juices by pulsed electric fields. *Food Science and Technology-LWT*, 31, 668-672.

Riener, J.; Noci, F.; Cronin, D.A.; Morgan, D.J.; Lyng, J.G. (2008). Combined effect of temperature and pulsed electric fields on apple juice peroxidase and polyphenoloxidase inactivation. *Food Chemistry*, 109, 402-407.

Rodrigo, D.; Barbosa-Cánovas, G.V.; Martínez, A.; Rodrigo, M. (2003a). Weibull distribution function based on an empirical mathematical model for inactivation of *Escherichia coli* by pulsed electric fields. *Journal of Food Protection*, 66, 1007-1012.

Rodrigo, D.; Barbosa-Cánovas, G.V.; Martínez, A.; Rodrigo, M. (2003b). Pectin methyl esterase and natural microflora of fresh mixed orange and carrot juice treated with pulsed electric fields. *Journal of Food Protection*, 66, 2336-2342.

Sánchez-Moreno, C.; Plaza, L.; Elez-Martínez, P.; De Ancos, B.; Martín-Belloso, O.; Cano, M.P. (2005). Impact of high-pressure and pulsed electric fields on bioactive compounds and antioxidant activity of orange juice in comparison with traditional thermal processing. *Journal of Agricultural and Food Chemistry*, 53, 4403-4409.

Tracy, R. L. (1932). Lethal effect of alternating current on yeast cells. *Journal of Bacteriology*, 24, 423-438.

Van Loey, A.; Verachtert, B.; Hendrickx, M. (2002). Effects of high electric field pulses on enzymes. *Trends in Food Science and Technology*, 12, 94-102.

Yeom, H. W.; Streaker, C. B.; Zhang, Q. H.; Min, D. B. (2000a). Effects of pulsed electric fields on the activities of microorganisms and pectin methyl esterase in orange juice. *Journal of Food Science*, 65, 1359-1363.

Yeom, H. W.; Streaker, C. B.; Zhang, Q. H.; Min, D. B. (2000b). Effects of pulsed electric fields on the quality of orange juice and comparison with heat pasteurization. *Journal of Agricultural and Food Chemistry*, 48, 4597-4605.

Yeom, H.W.; Zhang, Q.H.; Chism, G.W. (2002). Inactivation of pectin methyl esterase in orange juice by pulsed electric fields. *Journal of Food Science*, 67, 2154-2159.

Yin, Y.; Zhang, Q. H.; Sastry, S. K. (1997). High voltage pulsed electric field treatment chambers for the preservation of liquid food products. U.S. Patent n° 5,690,978.

Zárate-Rodríguez, E.; Ortega-Rivas, E.; Barbosa-Cánovas, G.V. (2000). Quality changes in apple juice as related to nonthermal processing. *Journal of Food Quality*, 23, 337-349.

Zhang, Q.; Monsalve-Gonzalez, A.; Qin, B.L.; Barbosa-Cánovas, G.V.; Swanson, B.G. (1994). Inactivation of E. coli and S. cerevisiae by pulsed electric fields under controlled temperature conditions. Transactions of the ASAE, 37, 581-587.

Zhang, Q.; Qin, B. L.; Barbosa-Cánovas, G. V.; Swanson, B. G.; Pedrow, P. D. (1996). Batch mode food treatment using pulsed electric fields. US Patent n° 5,549,041.

In: Fruit Juices: Properties, Consumption and Nutrition
Editor: Pauline G. Scardina

ISBN: 978-1-60741-505-3

Chapter 4

Impact of Harvesting and Storage on Bioactive Components in Varieties of Orange (*Citrus Sinensis* L.)

M.J. Esteve and A. Frigola

Área Nutrición y Bromatología. Facultad de Farmacia. Universitat de València. Avda. Vicent Andrés Estellés, s/n. 46100 Burjassot (Spain)

Abstract

Orange juice (*Citrus sinensis* L.) is probably the best-known and most widely consumed fruit juice all over the world, particularly appreciated for its fresh flavor and considered of high beneficial value for its high content in vitamin C and natural antioxidants such as carotenoids. Concentrations of bioactive compounds in oranges may depend on the variety, but also on the harvesting date and storage time. The aim of this work, therefore, was to determine the physical and chemical characteristics (juice/weight relationship, pH, °Brix, vitamin C, vitamin A, and carotenoids) of different varieties of orange and establish a relationship that would allow discrimination of oranges in terms of variety, harvesting date, and storage time. Three varieties of orange (Navelina, Navel, and Navel-Lane) were harvested randomly and directly in the field during their harvesting period. The harvesting was done on 3 different dates: 0 days (initial harvesting), 14 days later, and 28 days after the initial harvesting. Each of the harvested samples was stored at 4 ± 2 °C. To study the effect of storage, 3 determinations were made at 3 different times: 0 (initial), 15, and 30 days. A study was made of the evolution of the juice/weight relationship, pH, °Brix, vitamin C, vitamin A, and carotenoid profile of the different varieties of orange during harvesting and storage. The values of the juice/weight relationship, pH, °Brix, and vitamin C were in the ranges 46.30–57.81 mL/100 g, 3.31–4.01, 10.6–12.5, and 45.58–57.79 mg/100 mL, respectively, depending on the variety, harvesting date, and storage time. Fourteen carotenoids (including *cis* forms) were determined in the oranges analyzed, and the vitamin A (RAE) concentration obtained ranged between 2.93 and 29.44. A predictive model was obtained that could be used to differentiate the orange varieties analyzed. The model was verified with the results obtained for the Navel variety of orange harvested in the following season

Keywords: *Citrus sinensis*, bioactive compounds, storage, harvesting

Introduction

Citrus fruits are widely accepted all over the world because of their organoleptic characteristics and their nutritional value. Moreover, the citrus industry plays a very important role in Brazil, the United States, and Mexico, and also in Europe, where Spain is the largest producer, and in China (Señorans et al., 2001).

The growing interest in citrus products is partly due to the health benefits connected with their antioxidant properties, which are attributable to the ascorbic acid and carotenoids that they contain (Xu et al., 2008; Dhuique-Mayer et al., 2005; Morton et al., 2000; Pellegrini et al., 2003). These health benefits have prompted research into pre- and postharvest citrus fruit treatments to maintain or enhance their biological activity.

The physicochemical characteristics can vary significantly depending on a number of factors, such as orange variety, environmental factors (climate, soils, maturity at harvest, irrigation, fertilization, etc.), different processing procedures, and analytical methods. But the orange variety has a major influence on the characteristics of the juice (Li-ying et al. 2008; Barry et al. 2003; Lee and Castle 2001). The °Brix value is used to indicate the percentage of soluble solids and is one of the most important factors for grading the quality of a citrus juice (McAllister, 1980).

The variability of the bioactive compounds is connected with genetic and climatic factors. The vitamin C concentration in fruits and vegetables depends on various factors such as genotype, climatic conditions, and cultivation practices (Esteve et al., 1995; Lee and Kader, 2000). Oranges have high concentrations of violaxanthin, lutein, zeaxanthin, and β-cryptoxanthin (Kato et al., 2004; Meléndez-Martínez et al., 2005; Cortés et al., 2004, 2006). These concentrations depend on numerous factors, including growing conditions, geographical origin, degree of ripeness of the fruit, and variety (Mouly et al., 1999; Lee and Castle, 2001; Dhuique-Mayer et al, 2005; Lee, 2001). Goodner et al. (2001) report that mandarins, oranges, and their hybrids can be differentiated by their β-cryptoxanthin concentrations. Fanciullino et al. (2006) analyzed carotenoid concentrations in fruits of the *Citrus* genus to evaluate the influence of genetic factors including origin and cultivation characteristics. The results show that the variability in carotenoid concentration is more interspecific than intraspecific, and also that *cis*-violaxanthin and β-cryptoxanthin can be used to classify the data. Mouly et al. (1999) separated and quantified most of the carotenoids in Valencia variety orange juices from five countries. They were able to group the oranges by origin into two large groups on the basis of their total carotenoid contents: on the one hand, oranges from Israel and Spain, and on the other, oranges from Florida, Belize, and Cuba. Moreover, from the carotene profile they were able to differentiate the Valencia oranges grown in Israel from the ones from other origins. Cano et al. (2008) report that the most important parameters that can be used to classify different varieties of orange are the vitamin C and flavonoid concentrations. Dhuique-Mayer et al. (2005) compared the concentrations of carotenoids, vitamin C, and flavonoids in different varieties of orange (*Citrus* sp.) and found that the different varieties of orange could be classified in terms of their nutritional profile primarily on the basis of their carotenoid content. They also found strong correlations between β-cryptoxanthin and hesperidin, and between β-cryptoxanthin and β-carotene. The vitamin C concentration, however, did not correlate with carotenoids or with flavanone glycosides.

Oranges are considered to be non-climateric fruit, but storage treatment can increase fruit respiration because of possible chilling injury (Grierson and Ben-Yehoshua, 1986).

The aim of this work was to determine the physical and chemical characteristics (juice/weight relationship, pH, °Brix, vitamin C, vitamin A, and carotenoids) of different varieties of orange and establish a relationship that would allow discrimination of oranges in terms of variety, date of harvest, and storage time.

Methods

All the analyses were performed in triplicate, as was each of the determinations.

Juice/weight relationship. The juice/weight relationship was expressed in mL/100 g, the result being the quotient between the yield of juice from the oranges (total volume in mL) and their weight in grams. At the time of analysis the outer surface of the oranges that were to be used was cleaned with filter paper and they were weighed (analytical balance, Ultra Mark 500, BEL). After extraction of the juice with an electric extractor (UFESA, EX_7235), the total volume of the juice obtained was measured, always keeping the juice protected from the light. After homogenization, various aliquots were separated for determination of the remaining parameters.

pH determination was based on the potentiometric measurement at 20 °C. It was determined in a Crison GLP 21 pH meter equipped with a temperature compensation sensor.

°Brix was determined by measurement of the refraction index with an Atago model RX-1000 digital refractometer at 20°C.

Vitamin C. 5 mL of juice was diluted to 25 mL with the extraction solution: oxalic acid (Panreac, Barcelona, Spain) 1%, w/v, trichloroacetic acid (Baker, Deventer, Holland) 2%, w/v, sodium sulfate (Baker, Deventer, Holland) 1%, w/v. After vigorous shaking, the solution was filtered through a folded filter (Whatman no. 1). 9.5 mL of 1% (w/v) oxalic acid and 2 mL of 2M acetic acid/sodium acetate (Panreac, Barcelona, Spain) buffer (pH = 4.8) were added to an aliquot of 0.5 mL of filtrate and the solution was transferred to the polarographic cell. The following instrumental conditions were applied: DP_{50}, mode DME, drop size 2, drop time 1 s, scan rate 10 mV/s, initial potential –0.10 V. Determinations were carried out using the peak heights and standard additions method (Aparicio et al., 1992).

Carotenoids. The carotenoids (including geometrical isomers) were identified and quantified by LC with a UV-vis diode array detector (Hewlett-Packard, 1100 series) and a column thermostat (Agilent 1100 series). An extraction process (ethanol/hexane, 4:3, v/v) was performed, followed by saponification with diethyl ether/methanolic KOH (0.1%, w/v,

Table 1. Values of juice/weight relationship, pH, °Brix, vitamin C, and vitamin A obtained in the three varieties analyzed, by harvesting date and storage time. 2004–2005 season

	Storage (days)	**Harvesting** (days) **0**	**14**	**28**
		Juice/weight (mL/100 g)		
Navelina	0	50.0 ± 0.0^{a1}	46.3 ± 0.0^{a2}	49.3 ± 0.1^{a3}
	15	51.4 ± 0.0^{b1}	48.2 ± 0.0^{b2}	57.8 ± 0.0^{b3}
	30	51.1 ± 0.1^{c1}	53.5 ± 0.1^{c2}	56.4 ± 0.0^{c3}
Navel	0	56.1 ± 0.0^{a1}	57.0 ± 0.0^{a2}	51.0 ± 0.0^{a3}
	15	55.9 ± 0.0^{b1}	57.0 ± 0.0^{a2}	53.6 ± 0.0^{b3}
	30	55.7 ± 0.0^{c1}	56.6 ± 0.0^{c2}	53.9 ± 0.0^{c3}
Navel-Lane	0	55.5 ± 0.0^{a1}	55.9 ± 0.0^{a2}	56.8 ± 0.0^{a3}
	15	57.4 ± 0.0^{b1}	56.8 ± 0.0^{b2}	55.2 ± 0.0^{b3}
	30	58.1 ± 0.0^{c1}	56.9 ± 0.0^{c2}	55.1 ± 0.1^{c3}
		pH		
Navelina	0	3.41 ± 0.01^{a1}	3.31 ± 0.01^{a2}	3.49 ± 0.01^{a3}
	15	3.48 ± 0.01^{b1}	3.58 ± 0.01^{b2}	3.52 ± 0.01^{b1}
	30	3.75 ± 0.02^{c1}	3.78 ± 0.01^{c2}	3.56 ± 0.01^{c3}
Navel	0	3.48 ± 0.01^{a1}	3.64 ± 0.02^{a2}	3.72 ± 0.03^{a2}
	15	3.59 ± 0.01^{b1}	3.56 ± 0.01^{b2}	3.64 ± 0.01^{b3}
	30	3.63 ± 0.01^{c1}	3.76 ± 0.01^{c2}	4.01 ± 0.01^{c3}
Navel-Lane	0	3.43 ± 0.02^{a1}	3.63 ± 0.02^{a2}	3.59 ± 0.01^{a2}
	15	3.46 ± 0.01^{b1}	3.79 ± 0.01^{b2}	3.52 ± 0.02^{b3}
	30	3.50 ± 0.02^{b1}	3.69 ± 0.01^{c2}	3.68 ± 0.01^{c2}
			°Brix	
Navelina	0	11.2 ± 0.1^{a1}	10.8 ± 0.1^{a2}	11.2 ± 0.1^{a1}
	15	12.2 ± 0.0^{b1}	11.4 ± 0.0^{b2}	11.4 ± 0.2^{b2}
	30	12.2 ± 0.2^{b1}	11.0 ± 0.1^{c2}	11.8 ± 0.1^{c3}
Navel	0	11.8 ± 0.1^{a1}	11.6 ± 0.2^{a2}	10.8 ± 0.1^{a3}
	15	12.4 ± 0.2^{b1}	11.6 ± 0.2^{a2}	11.6 ± 0.2^{b2}
	30	12.2 ± 0.2^{c1}	11.6 ± 0.1^{a2}	11.6 ± 0.2^{c2}
Navel-Lane	0	10.8 ± 0.1^{a1}	11.0 ± 0.1^{a2}	11.8 ± 0.2^{a3}
	15	10.8 ± 0.1^{a1}	11.6 ± 0.1^{b2}	11.6 ± 0.1^{b2}
	30	10.6 ± 0.2^{b1}	12.5 ± 0.1^{c2}	11.6 ± 0.1^{b3}

Superscript: in the same column, identical letters indicate that there are no significant differences ($p < 0.05$); in the same row, identical numbers indicate that there are no significant differences ($p < 0.05$).

BHT) (1:1, v/v) for 0.5 h at room temperature. The injection volume used was 20 μL. A particle size of 5 μm and a Vydac 201TP precolumn (guard column) (4.6 mm i.d. cartridge with 5-μm particles) (Hesperia, CA) were used.

The mobile phase used was methanol (0.1 M ammonium acetate), tertbutyl methyl ether, and water (in a concentration gradient), and a temperature gradient was applied with retinol palmitate as an internal standard. Carotenoids were identified by UV-vis spectra and retention times in HPLC in the juices analyzed using the system HP Chemstation-A.06.03 (Cortes et al., 2004). Carotenoids were expressed as micrograms per 100 g.

Vitamin A. Vitamin A was expressed as retinol activity equivalents (RAE), using the following conversion (IOM, 2001; Trumbo et al, 2003):

RAE = (μg of β-carotene)/12 + (μg of β-cryptoxanthin + μg of α-carotene)/24.

Samples

The study was conducted on fresh citrus fruits. Three varieties of orange (*Citrus sinensis*) were chosen on the basis of their high production in the Valencian Community: Navelina, Navel, and Navel-Lane. They were picked directly and at random in three different fields, following statistical sampling procedures, in their respective harvesting periods (2003–2004 season). They were identified by type of sample, harvesting time, and period of storage at 4 ± 2 °C. The temperature selected (4 °C) was the temperature used for their storage until distribution. Each of the varieties was harvested on three different dates (0, 14, and 28 days), and each of the samples collected was stored in refrigeration for 15 and 30 days (Figure 1 gives a diagram of the process). In the following season (2004–2005) Navel variety oranges were harvested, the various physical and chemical parameters were determined, and the validity of the predictive model obtained was verified; the data corresponding to this season have already been published (Cortés et al., 2006a,2006b, 2007).

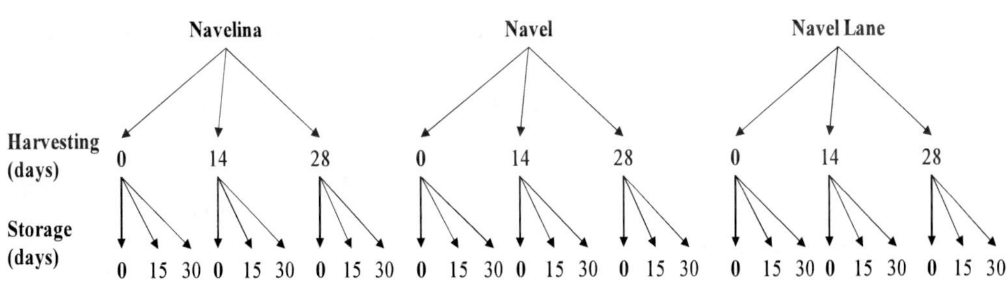

Figure 1. Diagram of sampling: variety, harvesting, and storage.

Sample Collection And Size

The oranges were picked at random in three different fields and mixed together.

Table 2. Concentrations of vitamin C and vitamin A during harvesting and storage. 2004–2005 season

	Storage (days)	Harvesting (days) 0	14	28
		Vitamin C (mg/100 mL)		
Navelina	0	47.0 ± 0.9^{a1}	57.8 ± 0.7^{a2}	55.9 ± 0.0^{a2}
	15	50.3 ± 0.4^{b1}	57.8 ± 0.1^{a2}	51.7 ± 1.5^{b1}
	30	54.9 ± 1.0^{c1}	51.8 ± 0.2^{b2}	50.2 ± 0.8^{b2}
Navel	0	52.3 ± 0.7^{a1}	53.3 ± 0.3^{a1}	47.8 ± 0.2^{a2}
	15	51.6 ± 0.3^{a1}	52.5 ± 1.7^{a1}	49.0 ± 0.1^{a1}
	30	52.0 ± 0.1^{a1}	50.4 ± 0.5^{a2}	48.6 ± 0.8^{a3}
Navel-Lane	0	51.8 ± 0.7^{a1}	49.8 ± 0.1^{a1}	45.6 ± 1.6^{a2}
	15	53.9 ± 0.7^{a1}	51.2 ± 0.4^{a2}	45.9 ± 0.8^{a3}
	30	53.2 ± 0.8^{a1}	56.2 ± 1.0^{b1}	45.6 ± 1.7^{a2}
		Vitamin A (RAE)		
Navelina	0	2.94 ± 0.16^{ab1}	2.71 ± 0.02^{a1}	5.11 ± 0.08^{a2}
	15	3.91 ± 0.35^{a1}	6.34 ± 0.36^{b1}	7.43 ± 1.88^{a1}
	30	6.38 ± 1.65^{b1}	5.73 ± 0.35^{b1}	5.53 ± 3.07^{a1}
Navel	0	8.63 ± 0.01^{a1}	6.01 ± 0.68^{a2}	10.84 ± 0.95^{a3}
	15	7.29 ± 0.09^{b1}	3.87 ± 0.75^{b2}	11.36 ± 0.34^{a3}
	30	11.71 ± 0.27^{c1}	10.92 ± 0.27^{c1}	10.15 ± 0.70^{a1}
Navel-Lane	0	6.23 ± 0.51^{a1}	7.96 ± 1.89^{a1}	14.67 ± 0.08^{a2}
	15	5.46 ± 0.27^{a1}	14.33 ± 0.54^{b1}	8.94 ± 4.14^{ab1}
	30	9.16 ± 0.70^{b1}	11.56 ± 0.46^{ab2}	8.31 ± 0.94^{a1}

Superscript: in the same column, identical letters indicate that there are no significant differences ($p < 0.05$); in the same row, identical numbers indicate that there are no significant differences ($p < 0.05$).

To obtain suitable precision in the results it was necessary first to establish the sample size, i.e., the number of oranges to be taken each time so that the results should be reliable and representative. Primo et al. (1963) established 21 units as the minimum orange sample size for the mean value to have a variation of ±3 mg, corresponding to 5% of the error with regard to the value found (depending on the vitamin C concentration). The evolution of analysis methods has made it possible to reduce the sample size and obtain results of equal reliability to those obtained with a larger sample, as confirmed by some more recent studies (Nagy, 1980; Ortuño et al., 1995).

The number of units taken in this study for each type of sample ranged between 9 and 12 oranges, depending on the volume of juice yielded. The harvesting of each variety of orange was also done on three different dates (Figure 1).

Storage

The outer surface of the oranges was cleaned with paper, and the oranges were weighed and placed in open plastic boxes that were numbered and marked with identification codes. They were then placed in a refrigerated chamber with controlled temperature (4 ± 2 °C) and humidity. The oranges were kept in the refrigerated chamber from their arrival at the laboratory until the time of their analysis, always occupying the same place in order to avoid possible temperature variations. Three determinations of each parameter were made with each sample at different storage times: 0 days (initial), 15 days, and 30 days (see Figure 1).

Statistical Analysis

An analysis of variance (ANOVA) of three factors was applied to the results obtained to verify whether there were significant differences in the parameters studied in relation to variety, harvesting time, and storage time, and the possible interactions between the factors. A multiple regression analysis was performed for each of the varieties and parameters to study the influence of harvesting date and/or storage time. To gain insight into the data structure a multivariate analysis called principal component analysis (PCA), a pure display method, was performed to detect the most important factors of variability and to describe the relations between variables and observations.

All statistical analyses were performed using Statgraphics Plus 5.0 (Statistical Graphics Corporation, Inc., Rockville, MD, USA).

Results

Tables 1 and 2 show the juice/weight relationship, pH, °Brix, vitamin C, and vitamin A values obtained in the three varieties of orange analyzed, by harvesting date and storage time.

By chromatographic analysis of the various samples studied, 10 carotenoids were identified and quantified. Tables 3–5 show the results for each of the varieties of orange analyzed and the variation during harvesting and storage.

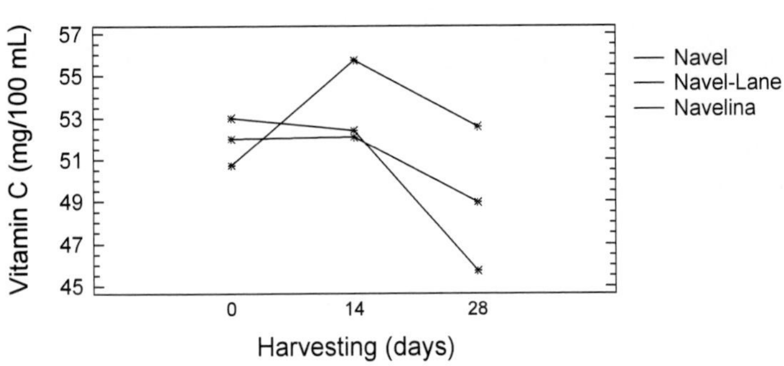

Figure 2. Continued on next page.

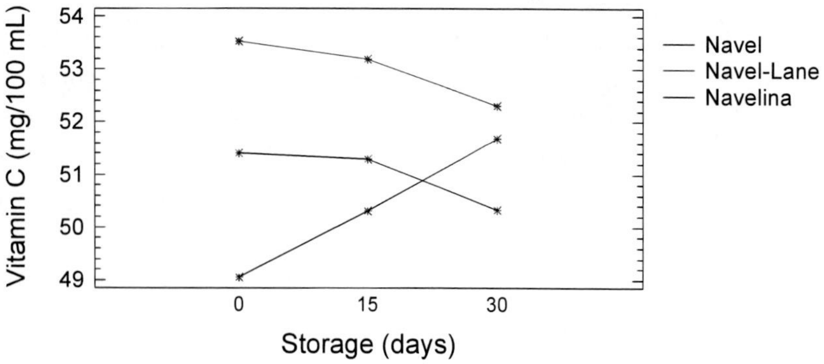

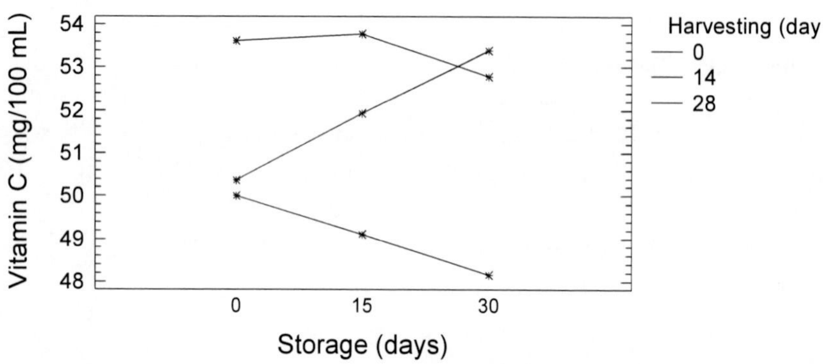

Figure 2. Influence of variety, harvesting date, and storage time on concentration of vitamin C.

The results are in agreement with those obtained by other authors (Cano et al, 2008; Dhuique-Mayer et al., 2005; Fanciullino et al, 2006; Meléndez-Martínez et al, 2005; Mouly et al, 1999; Rapisarda et al, 2008).

Vitamin C. Application of the analysis of variance to the results revealed significant differences ($p < 0.05$) between the vitamin C concentration in the Navelina variety oranges (53.0 ± 3.6 mg/100 mL, n = 27) and the concentrations in the other two varieties, Navel (51.0 ± 1.8 mg/100 mL, n = 27) and Navel-Lane (50.4 ± 3.9 mg/100 mL, n = 27), between which the differences were not significant. The oranges collected 28 days after the beginning of harvesting had a concentration (49.1 ± 3.3 mg/100 mL) significantly lower ($p < 0.01$) than that of the oranges collected during the first 14 days (51.9 ± 2.3 and 53.4 ± 3.0 mg/100 mL, for the oranges collected after 0 and 14 days, respectively). There were no significant differences in the various storage periods.

From the analysis of variance of more than one factor it was possible to show the existence of interactions between the effects of the factors studied: variety (Navel, Navelina, Navel-Lane), harvesting date (0, 14, and 28 days), and storage time (0, 15, and 30 days). The vitamin C concentration increased during storage of the oranges collected on the first date,

Table 3. Concentrations of carotenoids in Navelina variety oranges during harvesting and storage. 2004–2005 season

Carotenoids *(μg/100 g)*	Storage *(days)*	Harvesting *(days)* 0	14	28
9-*cis*-violaxanthin + neoxanthin	*0*	94.9 ± 12.7^{a1}	412.7 ± 25.9^{a2}	485.3 ± 31.2^{a2}
	15	578.6 ± 64.9^{b1}	516.2 ± 7.2^{b1}	608.6 ± 20.2^{a1}
	30	356.3 ± 83.9^{c1}	621.5 ± 38.3^{c1}	408.5 ± 14.4^{a1}
antheraxanthin	*0*	21.9 ± 1.7^{a1}	95.9 ± 3.6^{a2}	145.2 ± 7.4^{a3}
	15	144.9 ± 18.4^{b1}	181.4 ± 1.4^{b2}	183.2 ± 0.2^{a2}
	30	95.8 ± 29.7^{b1}	186.3 ± 17.8^{b1}	121.6 ± 43.1^{a1}
lutein	*0*	14.2 ± 0.3^{a1}	36.5 ± 0.3^{a2}	45.7 ± 1.8^{a3}
	15	50.2 ± 8.6^{b1}	47.4 ± 8.9^{a1}	48.5 ± 10.9^{a1}
	30	$31.8\ 11.1^{ab1}$	66.1 ± 6.2^{b2}	30.9 ± 7.8^{a1}
zeaxanthin	*0*	10.3 ± 0.1^{a1}	20.1 ± 0.4^{a2}	29.5 ± 1.8^{a3}
	15	23.4 ± 1.0^{b1}	32.0 ± 4.5^{b1}	32.0 ± 4.5^{a1}
	30	23.4 ± 4.5^{b1}	38.0 ± 4.1^{b2}	24.9 ± 3.4^{a1}
β-cryptoxanthin	*0*	29.7 ± 0.9^{a1}	45.1 ± 4.4^{a2}	64.8 ± 2.3^{a3}
	15	70.9 ± 5.5^{ab1}	101.7 ± 9.3^{b1}	111.3 ± 29.3^{a1}
	30	100.0 ± 28.1^{b1}	93.3 ± 3.4^{b1}	70.9 ± 3.1^{a1}
9-*cis*-α-carotene	*0*	28.0 ± 2.5^{a1}	35.1 ± 1.2^{a2}	35.2 ± 2.7^{a2}
	15	36.9 ± 1.9^{b1}	24.3 ± 1.6^{b2}	24.3 ± 4.4^{a2}
	30	37.2 ± 0.3^{b1}	20.7 ± 0.7^{b1}	40.5 ± 13.9^{a1}
α-carotene	*0*	10.4 ± 1.0^{a1}	9.3 ± 0.8^{a1}	19.0 ± 0.2^{a2}
	15	9.0 ± 0.9^{a1}	14.5 ± 2.3^{b12}	19.1 ± 4.6^{a2}
	30	15.1 ± 1.7^{b1}	10.8 ± 1.0^{a1}	17.3 ± 1.3^{a1}
phytoene + phytofluene	*0*	9.9 ± 0.2^{a1}	5.8 ± 0.4^{a2}	23.5 ± 0.6^{a3}
	15	8.1 ± 1.8^{a1}	28.1 ± 1.7^{b2}	31.1 ± 7.6^{a2}
	30	19.9 ± 0.1^{b1}	21.0 ± 1.7^{c1}	20.0 ± 5.4^{a1}
β-carotene	*0*	15.2 ± 1.0^{ab1}	5.2 ± 0.3^{a2}	19.4 ± 0.1^{a3}
	15	6.9 ± 1.0^{a1}	18.2 ± 1.0^{b2}	24.0 ± 5.6^{a3}
	30	19.0 ± 4.9^{b1}	16.6 ± 3.0^{b1}	22.3 ± 2.6^{a1}
9-*cis*-β-carotene	*0*	$19.2 + 0.2^{a1}$	8.9 ± 0.9^{a2}	21.4 ± 2.4^{a1}
	15	8.2 ± 0.2^{b1}	10.0 ± 0.9^{a1}	14.2 ± 3.4^{a1}
	30	24.6 ± 3.6^{a12}	8.8 ± 0.2^{a1}	29.1 ± 9.2^{a2}

Superscript: in the same column, identical letters indicate that there are no significant differences ($p < 0.05$); in the same row, identical numbers indicate that there are no significant differences ($p < 0.05$).

whereas in the oranges collected on the second date (14 days) and the third date (28 days) it decreased, more sharply in the latter case (Figure 2). The vitamin C concentration in the Navel and Navel-Lane varieties decreased to different extents, depending on the harvesting date, whereas in the Navelina variety it increased (Figure 2). The behavior during storage also varied: an increase in concentration in relation to storage time was seen only in the Navel-Lane variety. However, the only significant interaction detected was between storage time and variety.

Table 4. Concentrations of carotenoids in Navel variety oranges during harvesting and storage. 2004–2005 season

Carotenoids *(µg/100 g)*	Storage *(days)*	Harvesting *(days)*		
		0	14	28
9-*cis*-violaxanthin + neoxanthin	*0*	754.0 ± 47.2^{a12}	621.3 ± 6.0^{a1}	895.2 ± 96.4^{a2}
	15	817.2 ± 12.8^{a1}	723.1 ± 14.7^{b2}	642.8 ± 8.0^{b3}
	30	742.4 ± 11.3^{a1}	582.1 ± 9.4^{c2}	645.3 ± 35.8^{b2}
antheraxanthin	*0*	224.8 ± 9.3^{a1}	229.1 ± 4.5^{a1}	294.0 ± 30.6^{ab2}
	15	312.5 ± 9.2^{b1}	271.1 ± 11.7^{b2}	233.5 ± 12.1^{a3}
	30	240.8 ± 17.6^{a1}	217.8 ± 11.3^{a1}	350.9 ± 47.8^{b2}
lutein	*0*	53.6 ± 4.7^{a12}	43.6 ± 1.2^{a1}	60.9 ± 3.2^{a2}
	15	60.2 ± 6.4^{a1}	41.4 ± 7.8^{a1}	57.9 ± 5.1^{a1}
	30	54.4 ± 4.2^{a12}	44.6 ± 4.0^{a1}	65.3 ± 4.8^{a2}
zeaxanthin	*0*	36.9 ± 2.0^{a1}	36.6 ± 0.0^{a1}	53.9 ± 1.5^{a2}
	15	43.3 ± 3.4^{ab1}	43.7 ± 9.0^{a1}	37.8 ± 0.4^{b1}
	30	51.5 ± 6.3^{b1}	29.7 ± 1.3^{a2}	56.3 ± 1.9^{a1}
β-cryptoxanthin	*0*	120.1 ± 2.7^{a1}	86.0 ± 1.0^{a1}	103.1 ± 18.4^{a1}
	15	120.4 ± 2.5^{a1}	55.1 ± 1.0^{b2}	113.9 ± 5.2^{ab1}
	30	153.1 ± 14.9^{b1}	115.3 ± 0.4^{c1}	149.2 ± 15.7^{b1}
9-*cis*-α-carotene	*0*	35.4 ± 1.6^{a1}	42.6 ± 3.2^{a1}	52.1 ± 1.7^{a2}
	15	28.3 ± 0.7^{b1}	23.6 ± 0.6^{b1}	78.9 ± 5.4^{b2}
	30	68.3 ± 1.9^{c1}	63.9 ± 5.2^{c12}	22.1 ± 13.3^{a2}
α-carotene	*0*	20.5 ± 0.1^{a1}	20.5 ± 5.5^{a1}	34.8 ± 2.2^{a2}
	15	35.3 ± 3.9^{b1}	2.5 ± 0.8^{b2}	58.2 ± 1.8^{b3}
	30	13.4 ± 1.3^{a1}	50.2 ± 6.0^{c2}	35.8 ± 0.9^{a3}
phytoene + phytofluene	*0*	35.0 ± 0.1^{a1}	17.5 ± 7.1^{a2}	44.1 ± 4.1^{a1}
	15	14.3 ± 0.4^{b1}	10.5 ± 3.6^{a1}	52.1 ± 0.3^{b2}
	30	53.7 ± 10.0^{c1}	34.7 ± 1.0^{b2}	25.5 ± 0.3^{c2}
β-carotene	*0*	33.21 ± 1.1^{a1}	18.8 ± 7.4^{a2}	61.1 ± 1.15^{a3}
	15	9.7 ± 2.1^{b1}	17.6 ± 2.2^{a1}	50.2 ± 5.3^{b2}
	30	57.4 ± 3.5^{c1}	48.2 ± 0.3^{b2}	29.3 ± 0.2^{c3}
9-*cis*-β-carotene	*0*	22.0 ± 1.6^{a1}	25.6 ± 5.9^{ab1}	20.9 ± 5.0^{a1}
	15	11.8 ± 2.0^{a1}	16.1 ± 0.1^{a1}	35.5 ± 1.3^{b2}
	30	39.1 ± 3.5^{b1}	36.2 ± 5.5^{b1}	18.8 ± 0.5^{a2}

Superscript: in the same column, identical letters indicate that there are no significant differences ($p < 0.05$); in the same row, identical numbers indicate that there are no significant differences ($p < 0.05$).

Performance of a multiple regression analysis for each of the varieties studied yielded models that indicated the influence of the harvesting date and/or storage time. Only in the Navel-Lane variety did the harvesting date and storage time have a significant influence ($p < 0.05$) on the vitamin C concentration: vitamin C (mg/100 mL) = 52.7 – 0.26 R + 0.09 S (standard error = 1.6, $R^2 = 70.4$), where S the storage time (days). In the Navel variety it was the harvesting date that had a statistically significant influence ($p < 0.05$) on the vitamin C

Table 5. Concentrations of carotenoids in Navel-Lane variety oranges during harvesting and storage. 2004–2005 season

Carotenoids *(μg/100 g)*	Storage *(days)*	Harvesting *(days)*		
		0	14	28
9-*cis*-violaxanthin + neoxanthin	*0*	693.8 ± 97.0^{ab1}	736.5 ± 18.4^{a1}	663.0 ± 1.1^{a1}
	15	532.9 ± 61.1^{a1}	816.0 ± 5.3^{b2}	711.3 ± 19.8^{a2}
	30	806.4 ± 60.8^{b1}	554.7 ± 18.8^{c2}	787.7 ± 34.9^{b1}
antheraxanthin	*0*	206.2 ± 25.7^{ab1}	266.3 ± 0.2^{a2}	193.7 ± 3.5^{a1}
	15	148.4 ± 18.7^{a1}	268.8 ± 11.5^{a2}	229.6 ± 14.4^{a2}
	30	246.7 ± 37.4^{b12}	185.2 ± 24.1^{b1}	310.4 ± 19.7^{b2}
lutein	*0*	44.2 ± 2.4^{a1}	51.6 ± 0.7^{a2}	41.0 ± 1.1^{a1}
	15	40.0 ± 11.7^{a1}	44.4 ± 3.8^{ab1}	39.0 ± 3.6^{a1}
	30	48.6 ± 7.7^{a1}	37.3 ± 4.7^{b1}	49.1 ± 1.5^{b1}
zeaxanthin	*0*	32.6 ± 0.2^{a1}	45.3 ± 1.0^{a2}	41.8 ± 3.0^{a2}
	15	29.3 ± 4.1^{a1}	45.6 ± 2.9^{a2}	39.0 ± 7.1^{a12}
	30	33.1 ± 2.0^{a1}	34.0 ± 2.5^{b1}	44.7 ± 0.3^{a2}
β-cryptoxanthin	*0*	91.4 ± 1.1^{a1}	131.2 ± 26.4^{a1}	134.4 ± 4.0^{a1}
	15	79.3 ± 16.2^{a1}	174.2 ± 2.8^{a2}	97.1 ± 4.8^{a1}
	30	95.6 ± 13.4^{a1}	138.3 ± 1.9^{a2}	126.1 ± 0.8^{a2}
9-*cis*-α-carotene	*0*	34.5 ± 3.5^{a1}	23.6 ± 3.8^{a1}	104.6 ± 5.5^{a2}
	15	20.3 ± 1.0^{b1}	38.8 ± 6.6^{ab1}	33.6 ± 5.3^{b1}
	30	50.5 ± 5.4^{c12}	77.1 ± 2.4^{b1}	26.1 ± 4.7^{b2}
α-carotene	*0*	9.0 ± 2.7^{a1}	13.1 ± 3.0^{a1}	75.5 ± 4.0^{a2}
	15	14.6 ± 4.1^{a1}	44.1 ± 6.9^{b1}	41.5 ± 2.7^{a1}
	30	37.9 ± 3.0^{b1}	49.7 ± 7.5^{b1}	33.3 ± 2.1^{a1}
phytoene + phytofluene	*0*	24.3 ± 5.7^{a1}	36.8 ± 10.9^{a1}	72.1 ± 2.1^{a2}
	15	31.6 ± 4.2^{a1}	62.0 ± 0.0^{b1}	31.4 ± 7.0^{b1}
	30	43.7 ± 0.9^{b1}	37.1 ± 1.7^{a1}	18.1 ± 3.3^{b2}
β-carotene	*0*	24.6 ± 8.0^{a1}	23.3 ± 8.0^{a1}	71.1 ± 1.1^{a2}
	15	18.6 ± 2.8^{a1}	62.7 ± 1.6^{b2}	37.9 ± 2.0^{ab12}
	30	43.1 ± 3.3^{b1}	44.7 ± 2.7^{c1}	19.9 ± 4.3^{b2}
9-*cis*-β-carotene	*0*	7.6 ± 1.6^{a1}	11.1 ± 2.6^{a1}	30.6 ± 3.9^{a2}
	15	6.3 ± 1.8^{a1}	23.3 ± 5.1^{b2}	19.9 ± 1.5^{ab12}
	30	14.3 ± 0.8^{b12}	18.9 ± 2.6^{ab1}	10.0 ± 0.3^{b2}

Superscript: in the same column, identical letters indicate that there are no significant differences ($p < 0.05$); in the same row, identical numbers indicate that there are no significant differences ($p < 0.05$).

concentration: vitamin C (mg/100 mL) = 52.5 – 0.11 H (standard error = 1.3, $R^2 = 50.6$), where H is the harvesting date (days).

Vitamin A (RAE). There were significant differences ($p < 0.05$) in vitamin A concentration between the Navel (9.0 ± 2.7) and Navel-Lane (9.6 ± 3.4) varieties and the Navelina variety, which had a much lower concentration (5.1 ± 1.8). As the harvesting date advanced there was an increase in the vitamin A concentration, although no significant differences were observed, and there were also no differences during storage.

The analysis of variance of more than one factor indicated that there were significant interactions ($p < 0.01$) between harvesting date and storage time. In the oranges collected on the first and second harvesting dates there was an increase in the vitamin A concentration during storage, whereas in the oranges collected on the third harvesting date (28 days) the vitamin A concentration decreased (Figure 3). When a multiple regression analysis was performed for each of the varieties of orange studied, the vitamin A of the Navelina and Navel-Lane varieties was fitted significantly ($p < 0.05$) to a linear model and it was seen that only the harvesting date increased the vitamin A concentration significantly ($p < 0.05$): vitamin A (RAE) = 3.97 + 0.08 S (standard error = 1.63, R^2 = 27.2) and vitamin A (RAE) = 7.78 + 0.13 H (standard error = 3.09, R^2 = 21.1), where H is the harvesting date (days) and S the storage time for the Navelina and Navel-Lane varieties, respectively.

Navelina variety, whereas in the other two varieties it increased. During storage, pH increased in the three varieties, although to different extents.

The multiple regression analysis performed for each of the varieties showed that the variations in pH followed a linear model. In the Navel variety both harvesting date and storage time had a significant influence on the pH value (pH = 3.47 + 0.0077 H + 0.0061 S (standard error = 0.09, R^2 = 68.1), where H is the harvesting date (days) and S the storage time (days). In the Navelina variety, however, only storage time had an influence (pH = 3.40 + 0.0099 S, standard error = 0.08, R^2 = 70.6), and in the Navel-Lane variety only harvesting date had an influence (pH = 3.52 + 0.005 H, standard error = 0.11, R^2 = 24.3)

°Brix. No significant differences were seen between the three varieties of orange studied, although the value was slightly higher in the Navel oranges (11.69 ± 0.44) than in the Navelina oranges (11.47 ± 0.49) and the Navel-Lane oranges (11.37 ± 0.59). There were also no significant differences between the various harvesting dates. However, after 15 days of storage there was generally a significant increase ($p < 0.05$) in °Brix. The multifactor analysis of variance showed the existence of interactions ($p < 0.01$) only between harvesting date and variety, with °Brix decreasing in the Navelina and Navel varieties as harvesting advanced, whereas in the Navel-Lane variety it increased (Figure 5). The performance of a multiple regression analysis enabled us to predict the °Brix on the basis of harvesting date and storage time according to the variety. In the Navelina variety, only storage had a significant influence ($p<0.01$): °Brix = 11.2 + 0.02 S (standard error = 0.43, R^2 = 27.0); in the Navel-Lane oranges, the significant factor ($p < 0.01$) was storage time: °Brix = 10.9 + 0.03 H (standard error = 0.46, R^2 = 43.6); and in the Navel oranges the °Brix depended on harvesting date ($p < 0.0$) and storage time ($p < 0.01$): °Brix = 11.9 – 0.03 H + 0.01 S (standard error = 0.23, R^2 = 74.6).

Juice/weight relationship (v/w). In the Navel (55.2 ± 1.9 mL/g) and Navel-Lane (56.4 ± 1.0 mL/g) varieties the juice/weight relationship was significantly higher ($p < 0.01$) than in the Navelina variety (51.6±3.6 mL/g), although no differences were found according to harvesting date and storage time. There were statistically significant interactions ($p < 0.01$) between variety and harvesting date, and also with storage time. Figure 6 shows in the Navelina variety the juice/weight relationship increased with harvesting date, whereas in the other two varieties it decreased. During storage, however, it increased in all three varieties, although in different proportions. There was a statistically significant relation ($p < 0.01$) between juice/weight relationship and harvesting date: juice/weight relationship = 56.7 – 0.11 H (standard error = 1.48, R^2 = 44.4) and juice/weight relationship = 57.1 – 0.05 H (standard error = 0.89, $R^2 = 28.6$) for the Navel and Navel-Lane varieties, respectively. In the Navelina variety, however, both harvesting date and storage time had a significant influence ($p < 0.01$): juice/weight relationship = 47.2 + 0.13 H + 0.17 S (standard error = 2.66, $R^2 = 52.9$).

Carotenoids. The Navelina variety had the lowest concentration of each of the carotenoids, and the differences in comparison with the other two varieties were significant ($p < 0.01$) except for lutein and 9-*cis*-β-carotene. The concentrations of zeaxanthin and 9-*cis*-α-carotene were significantly higher ($p < 0.01$) in the oranges collected 28 days after the start of harvesting. However, storage time did not produce changes in the concentrations of the various carotenoids, except for β-cryptoxanthin, the concentration of which increased ($p < 0.01$). The multifactor analysis of variance showed that there were no interactions between the various factors (harvesting, storage, and variety) and the concentration of antheraxanthin, but the same factors had varying degrees of influence on the other carotenoids, producing a significant presence of interactions ($p < 0.05$). Variety, harvesting date, and storage time **pH**. The pH of the Navel variety oranges (3.67 ± 0.14) was significantly higher ($p < 0.01$) than that of the Navelina oranges (3.54 ± 0.15) and the Navel-Lane oranges (3.59 ± 0.12), between which there were no differences. There were also significant differences ($p < 0.01$) according to the harvesting date, with an increase in pH between the first date (3.53 ± 0.11) and the following dates (3.54 ± 0.15, in both cases) and during storage, when there was a significant increase ($p < 0.01$) in the pH with time (3.52 ± 0.13, 3.57 ± 0.10, and 3.71 ± 0.14 for 0, 15, and 30 days of storage, respectively).

There was a significant interaction ($p < 0.01$) between variety and harvesting date, and between variety and storage time (Figure 4). At the end of harvesting the pH decreased in the influenced the concentration of phytoene+phytofluene, and there were interactions between the factors (Figure 7). In the other carotenoids there were interactions between variety and harvesting date, except in 9-*cis*-α-carotene, α-carotene, and β-carotene, for which there was only an interaction between harvesting date and storage time. Also, the variation in the concentrations of 9-*cis*-violaxanthin+neoxanthin and β-cryptoxanthin during storage depended on the variety. The variation in the concentrations of zeaxanthin and 9-*cis*-β-carotene during storage also depended on the harvesting date.

In order to be able to predict the changes in the various carotenoids in the different varieties of orange in relation to harvesting date and storage time we performed a multiple regression analysis. Table 6 shows the statistically significant ($p < 0.05$) models obtained. To study the data and group them naturally in accordance with their characteristics (vitamin C, vitamin A, pH, ºBrix, juice/weight relationship, and carotenoid profile), we performed a principal component analysis and a discriminant analysis of the results.

The principal component analysis was used to examine the structure of the data. Table 7 shows the contributions of the components. In this case, 4 components were extracted, which accounted for 80.7% of the variability in the original data. This analysis does not permit satisfactory differentiation of the varieties of orange, and we therefore performed a discriminant analysis. To trace the discriminant functions with which to develop a model for differentiating the three varieties of orange we used 54 cases. By using a stepwise selection algorithm we found that 6 variables were predictors (antheraxanthin, lutein, 9-*cis*-β-carotene vitamin A, pH, and juice/weight relationship). Table 8 shows the two statistically significant ($p < 0.05$) discriminant functions, and Figure 8 shows the two functions verifying the ability to differentiate the varieties studied. By applying these functions we obtained a model with which it was possible to classify 96% of the cases correctly. The predictive model was applied to oranges harvested in the 2004/05 season (data in Table 9) and we confirmed that the oranges were of the Navel variety. The same study was applied to each of the varieties to establish a model that could be used to differentiate the harvesting date and storage time of the oranges. We first studied the data to see the ability to predict the harvesting date. The discriminant analysis showed that the predictor variables depended on the variety (Table 10), classifying 100% of the cases correctly (in the three varieties of orange). Given that the oranges from the 2004/05 season were of the Navel variety, by applying the model obtained we found that the oranges corresponded to the end of the harvesting period (28 days). The factors that permitted classification of the oranges by storage time were 9-β-carotene, pH, and °Brix for the Navel oranges, pH and β-cryptoxanthin for the Navelina oranges, but no factor for the Navel-Lane oranges. In the first two cases the percentages of correct classifications were 83 and 78%, respectively. The oranges analyzed from the 2004/05 season were of the Navel variety, and according to the predictive model the storage time was either zero or, with almost the same probability, 15 days.

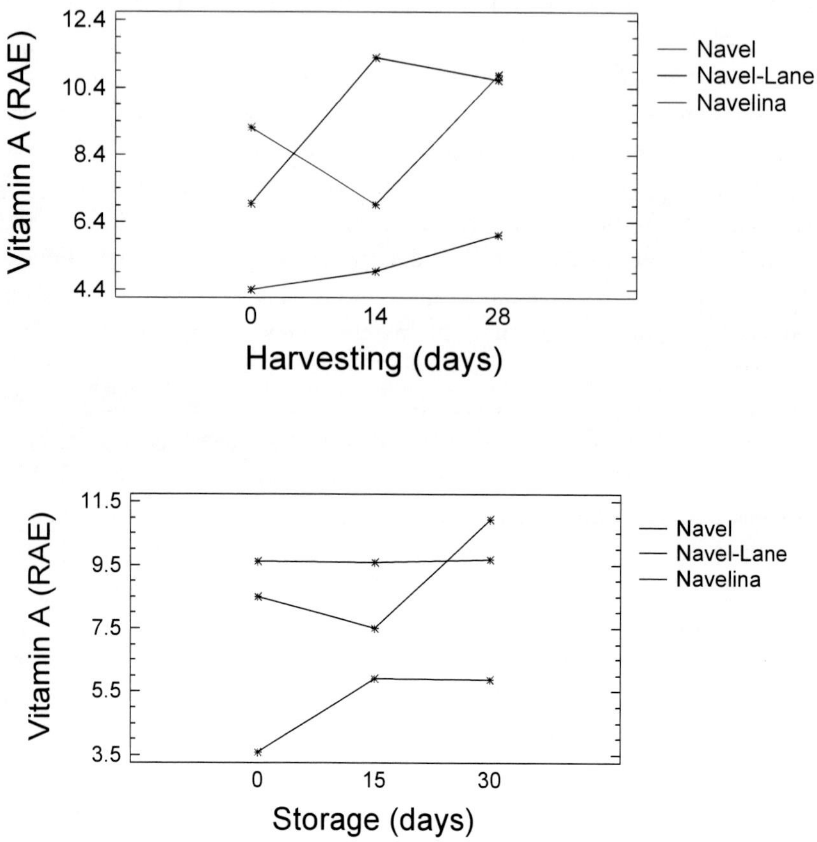

Figure 3. Influence of variety, harvesting date, and storage time on concentration of vitamin A.

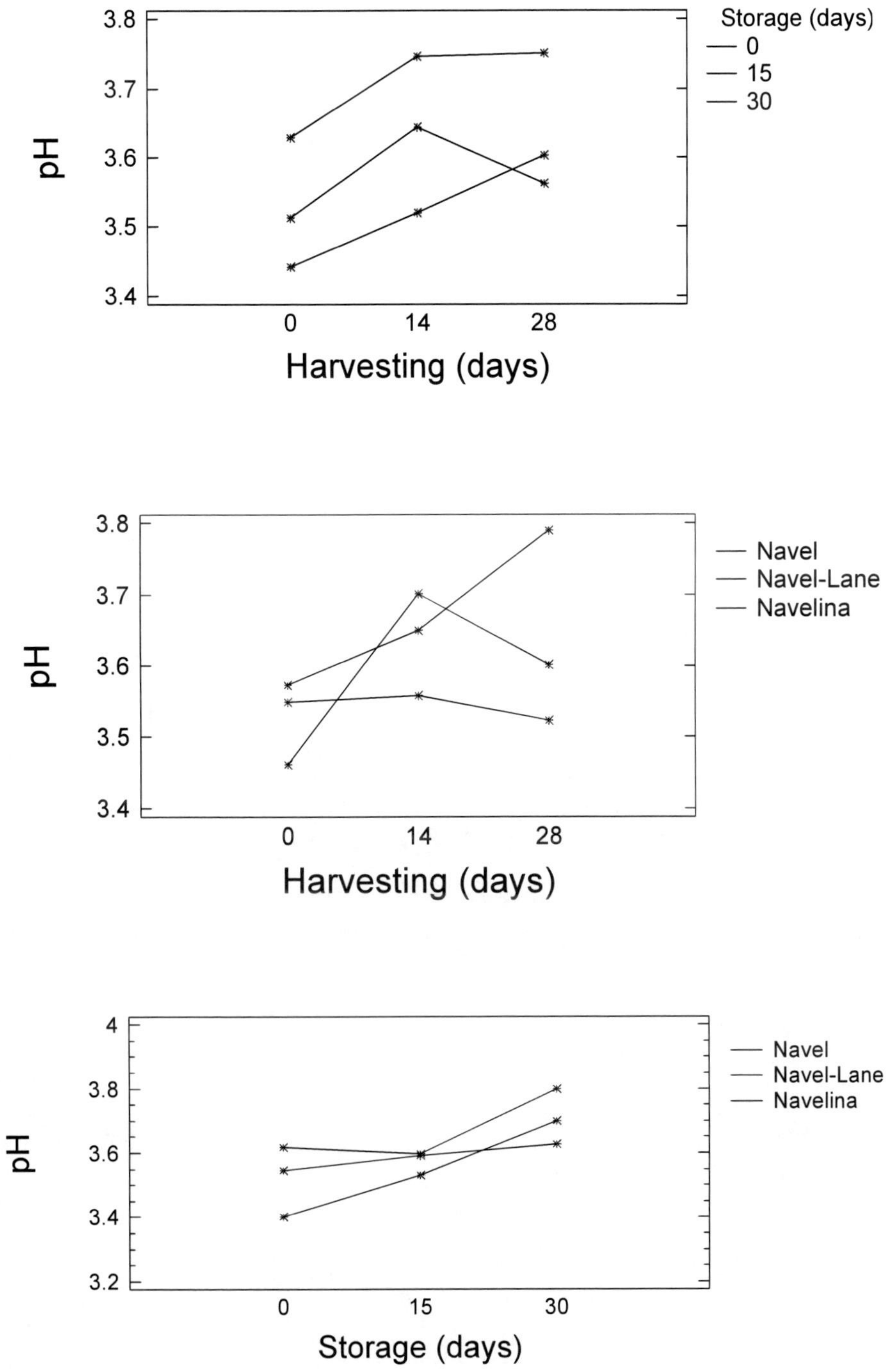

Figure 4. Influence of variety, harvesting date, and storage time on pH.

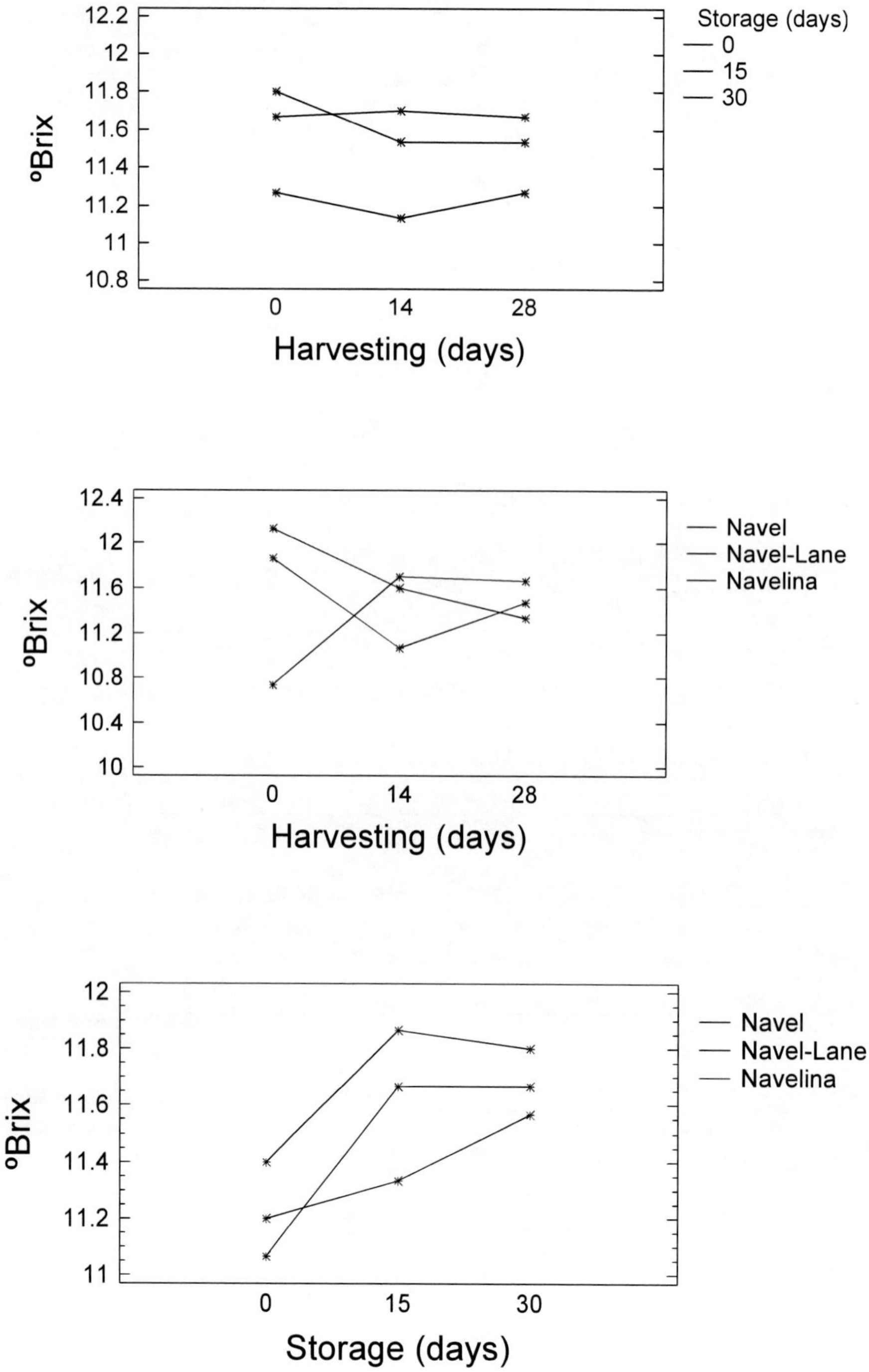

Figure 5. Influence of variety, harvesting date, and storage time on °Brix.

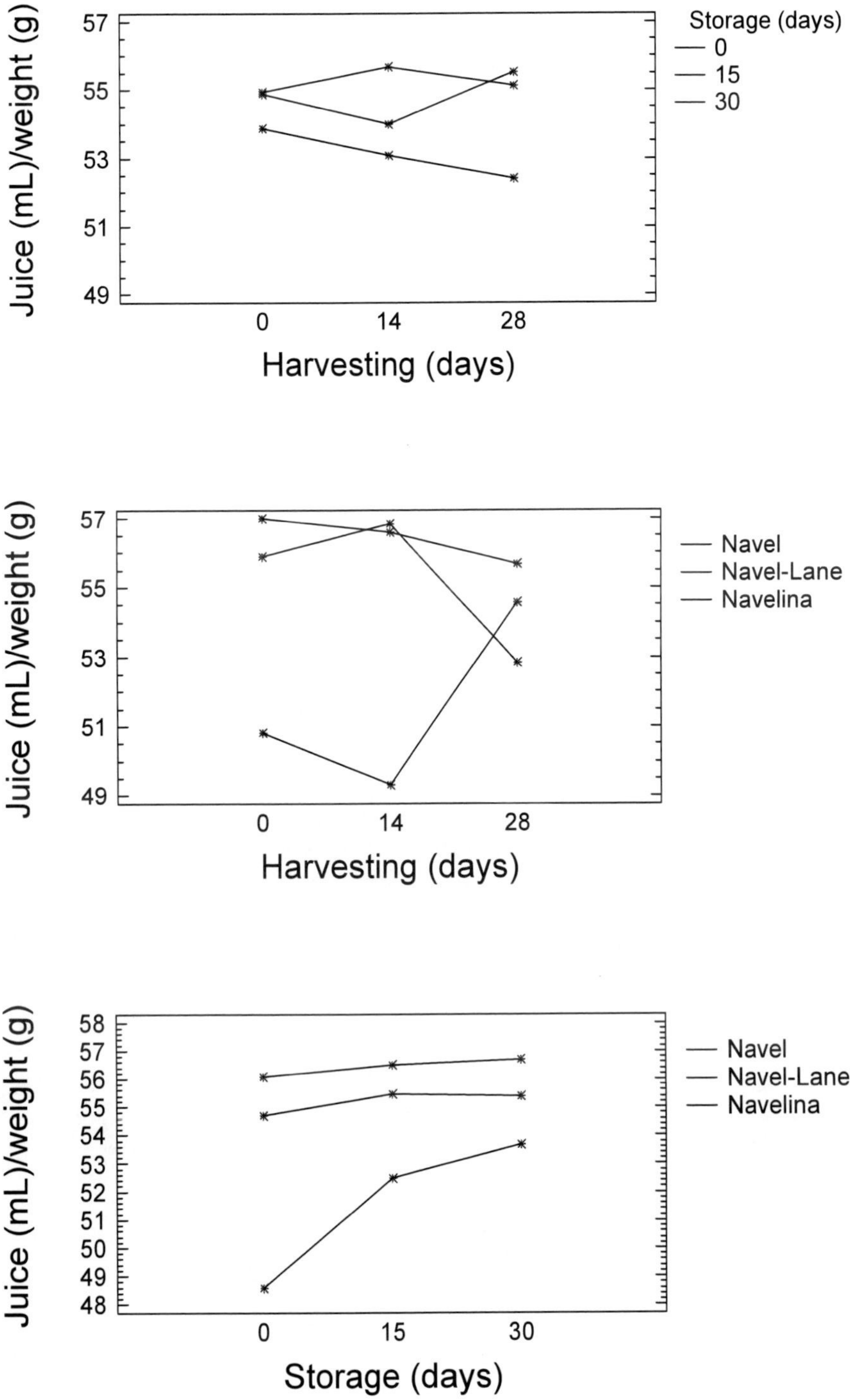

Figure 6. Influence of variety, harvesting date, and storage time on juice/weight relationship.

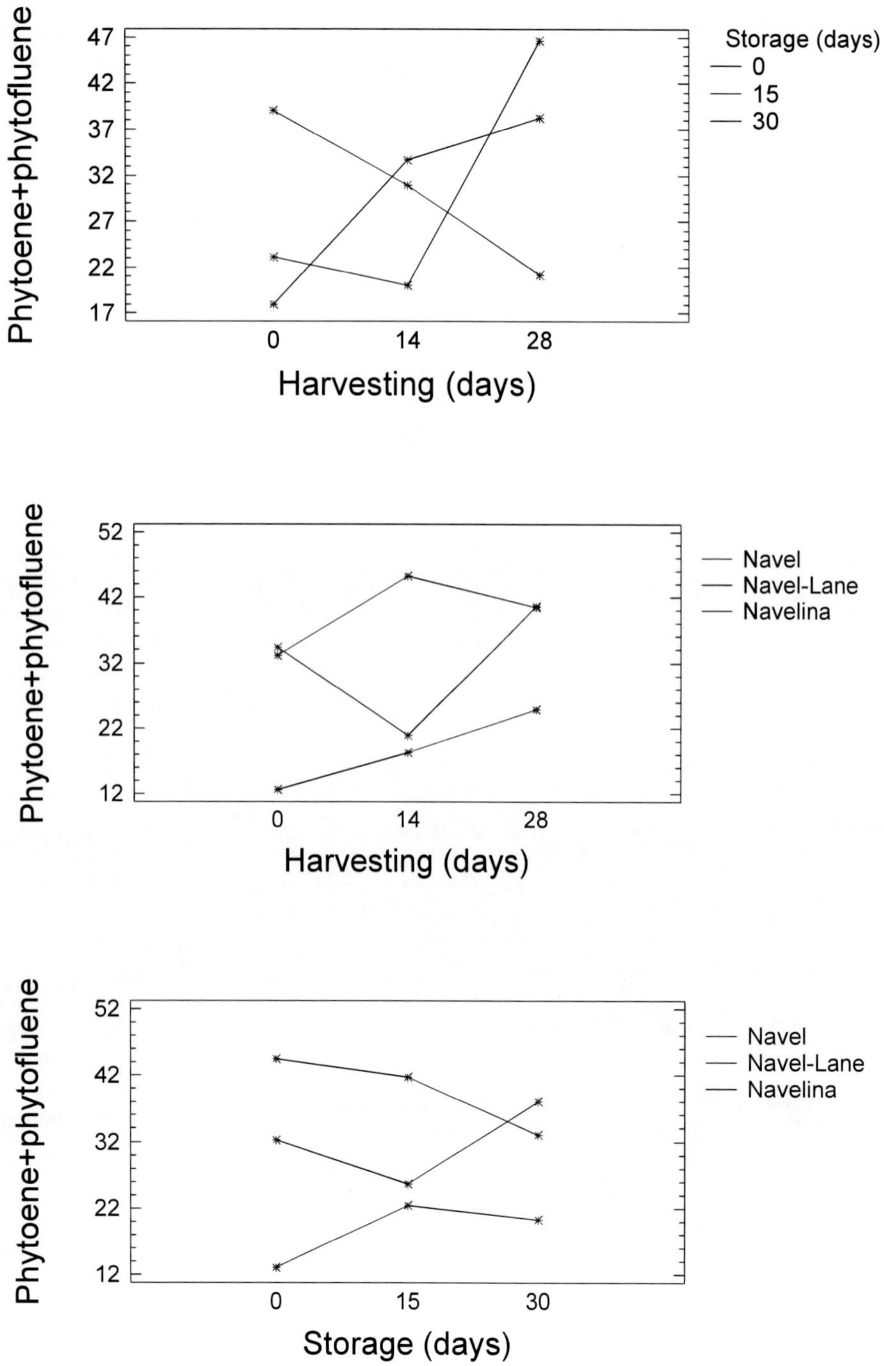

Figure 7. Influence of variety, harvesting date, and storage time on concentration of phytoene+phytofluene (mg/100mL).

Table 6. Multiple regression analysis for each of the varieties and carotenoids studied

	Equation *Standard error, R^2*		
	Navel	**Navelina**	**Navel-Lane**
antheraxanthin	-	y= 99.7 + 2.18 H *48.6, 22.8*	-
zeaxanthin	-	y= 16.7 + 0.35 H + 0.29 S *6.4, 45.9*	y= 33.3 + 0.36 H *5.1, 42.8*
β-cryptoxanthin	y= 94.8 + 1.20 S *26.6, 25.64*	y= 55.6 + 1.31 S *24.9, 34.3*	-
α-carotene	y= 20.2 + 0.71 H *15.6, 23.2*	y= 10.3 + 0.25 H *4.4, 32.6*	y= 20.6 + 1.06 H *18.3, 32.9*
phytoene + phytofluene	-	y= 12.5 + 0.44 H *8.4, 28.7*	-
β-carotene	-	y= 12.2 + 0.29 H *6.5, 22.7*	-
9-*cis*-β-carotene	-	-	y= 10.4 + 0.39 H *7.0, 30.6*

y: concentration of carotenoid (μg/100 g)
H: harvesting date (days)
S: storage time (days)

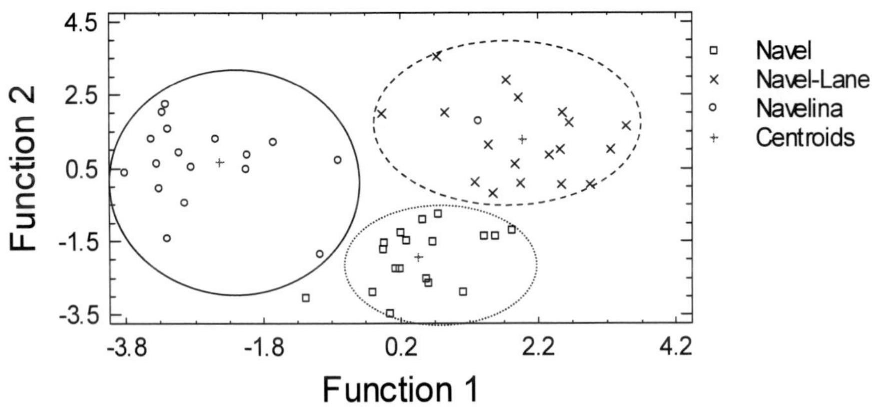

Figure 8. Differentiation of citrus using PCA (principal component analysis).

Table 7. Equations of principal components

	Component 1	Component 2	Component 3	Component 4
°Brix	0.096631	0.175569	0.724526	-0.178299
pH	0.248375	-0.0797832	0.436104	0.096048
v/w relationship	0.206408	-0.0020624	-0.076062	-0.553779
vitamin C	-0.156465	-0.079604	0.138871	0.679216

Table 7. (Continued)

vitamin A	0.361228	0.191781	-0.057335	0.119424
9-*cis*-violaxanthin + neoxanthin	0.287191	-0.340725	-0.183667	-0.062828
antheraxanthin	0.293045	-0.371868	0.033496	-0.126798
lutein	0.211846	-0.433149	0.059980	0.255225
zeaxanthin	0.314006	-0.296869	0.035142	0.024046
β-cryptoxanthin	0.338492	-0.006529	0.165609	0.125478
phytoene + phytofluene	0.306366	0.235623	-0.302443	0.219785
β-carotene	0.315411	0.280761	-0.240047	0.145681
9-*cis*-β-carotene	0.183739	0.422852	0.183911	0.073467

Table 8. Standardized coefficients of statistically significant discriminant functions ($p < 0.05$)

	Function 1	Function 2
antheraxanthin	1.09069	-0.847851
lutein	-0.925756	-0.539785
9-*cis*-β-carotene	-0.559976	-1.66502
vitamin A	1.05061	1.24113
pH	-0.582712	0.00667418
juice volume/weight	0.486999	0.135636

Table 9. Standardized coefficients of statistically significant discriminant functions ($p < 0.05$) by variety. Harvesting

	Function 1	Function 2
Navelina		
antheraxanthin	-1.27434	0.45347
9-*cis*-β-carotene	-0.40511	1.06597
°Brix	1.26884	0.00191
Navel		
9-*cis*-violaxanthin + neoxanthin	2.60516	1.01936
provitamin A	1.44022	0.62778
°Brix	-0.54563	1.30106
v/w relationship	3.07791	-0.40654
Navel-Lane		
zeaxanthin	0.22041	1.32729
°Brix	1.69630	0.405815
vitamin C	-1.60034	1.04193

Table 10. Navel oranges. 2005–2006 season

°Brix	11.8±0.0
pH	3.35±0.00
v/w relationship	52
vitamin C (mg/100 mL)	47.56±1.36
vitamin A (RAE)	14.63±0.65
9-*cis*-violaxanthin + neoxanthin (mg/100 mL)	444.57±23.21
antheraxanthin (mg/100 mL)	161.93±10.14
lutein (mg/100 mL)	27.28±1.89
zeaxanthin (mg/100 mL)	68.26±0.95
β-cryptoxanthin (mg/100 mL)	206.42±14.35
9-*cis*-α-carotene (mg/100 mL)	30.81±1.03
α-carotene (mg/100 mL)	49.91±1.82
phytoene + phytofluene (mg/100 mL)	23.34±0.19
β-carotene (mg/100 mL)	37.21±1.44
9-*cis*-β-carotene (mg/100 mL)	12.61±0.55

Conclusion

The results show that the concentrations/values of the parameters determined depend on various factors such as variety, harvesting date, and postharvest storage time. A predictive model that could be used to determine each of the factors was obtained and it was verified with oranges harvested in a subsequent season.

Acknowledgments

This research was supported by the Spanish Ministry of Science and Technology and European Regional Development Funds (Project AGL-2006-13320-C03-03) and the Generalitat Valenciana's Aid for Research Groups 3/147 and GV/2007/ 048.

References

Aparicio, P., Farré, R. & Frígola, A. (1992) Determinación del ácido ascórbico en vegetales por polarografía diferencial de impulsos. *Anales de Bromatología, 44*, 257-261.

Barry, G. H., Castle, W. S. & Davies, F. S. (2003) Variability in juice quality of Valencia Sweet orange and sample size estimation for juice quality experiments. *Journal of the American Society for Horticultural Science, 128*, 803-808.

Cano, A., Medina, A. & Bermejo, A. (2008) Bioactive compounds in different citrus varieties. Discrimination among cultivars. *Journal of Food Composition and Analysis, 21*, 377-381.

Cortes, C., Esteve, M. J., Frigola, A. & Torregrosa, F. (2004) Identification and quantification of carotenoids including geometrical isomers in fruit and vegetable juices by liquid chromatography with ultraviolet-diode array detection. *Journal Agricultural and Food Chemistry, 52*, 2203-2212.

Cortés, C., Esteve, M. J., Rodrigo, D., Torregrosa, F. & Frigola, A. (2006a) Changes of colour and carotenoids during high intensity pulsed electric treatment in oranges juices. *Food and Chemical Toxicology, 44*, 1932-1939.

Cortés, C., Esteve, M. J., Torregrosa, F., Frigola, A. (2006b) Carotenoid profile modification refrigerates storage in untreated and pasteurized orange juice and orange juice treated with high intensity pulsed electric fields. *Journal of Agricultural and Food Chemistry, 54*, 6247-6254.

Cortés, C., Esteve, M. J. & Frigola, A. (2007) Effect of refrigerated storage on ascorbic acid content of orange juice treated by pulsed electric fields and termal pasteurization. *European Food research and Technology, 227*, 629-635.

Dhuique-Mayer, C., Caris-Veyrat, C., Ollitrault, P., Curk, F. & Amiot, M. J. (2005) Varietal and interspecific influence on micronutrient contents in citrus from the Mediterranean area. *Journal of Agricultural and Food Chemistry, 53*, 2140-2145.

Esteve M. J, Farre R., Frigola A. & Clemente, G. (1995) Changes in ascorbic-acid content of green asparagus during the harvesting period and storage. *Journal of Agricultural and Food Chemistry, 43*, 2058-2061.

Fanciullino, A.L., Dhuique-Mayer, C., Luro, F., Casanova, J., Morillon, R. & Ollitrault, P. (2006) Carotenoid diversity in cultivated citrus is highly influenced by genetic factors. *Journal of Agricultural and Food Chemistry, 54*, 4397-4406.

Goodner, K. L., Rouseff, R. L. & Hofsommer, H. J. (2001) Orange, mandarin, and hybrid classification using multivariate statistics based on carotenoid profiles. *Journal of Agricultural and Food Chemistry, 49*, 1146-1150.

Grierson, W. & Ben-Yehoshua S. Storage of Citrus fruits. In: Wardowski, V. F, Nagy, S. & Grierson, W. editors. *Fresh Citrus Fruits*. Westport, CT: Avi Publising Co. Inc.; 1986; 479-507.

Institute of Medicine (IOM), Food and Nutrition Board. *Dietary Reference Intakes for Vitamin A, Vitamin K, Arsenic, Boron, Chromium, Copper, Iodine, Iron, Manganese, Molybdenum, Nickel, Silicon, Vanadium, and Zinc*. Washington, DC: National Academy Press; 2001.

Kato, M., Ikoma, Y., Matsumoto, H., Sugiura., Hyodo, H. & Yano, M. (2004) Accumulation of carotenoids and expression of carotenoid biosynthethic genes during maturation in citrus fruit. *Plant Physiology, 134*, 1-14.

Lee, H. S. (2001) Characterization of carotenoids in juice of red Navel orange (Cara Cara). *Journal of Agricultural and Food Chemistry, 49*, 2563-2568.

Lee, H. S. & Castle, W. S. (2001). Seasonal changes of carotenoid pigments and color in Hamlin, Earlygold, and Budd Blood orange juices. *Journal of Agricultural and Food Chemistry, 49*, 877-882.

Lee, S. K. & Kader, A. A. (2000) Preharvest and postharvest factors influencing vitamin C content of horticultural crops. *Postharvest Biology and Technology, 20*, 207-220.

Li-Ying, N., Ji-Hong, W., Xiao-Jun, L., Fang, C., Zheng-Fu, W., Guang-Hua, Z. & Xiao-Song, H. (2008) Physicochemical Characteristics of Orange Juice Samples From Seven Cultivars. *Agricultural Sciences in China, 7*, 41-47

Marsh, K., Attanayake, S., Walker, S., Gunson, A., Boldingh, H. & MacRae, E. (2004) Acidity and taste in kiwifruit. *Postharvest Biology and Technology, 32*, 159-168.

McAllister, J. W. (1980) *Citrus Nutrition and Quality*. Washington DC: American Chemical Society.

Meléndez-Martínez, A. J., Britton, G., Vicario, I. M. & Heredia, F. J. (2005) Color and carotenoid profile of Spanish Valencia late ultrafrozen orange juice. *Food Research International, 38*, 931-936.

Morton, L.W., Caccetta, R. A., Puddey, I. B. & Croft, K. D. (2000) Chemistry and biological effects of dietary phenolic compounds: Relevance to cardiovascular disease, *Clinical and Experimental Pharmacology and Physiology, 27*, 152-159.

Mouly, P. P., Gaydou, E. M., Lapierre, L. & Corsetti, J. (1999) Differentiation of several geographical origins in single-strength Valencia orange juices using quantitative comparison of carotenoid profiles. *Journal of Agricultural and Food Chemistry, 47*, 4038-4045.

Pellegrini, N., Serafini, M., Colombi, B., Del Rio, D., Salvatore, S. & Bianchi M. (2003) Total antioxidant capacity of plant foods, beverages and oils consumed in Italy assessed by three different in vitro assays, *Journal of Nutrition 133*, 2812-2819.

Rapisarda, P., Lo Bianco, M., Pannuzzo, P. & Timpanaro, N. (2008) Effect of cold storage on vitamin C, phenolics and antioxidant activity of five orange genotypes [*Citrus sinensis* (L.) Osbeck]. *Postharvest Biology and Technology, 49*, 348-354.

Señoráns, F. J., Ruiz-Rodriguez, A., Cavero, S., Cifuentes, A., Ibañez, E. & Reglero, G. (2001) Isolation of antioxidant compounds from orange juice by using countercurrent supercritical fluid extraction (CC-SFE), *Journal of Agricultural and Food Chemistry, 49*, 6039-6044.

Trumbo, P. R., Yates, A. A., Schlicker-Renfo, S. & Suitor, C. (2003) Dietary reference intakes: revised nutritional equivalents for folate, vitamin E and provitamin A carotenoids. *Journal of Food Composition Analysis, 16*, 379-382.

Xu, G., Liu, D., Chen, J., Ye, X., Ma, Y. & Shi, J. (2008) Juice components and antioxidant capacity of citrus varieties cultivated in China. *Food Chemistry, 106*, 545-551.

In: Fruit Juices: Properties, Consumption and Nutrition
Editor: Pauline G. Scardina
ISBN: 978-1-60741-505-3

Chapter 5

Reduction in Reovirus Infectivity by Pure and Store-Purchased Cranberry and Grape Juice Drinks

Steven M. Lipson [a*], ***Angelika Sobilo*** [a], ***Maria Adragna*** [a], ***Martin Roy*** [b], ***Allen Burdowski*** [a], ***Ben Collins*** [c] ***and Guenther Stotzky*** [c]

[a] Department of Biology, St. Francis College., Brooklyn Heights, NY
[b] Department of Basic Science and Craniofacial Biology, New York University College of Dentistry, New York, NY
[c] Department of Biology, New York University, New York, NY

Abstract

Antimicrobial/antiviral activity by grape (*Vitis labrusca*) and cranberry (*Vaccinium macrocarpon*) species remains an area of interest among food scientists. The purpose of this study accordingly, was to investigate the effect of pure and store-purchased grape and cranberry drinks on the infectivity/inactivation of the reovirus, a mammalian enteric infectious agent. Infectivity titrations were performed by a cell culture based immunofluorescence focus assay. Polyacrylamide gel electrophoresis was used to determine the integrity of the viral dsRNA in cell-free suspensions. Cytotoxicity testing was performed in part, using an adenylate kinase – bioluminescence assay. Animal studies employed athymic mice. Treatment of cell cultures with concentrations of 2 to 16% pure or store purchased cranberry and grape juice drinks prior to virus

* *Correspondence author: Department of Biology, St. Francis College, 180 Remsen Street, Brooklyn Heights, New York 11201, U.S.A. Tel: +1 718 489 5210; fax: +1 718 522- 1274, E-mail address: slipson@stfranciscollege.edu

inoculation reduced infectivity titers by approximately one order of magnitude. Neither juice affected a monolayer toxicity. The

vitamin C supplement in store-purchased cranberry juice cocktail (CJC) drink displayed no adverse effect on viral titers. A synergistic effect between store-purchased grape (CGJ) and CJC drinks was not observed. A proanthocyanidin-enriched cranberry concentrate (PACran™) of <1% reduced virus infectivity titers by ca. 95%. Reovirus dsRNA was not detected in virus-juice cell-free suspensions. Clinical disease was not apparent in mice after oral administration of juice-reovirus suspensions. Mice treated with CJC-reovirus suspensions displayed normal colon histology. These data suggest that the viral inhibitory effects may be associated with a blockage of virus receptor sites, a direct inactivation of the infectious particles *per se*, or a combination of both. *In vivo* studies supported the *in vitro* antiviral activity by grape and cranberry juices.

Introduction

The health benefits of "medicinal" phytochemicals [e.g., flavonols (including flavan-3-ols)] and potable fruit juices prepared from grape (*Vitis labrusca*), and cranberry *(Vaccinium macrocarpon Ait.*) species have been the focus of numerous anecdotal and prospective studies (Aron and Kennedy, 2008; Dixon et al., 2005; Espin et al., 2007; Jassim and Naji, 2003). *In vitro* and *in vivo* studies have suggested for example, improved health benefits through the consumption/administration of grape and cranberry juices or their extracts/concentrates on cholesterol levels, cardiac circulation after ischemia, atherosclerosis, the inflammatory response, periodontal disease, and urinary tract infections in women (Dixon et al., 2005; Kontiokari, 2003, 2004). Proanthocyanidins, major phenolic phytochemical components in the berry, grape, and other plant species, have been associated with a reduction of urinary tract infections in women (Howell, 2007). The effects of grape and cranberry juice/extracts as antiviral agents to herpes simplex virus, influenza virus, and perhaps most extensively studied, the human immunodeficiency virus type 1 have been reported (Chung et al., 1998; Docherty et al., 2005; Khan and Ather, 2007; Weiss et al. 1998, 2005). Except for the studies of Lipson and co-workers, the antiviral efficacy of cranberry juice cocktail drink, grape juice drink, and their concentrates or extracts on enteric (rotavirus, reovirus) viral infections have not been addressed (Lipson et al., 2007a,b)

In vitro cell culture studies suggested an antiviral effect of store-purchased grape juice drink, cranberry juice cocktail drink, and manufacturer supplied cranberry extracts (viz., NC-90, NC-100) (Burdowski et al., 2007; Lipson et al. 2007a,b). These studies, however, utilized store-purchased juices and were limited to cell culture infectivity titer assays. Consequently, the purpose of this study was to evaluate and compare the efficacy of unadulterated or pure cranberry and grape juices with store-purchased juice drinks as inhibitory agents of viral infectivity titers. Juice-virus cell-free suspension studies were performed to determine whether cranberry and grape juice drinks *per se*, might serve as natural products to directly affect a loss of viral infectivity. A proanthocyanidin (PAC)-enriched cranberry extract – PACran™, was tested as well. Athymic mice were used to determine the efficacy of cranberry and grape juice drinks as antivirals in the animal model. The reovirus was used as a model enteric infectious agent throughout this study.

Materials And Methods

Virus and cell culture.

The bovine reovirus type 3 [American BioResearch Laboratories (ABL;Sevierville, TN)] was used as a model enteric virus. The cell host system was Rhesus monkey kidney epithelial-like (MA-104) cells which were grown on 12 mm circular glass cover slips in 40 X 13 mm^2 capped glass vials [ViroMed Laboratories (Minnetonka, MN)]. Reovirus stock aliquots were prepared in MA-104 cell cultures grown in T25 cm^2 flasks. Cell growth medium consisted of Earle's minimal essential medium supplemented with L-glutamine, penicillin/streptomycin, amphotericin B, and 10% heat-inactivated fetal bovine serum (FBS). Maintenance medium was identical to the growth medium but contained 2% FBS (Lipson et al., 1992).

Infectivity titration.

Virus quantitation was performed by antigen detection-cell culture amplification. Briefly, 0.2 ml experimental preparations were inoculated into MA-104 monolayers in glass vials and incubated at 36.5°C for 50 min. Monolayers were washed with phosphate-buffered saline (PBS), incubated overnight (16 to 20 h), and immunostained with a fluorescein isothiocyanate (FITC)-conjugated caprine polyclonal antibody to the reovirus. Titers were expressed as fluorescent focus units (FFU) per ml, as described previously (Lipson et al. 2007b). Fluorescent signals were viewed using a Nikon Eclipse FA microscope equipped with a 100 W halogen bulb.

Manufacturer supplied and store-purchased products.

Pure cranberry juice (pure CJ) and pure purple grape juice (pure GJ) were supplied by Ocean Spray Cranberries, Inc. (Lakeville-Middleboro, MA) and Welch Foods, Inc. (Concord, MA), respectively. Cranberry Juice Cocktail from Concentrate (CJC, Ocean Spray) and Welch's 100% Grape Juice From Concentrate With Vitamin C, "From Welch's Own Concord Grape" (commercial GJ; Welch Foods, Inc.) were purchased from a local food store. Vitamin C (ascorbic acid) powder was supplied by Welch Foods, Inc., and was identical to that present in store-purchased CGJ. PACran™ whole cranberry powder, manufactured to contain 1.5% proanthocyanidins (PACs), was supplied by Decas Botanical Synergies (Carver, MA).

Dose response curves.

Dose response curves were generated by pretreatment of MA-104 cell culture monolayers for 3 to 5 min with varying concentrations of pure and store-purchased fruit drinks, PACran^{TM}, and vitamin C. The diluent was phosphate-buffered saline (PBS) without Ca^{2+} and Mg^{2+} . After washing of the monolayers with PBS, reovirus was added, the monolayers incubated 50 min at 36.5°C, followed by washing with PBS. Maintenance medium (1 ml) was added to each vial, followed by incubation for 16 to 20 h at 36.5°C. Monolayers were then immunostained to determine viral infectivity titers. Experiments were performed in triplicate or quadruplicate.

Effect of combined CGJ and CJ on the reduction of reovirus infectivity titers.

Three per cent pure CGJ and CJ suspensions (in PBS) were combined equally into a single solution. MA-104 culture monolayers were inoculated with 0.2 ml of the juice preparation, and incubated for 3 to 5 min at 23°C. The monolayers were washed with PBS, followed by inoculation of 0.2 ml reovirus. Viral incubation, monolayer processing, and immunofluorescent testing were performed as described and expressed as per cent of control. Additional monolayers were pretreated in parallel with individual juice preparations followed by virus infection. Positive control monolayers were inoculated with virus only. Negative controls consisted of monolayers inoculated with PBS. Suboptimal doses of each juice drink were used to determine a synergistic effect. Experiments were performed in triplicate or quadruplicate.

Cytotoxicity testing.

Cell viability/cytotoxicity was evaluated by trypan blue exclusion, as described previously (Lipson et al. 2007b). Briefly, 1 ml of a 25% solution of store-purchased CJ and CGJ drinks was added to MA-104 cultures in T25 cm^2 flasks. After a 3 to 5 min incubation at 23°C, the juice was removed followed by washing with PBS. The monolayer was trypsinized, washed, and 0.5 ml of a 0.4% trypan blue reagent (Sigma-Aldrich, St. Louis, MO) was added to an equal volume of cell suspension. The suspensions were incubated for 5 min at 23°C, and the per cent viable cells (unstained cells) were determined. Suspended cells were additionally examined by light microscopy for any overt morphological aberrancy (e.g., cytoplasmic projections/bleb formation; Kawai and Fujita, 2007). The control consisted of monolayers treated with the PBS, alone.

Cell growth was determined following monolayer pretreatment with CGJ drink. Briefly, monolayers were pretreated with CGJ at 23°C for 3 to 5 min. The monolayers were subpassaged and maintained for a period of 9 days in culture (with appropriate medium changes), followed by trypsinization and cell quantitation. Cells were counted using a hemocytometer. Control cultures were treated exactly as the experimentals but PBS was utilized in place of the juice drinks.

The ToxiLight[R] BioAssay (Cat. No. LT17-217; Lonza Rockland, Inc., Rockland, ME), a non-destructive bioluminescent cytotoxicity assay, was used to measure quantitatively the release of adenylate kinase (AK) from damaged cells in monolayer culture. Confluent MA-104 monolayers were washed with PBS, followed by the addition of 10% suspensions of manufacturer-supplied pure CGJ and CJ. Monolayers were incubated for a period of 5 min at 23°C followed by the addition of the adenylate kinase detection reagent (AKDR) for an additional 5 min. Emitted light was measured on a beta counter (Model LS6000LL; Beckman Instruments, Inc., Fullerton, CA) set to a read-time of 1 sec. Readings were expressed as counts per min. The negative control consisted of monolayers treated with PBS. The positive control consisted of monolayers treated with ToxiLight[R] 100% Lysis Reagent(Cat. No. LT07-517; Lonza Rockland, Inc.). The controls were treated exactly as the experimentals. Experiments were performed in triplicate.

Virus infectivity testing in mice.

All mice studies were approved by the University Animal Welfare Committee (UAWC; New York University - Washington Square Campus, New York, NY). CD-1 (Crl:CD-1-nuBR) T-cell deficient female nude mice were utilized in these studies (Charles River Laboratories, Wilmington, MA). The testing of store-purchased CJ cocktail and CGJ drinks in mice was performed as follows. Briefly, 0.2 ml of virus plus CJ cocktail drink or CGJ drink (40% juice concentration at a 1:1 juice-virus ratio) were inoculated into mice by gavage. The positive control consisted of virus plus PBS. The negative control consisted of PBS alone. Noninoculated mice were maintained during the experimental period to eliminate the possibility of a confounding effect on data interpretation by endogenous or exogenous pathogens. All mice experiments were performed in pentuplicate. Upon mortality of the positive control mice, experimentals, negative controls, and non-inoculated mice were euthanized and examined by dissection and colon histology. Distal-colon sections were placed into10% neutral buffered formalin, dehydrated in a graded series of ethanol, placed into xylene, embedded in paraffin, sectioned (5 um), rehydrated in a graded series of ethanols, and stained with hematoxylin and eosin (Klatt, 2008). The tissue specimens were analyzed at magnifications of 100, 200, and 400X. Colon specimens for viral isolation testing were placed into PBS supplemented with 2% FBS and temporarily frozen at -50°C before testing.

Polyacrylamide gel electrophoresis (PAGE) of viral dsRNA and detection of viral infectivity.

Virus-juice suspensions were prepared to identify whether pure CJ and pure CGJ were capable of directly inactivating reovirus particles. Briefly, two ml of an undiluted virus stock suspension was added to an equal volume of pure CJ and CGJ diluted to 10% in PBS. The positive control consisted of virus plus an equal volume of PBS. The negative control consisted of pure CJ and CGJ plus an equal volume of PBS. Both negative and positive controls were tested in parallel with experimentals. Juices were filter-sterilized (0.2 um filter) to eliminate microbial contamination of the cell cultures (see below). After a 60 min incubation at 23°C, experimental and control preparations were concentrated using a polyacrylamide absorbent gel (Cat. No. 81128; Sigma-Aldrich, St. Louis, MO). Viral RNA was extracted from equal volumes (300 ul) of experimental and control concentrates using the AquaPure RNA isolation kit (Cat. #732-6370; BioRad Laboratories, Hercules, CA) as per manufacturer's instructions). The extracted viral RNA was suspended in Laemli sample buffer for loading onto polyacrylamide gels (Precast PAGEr 4-12% T-G) for analysis. Electrophoresis was run for 50 min at 70 V. RNA segments were visualized by silver staining, as described previously (Lipson and Kaplan, 1992). Experiments were performed in triplicate. Virus detection in cell culture was determined by immunoflourescence, as described above.

Statistics.

Cell culture based experiments were performed in triplicate or quadruplicate. The reading of slides was performed by at least three individuals. The data are presented as the arithmetic +/- standard error of the mean. Control and experimental means were compared by the Student's "*t*" test where $P < 0.05$ was assumed to be statistically significant.

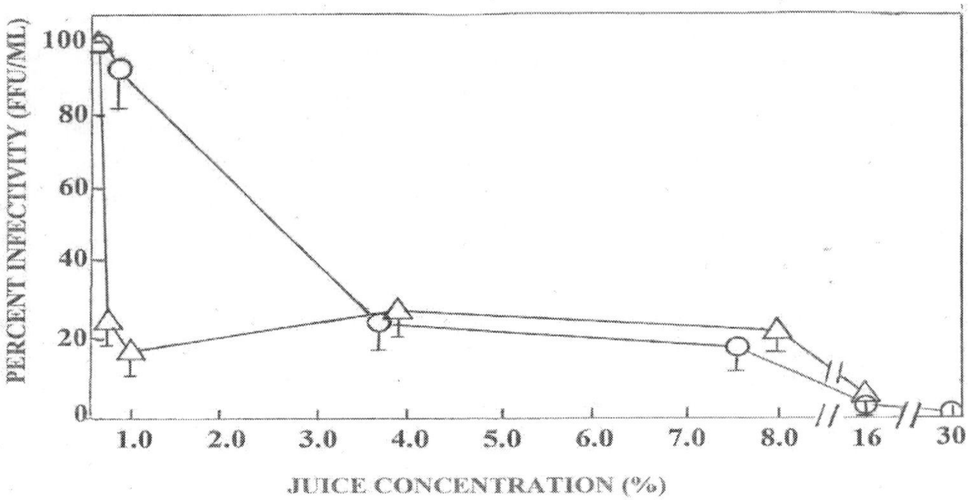

Fig. 1. Effect of pure (manufacturer-supplied) cranberry (CJ) and grape juices (GJ) on the infectivity titer of reovirus. Cell culture monolayers were pretreated for 3 to 5 min with each juice, followed by viral inoculation. Cultures were incubated for 16 to 20 h, followed by the determination of viral infectivity titers by immunostaining. Input viral titer: 2 X 10^6 FFU/ml. Data points represent mean +/- standard error of the mean.

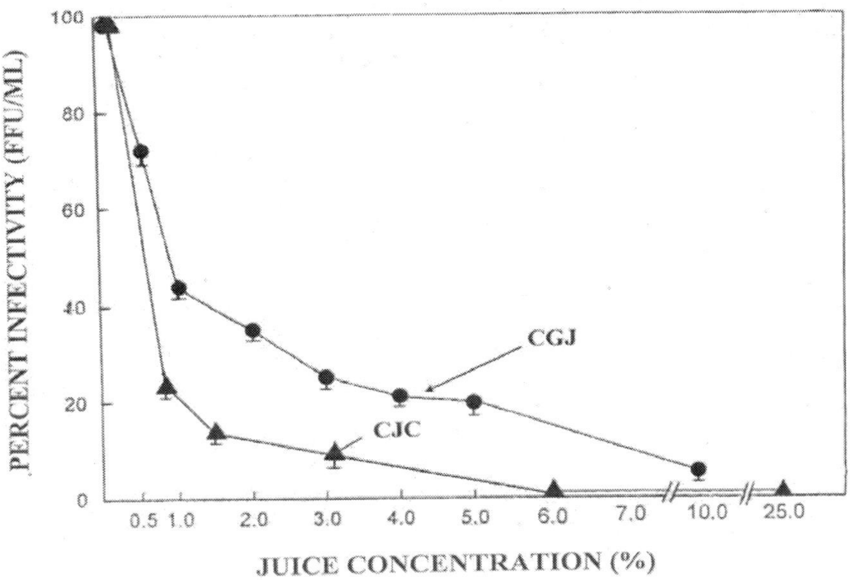

Fig. 2. Comparison of store-purchased cranberry juice cocktail (CJC) and grape juice (CGJ) drinks on the reduction of reovirus infectivity titers in MA-104 cell cultures. Monolayers were pretreated with each store-purchased juice for 3 to 5 min followed by inoculation of reovirus. Cultures were incubated for 16 to 20 h, followed by immunostaining to determine viral infectivity titers. Input viral titer: 2 X 10^6 FFU/ml. Mean +/- standard error of the mean.

Results And Discussion

Studies were conducted to determine the effects of manufacturer-supplied pure and store- purchased grape and cranberry drinks and a PAC-enriched cranberry extract (PACran^{TM}) on the loss of reovirus infectivity and/or reduction of infectivity titers in host cell cultures. Concentrations of 2.0 to 16% pure CJ reduced reovirus infectivity titers in MA-104 cell culture monolayers by 75 to 95%, respectively. Similar viral inactivation curves, reflecting reductions in infectivity titers starting at ca. 4%, were observed using pure GJ (Fig. 1). Reduction in reovirus infectivity titer after pre-treatment of cell culture monolayers with store-purchased CGJ or CJC drinks were similar to that identified using manufacturer-supplied pure juices (Fig. 2). Neither store-purchased CGJ nor CJC drinks contains artificial flavorings or colorings (manufacturer label specifications). Both store-purchased drinks in question however, contain approximately 30 mg vitamin C (ascorbic acid) per 100 ml serving (Mullen et al., 2007; Dr. J. Wightman, personal communication). Experiments were performed accordingly, to determine whether a concentration of vitamin C equal to that present in the store-purchased juice drinks might be responsible for reductions in viral infectivity titers. Compared to GJ drink, vitamin C at concentrations $\geq$ 30 mg per 100 ml had no inhibitory effects on reovirus infectivity titers (Fig. 3).

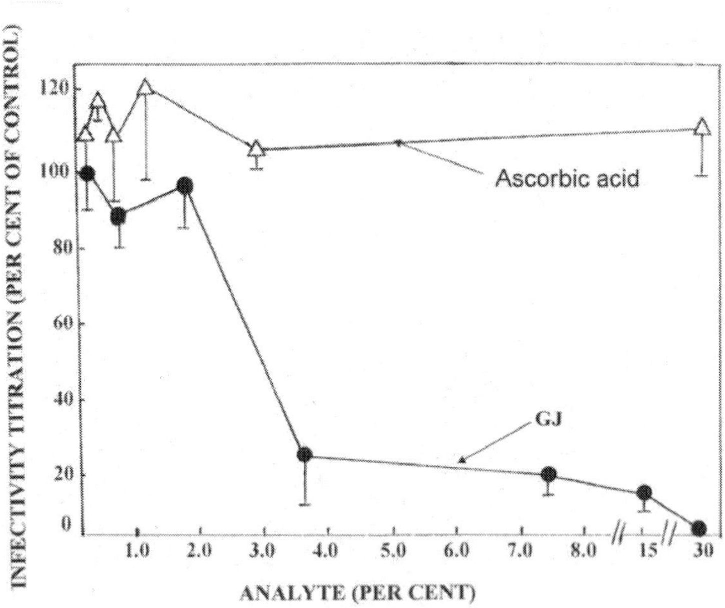

Fig. 3. Comparison of pure grape juice (GJ) and ascorbic acid on reovirus infectivity titration in MA-104 cell cultures. MA-104 cell cultures were pretreated for 3 to 5 min with varying concentrations of pure grape juice or ascorbic acid (vitamin C). The monolayers were washed with PBS, followed by the addition of the reovirus. Viral infectivity titers were determined by immunofluorescence staining. Input viral titer: 2 X 10^6 FFU/ml. Mean +/- standard error of the mean.

There was no cytotoxicity to the MA-104 cells by pure CJ or GJ drinks, as performed by a non cellular-destructive bioluminescent assay. These findings concur with trypan blue exclusion testing and cell quantitation determinations following monolayer subpassage.

In general, synergistic effects between phenolic compounds in cranberry, grape, and other plant species, especially at increased concentrations present in nutraceuticals, remains poorly defined (Chung et al., 1998; Espin et al., 2007). Synergistic effects between mixed phytochemicals in whole fruits and vegetables as antioxidants and antitumor agents however, have been studied (Liu 2004). In the current study, a combination of store-purchased CJC and CGJ drinks displayed no synergistic effect on viral infectivity titer reductions compared to either juice alone (Fig. 4). These data might be explained by relatively low levels of naturally occurring phytochemicals in each drink [e.g., CJC (51 mg PACs/L) and CGJ (524 mg PACs/L)] or to a redundancy of antiviral phytochemicals (e.g., proanthocyanidins) (Amoros et al., 1992; Chen et al., 2001; Gu et al., 2004; Krenn et al., 2007; Lipson et al., 2007; Liu, 2004). PACran™ whole cranberry powder reduced reovirus infectivity titers by ca. 95% at concentrations <1% (Fig. 5). These findings probably reflect the extract's increased PAC content of 1.5%. PACran™ cranberry powder is potentially unique among the multitude of phytochemicals available in the nutraceutical market. According to the manufacturer's product description, PACran™ is the first PAC-containing product employing a USDA-approved high performance liquid chromatography preparative method (Document #RF5013, Decas Botanical Synergies, Carver, MA). The PACran® whole cranberry powder may represent an early manufacturing trend to fulfill the need for product standardization, critical to attain reproducible product evaluation testing within the same and between independent laboratories (Chung et al., 1998; Espin et al., 2007).

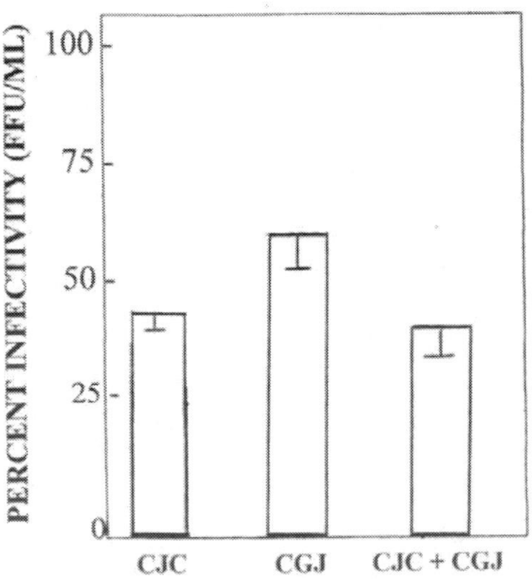

Fig. 4. Effect of combined cranberry juice cocktail and grape juice drinks on reovirus infectivity titers in MA-104 cells. Cell monolayers were pretreated with 3% concentrations of store-purchased CJC and CGJ drinks for 3 to 5 min, followed by inoculation of virus. The cell cultures were incubated for 16 to 24 h and then immunostained to determine viral titers. The positive control consisted of reovirus plus PBS. Data points represent mean +/- standard error of the mean. CJC vs. CGJ: $p = 0.07$; CJC vs. CJC/CGJ: $p = 0.51$; CGJ vs. CJC/CGJ: $p = 0.58$; CGJ, CJC, or CJC/CGJ vs. positive control: $p < 0.05$. Input viral titer: 2×10^6 FFU/ml.

Reovirus dsRNA was not detected in virus-CJC or virus-CGJ drink cell-free suspensions by PAGE testing for the presence of the viral dsRNA (Fig. 6, 7). Virus was not isolated from virus-juice suspensions following inoculation of MA-104 cell cultures, underscoring the absence of infectious particles. Inhibitory effects by CJC of reovirus infectivity titers in cell cultures were previously identified utilizing PAGE analysis and by transmission electron microscopy (Lipson et al., 2007a; Lipson et al., 2007b). These earlier studies coupled with that currently reported suggest a cranberry and grape juice-associated blockage of host-cell receptor site(s) and/or a direct inactivation of virus infectivity *per se*. Importantly, transport of PAC oligomers across epithelial cells in culture occur, but is not attained until ca. 15 min after cell treatment (Deprez et al., 2001). The 3 to 5 min monolayer pretreatment by juices of MA-104 cells in the current study suggests accordingly, an effect associated with an early event in viral adsorption and/or penetrations at the particle-cell interface.

Efficacy i*n vitro* does not necessarily predict that which will occur *in vivo*. Consequently, antiviral testing was extended to the animal model. Clinical disease was absent in mice 4 days after oral administration of reovirus-CJC or reovirus-CGJ drinks. Positive control mice inoculated with virus plus FBS displayed systemic hemorrhage, diarrhea, dehydration, and death 3 to 4 days after inoculation (Fig. 8). Histological analysis of mouse colon revealed normal mucosa, intact goblet cells, and dense feces among animals treated

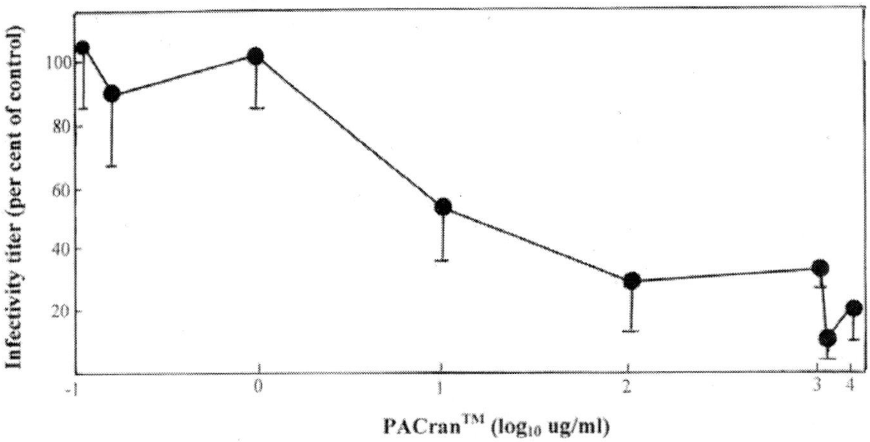

Fig. 5. Effect of PAC-standardized PACran[R] powder on reovirus infectivity titration in MA-104 cell cultures. Monolayers were pretreated with varying concentrations of PACran[R]. After 3 to 5 min, virus was inoculated into monolayers with subsequent determination of infectivity titers. Input viral titer: 2 X 10^6 FFU/ml. Mean +/- standard error of the mean.

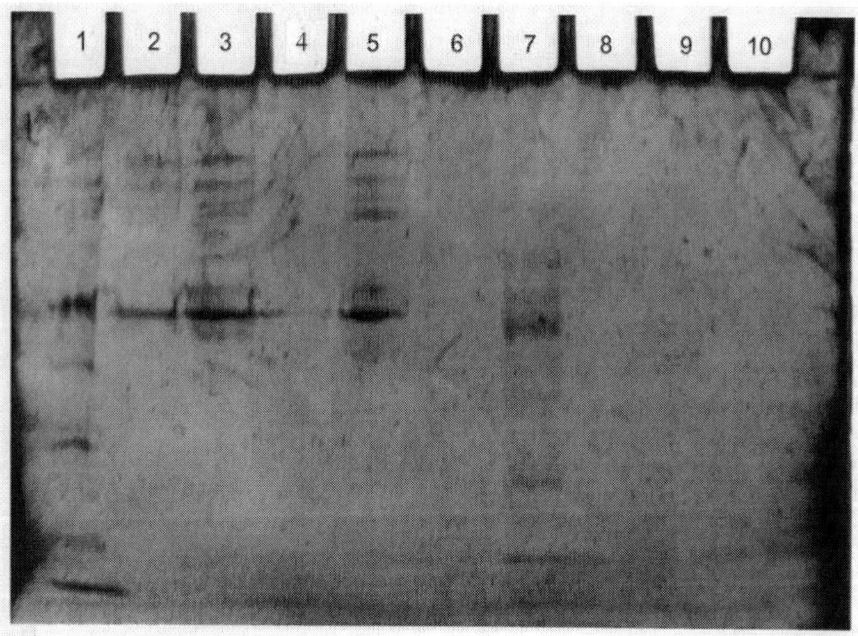

Fig. 6. Effect of cranberry juice cocktail (CJC) drink on the integrity of reovirus genomic RNA. Reovirus was added to equal volumes of undiluted filter-sterilized CJC drink. After 30 min at 23°C, preparations were subjected to RNA extraction and PAGE analysis. Lane 1, 7: ProSieve[R] 11-190 kDa protein marker: Lane 2, 3, 5: Positive control [reovirus (2 X 10^7 FFU/ml) + PBS); Lane 4,6: Empty (no inocula); Lane 8, 9, 10: Reovirus (2 X 10^7 FFU/ml) + CJC.

with virus-CJC drink. Colon specimens obtained from mice inoculated with virus-CGJ drinks had shrunken mucosa, mucin-depleted goblet cells, large inflammatory foci, and debris in the lumen. Markedly damaged mucosa with thinned muscularis externa was observed upon histological examination of positive but not negative control mice (Fig. 8). The CJC drink and to a lesser extent, the CGJ drink, effected antiviral inhibitory activity in the mouse model. The athymic nude mouse was chosen as a model system to control for a potential masking of results by the animals' cell mediated immune response

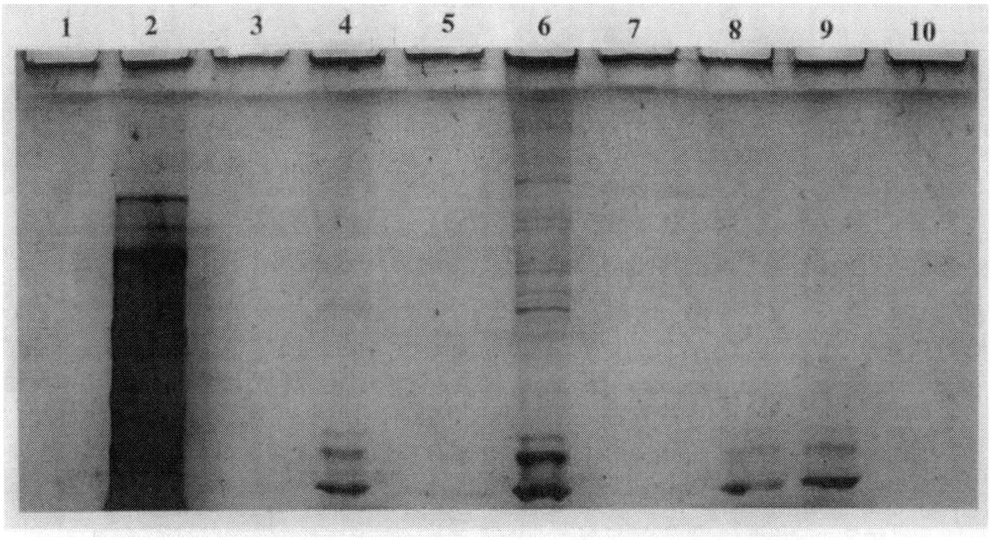

Fig. 7. Effect of grape juice (CGJ) drink on the integrity of reovirus genomic RNA. Reovirus was added to equal volumes of a 10% filter-sterilized concentration of CGJ drink. After 60 min at 23°C, preparations were subjected to RNA extraction and PAGE analysis. Lane 1, 10: Empty (no inocula); Lane 2: ProSieve[R] 11-190 kDa protein marker; Lane 3, 5, 7: CGJ + PBS; Lane 4: Reovirus (2 X 10^4 FFU/ml) + PBS; Lane 6: Reovirus (2 X 10^7 FFU/ml) + PBS; Lane 8, 9: Reovirus (2 X 10^7 FFU/ml) + CGJ drink.

Antimicrobial (antibacterial/antifungal) mechanisms of polyphenolics in edible plants (e.g., grapes, cranberries, pears, tea, cacao) have been investigated; some of the more substantive work has addressed the effects of tannins (e.g., PACs) as antimicrobial agents (Cos et al., 2003; Puupponen-Pimia et al., 2001). It has been proposed, for example, that PACs express their antimicrobial activity through an inhibition of microbial extracellular enzymes and oxidative phosphorylation, as well as a chelation of metal ions important to growth (Scalbert, 1991). Reduction of urinary tract infections in women by PACs in cranberry juice have been ascribed to a blockage of adhesion of P-fimbriated *Escherichia coli* adhesion to uroepithelial cells (Howell et al., 2005). Alteration of bacterial cell zeta potential, conformational changes in fimbrial structure, or a reduction in fimbrial expression at the genetic level have also been proposed as antiadhesion mechanisms (Habash et al., 2000; Liu et al., 2006). The use of polyphenols [encompassing tannins, flavan-3-ols (e.g., PACs)] as antiviral agents has been reported (Aron and Kennedy, 2007; Cos et al., 2003). Studies describing the antiviral effects of plant compounds on the human immunodeficiency virus type 1(HIV-1) targeting for example, virus penetration, cell fusion, and the inhibition of protease, intergrase, and/or reverse transcriptase have been published (Khan and Ather, 2007;

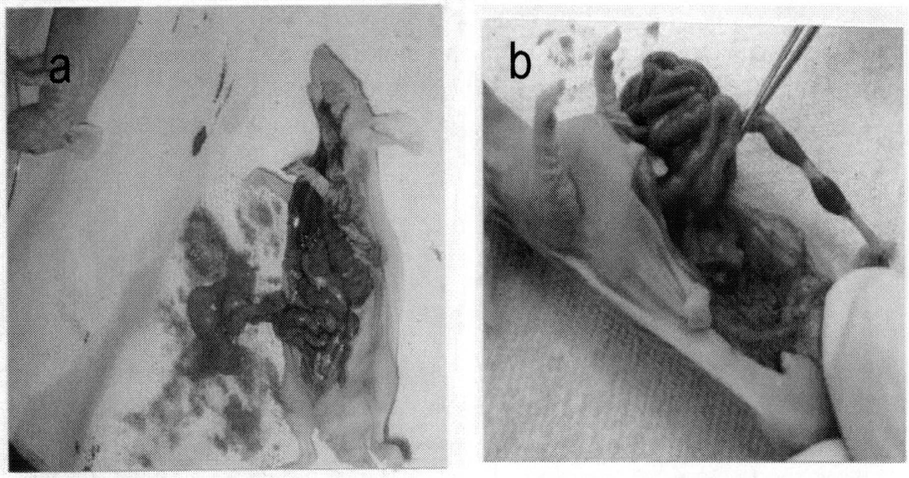

Fig. 8. Antiviral effect of cranberry juice (CJ) cocktail and CGJ drinks in athymic mice. a, Positive control. Mice were inoculated with CJ cocktail drink or CGJ drink + reovirus. No overt indication of disease was recognized on autopsy. Note normal (pelleted) stool in the colon. Input viral titer: 2 X 10^6 FFU/ml. Experiments were performed in pentuplicate.

Lin et al., 2004). Although promising *in vitro*, detrimental health effects (e.g., activation of procarcinogens, hepatotoxicity, digestive disorders, etc.) have been described in studies with animals (including human beings) from the administration or ingestion of large amounts of tannins (e.g., PACs, flavan-3-ols) (Aron and Kennedy, 2007; Chung et al., 1998). Significantly, the consumption of store-purchased fruit juice drinks (viz., those described in the current study) rejects a suggestion of ill effects imparted by the normal intake of these drinks for their potential health benefit effects.

In conclusion, CJ cocktail and CGJ drinks reduced reovirus titers in cell culture and affected a loss of viral infectivity in cell-free suspensions. In cell culture, reduced infectivity titers occurred following a relatively brief (i.e., $\leq$ 5 min) contact between both juices and host cell monolayers.

These data suggest an inhibitory effect at an early stage in the virus multiplication cycle (e.g., viral adsorption, attachment). Loss of viral infectivity and failure to detect the viral RNA by PAGE in cell-free suspensions, may be ascribed to a CJC or CGJ-associated loss of viral coat protein integrity and, in turn, a ready degradation of the RNA. Due to the astringency of plant "tannins", these phytochemicals precipitate proteins to which they come in contact (Scalbert, 1991). A reduction of reovirus virulence in the juice suspensions or an alteration of viral receptor sites on pretreated host cells by one or more phytochemical components may not be ruled out.

Inoculation of virus-CJC and virus-CGJ suspensions into mice resulted in a clinically benign effect. Mouse autopsy confirmed clinical observations. Histologic testing of colon autopsy tissue confirmed gross anatomical findings, specifically among mice inoculated with virus-CJC suspensions. These data report for the first time a clinical protective effect by CJC or CGJ to an enteric viral agent in an animal model.

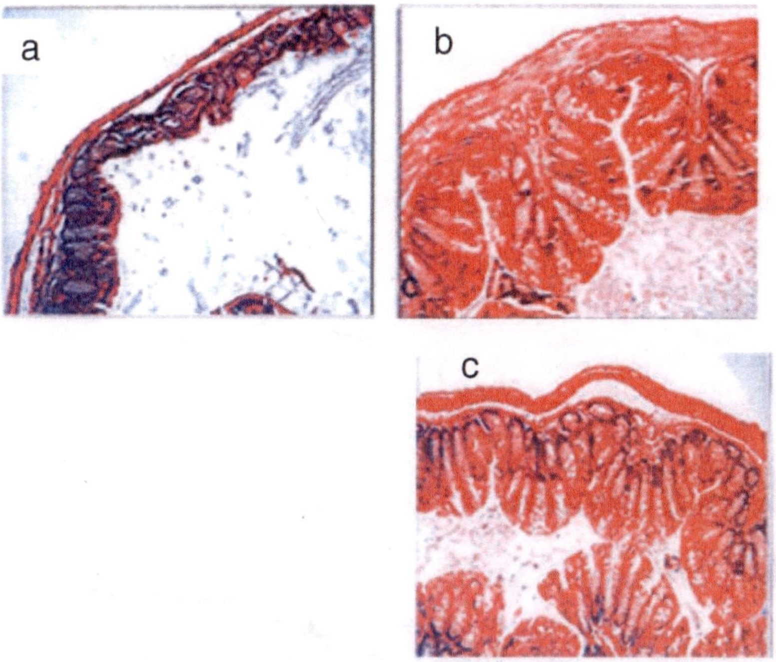

Fig. 9. Effect of cranberry juice (CJ) cocktail and grape juice (CGJ) drinks on the histologic integrity of mouse colon. Mice were inoculated with juice-reovirus (2 X 10^4 FFU/ml) suspensions at a ratio of 1:1. After nine days, animals were euthanized, subjected to autopsy, followed by removal of colon sections for histological examination. a, Positive control. Mice inoculated with virus plus PBS. Note damage to mucosa and muscularis thinned in some areas. The positive control mice presented with loose stools on autopsy. Distal colon histology among CGJ-virus inoculated mice showed shrunken mucosa, mucin depleted goblet cells, large inflammatory foci, and debris in lumen (not shown); b, Colon specimens prepared from mice inoculated with CJ-reovirus suspension. Note relatively intact goblet cells and normal mucosa; c, Negative control. Mice inoculated with juice-PBS suspension. Note normal mucosa (full height) and muscularis externa. Testing was performed in pentuplicate.

Prior studies in our laboratory have shown low concentrations (i.e., 5%) of grape and cranberry PACs reduced reovirus infectivity titers in MA-104 monolayers to undetectable levels (Lipson et al., 2007b). It would not be unreasonable to suggest that the same phytochemical in pure and store-purchased CJC and CGJ drinks might be responsible for the loss of viral infectivity titers reported herein. The data reported in the current study coupled with studies utilizing the [PAC-enhanced] PACran^R cranberry supplement, suggests an association between PACs and reduced viral infectivity titers. Flavan-3-ols, the major constitutive component of PACs, are the most common flavonoid in the diet (Gu et al., 2004; Santos-Buela and Scalbert, 2000).

A continuing need exists to identify new antiviral agents which are efficacious, have limited to no side effects, and do not select for mutant [viral] strains. *In vitro* testing of cranberry and grape juices (or flavonoid extracts from these plant species) utilizing different enteric viral groups in concert with studies in animal models are warranted.

Acknowledgments

This work was supported by grants from the Cranberry Institute and Welch Food, Inc. Additional support was obtained from St. Francis College Faculty Research and Development Grants. We thank Joseph Burdowski and Nicole Bresese for their technical assistance and Andrea Grappone and Wendy Hughes for their assistance in the handling and maintenance of the mice. We appreciate H. P. Lipson for proofreading the manuscript.

References

Amoros, M., Simoes, C.M. & Girre, L. (1992). Synergistic effect of flavones and flavonols against herpes simplex virus type 1 in cell culture. Comparison with the antiviral activity of propolis. J. Nat. Prod. *55*, 1732-1740.

Aron, M. & Kennedy, J. A. (2008). Flavan-3-ols: Nature, occurrence and biological activity. Mol. Nutr. Food Res. *52*, 79-104.

Burdowski, J., Roy, M., Burdowski, A., Stotzky, G. & Lipson, S.M. (2007). Inhibitory effects on reovirus infectivity and viral-induced gastroenteritis in athymic mice by cranberry cocktail and Concord grape juice drinks. Abstr. 107th Gen. Mtg. Amer. Soc. Microbiol. Abstr. 07-GM-A-2639-ASM, P-075.

Chen. H., Zuo, Y. & Deng, Y. (2001). Separation and determination of flavonoids and other phenolic compounds in cranberry juice by high-performance liquid chromatography. J. Chromatog. A. *913*, 387-395.

Chung, K.-T., Wong, T.Y., Wei, C.I., Huang, Y.-W. & Lin, Y. (1998). Tannins and human health: A review. Crit. Rev. Food Sci. Nutr. *38*, 41-464.

Cos, P., De Bruyne, T., Hermans, N., Apers, S., Vanden Berghe, D. & Vlietnick, A.J. (2003). Proanthocyanidins in health care: Current and new trends. Cur. Med. Chem. *10*, 1345-1359.

Deprez, S., Mila, I., Huneau, J.F., Tome, D. & Scalbert, A. (2001). Transport of proanthocyanidin dimer, trimer, and polymer across monolayers of human intestinal epithelial Caco-2 cells. Antiox. Redox Signal. *3*, 957-967.

Dixon R.A., Xie, D.-Y., Sharma, S.B. & Shashi, B. (2005). Proanthocyanidins – a final frontier in flavonoid research? New Phytol. *165*, 9-28.

Docherty J.J., Fu, M.M., Hah, J.M., Sweet, T.J., Faith, S.A. & Booth, T. (2005). Effect of resveratrol on herpes simplex virus vaginal infection in the mouse. Antiviral Res. *67*, 155-162.

Espin, J. C., Garcia-Conesa, M.T. & Tomas-Barberian, F.A. (2007). Nutraceuticals: facts and fiction. Phytochemistry *68*, 2986-3008.

Gu, L, Kelm, M.A., Hammerstone, J.F., Beecher, G., Holden, J., Haytowitz, D., Gebhardt, S. & Prior, R.L. (2004). Concentrations of proanthocyanidins in common foods and estimations of normal consumption. J. Nutr. *134*, 613-617.

Habash, M.B., van der Mei, H.C., Busscher, H.J. & Reid, G. (2000). Adsorption of urinary components influences the zeta potential of uropathogen surfaces. Colloid. Surf. B *19*, 13-17.

Howell, A. B. (2007). Bioactive compounds in cranberries and their role in prevention of urinary tract infections. Mol. Nutr. Food Res. *51*, 732-737.

Howell, A.B., Reed, J.D., Krueger, C.G., Winterbottom, R, Cunningham, D. G. & Leahy, M. (2005).

A-type cranberry proanthocyanidins and uropathogenic bacteria anti-adhesion activity. Phytochemistry. *66,* 2281-2291.

Jassim, S.A. & Naji, M.A. (2003). Novel antiviral agents: A medicinal plant perspective. J. Appl. Microbiol. *93*, 412-427.

Kawai, A. & Fujita, K. (2007). Small red bean (Azuki) sheds biologically active substances as a prerequisite for germination, one of which displays the antiviral activity against the rabies virus infectivity and infections in culture. Microbiol. Immunol. *51*, 1071-1079.

Khan, H. Ather, A., 2007. Potentials of phenolic molecules of natural origin and their derivatives as anti-HIV agents. Biotechnol. Annu. Rev. 13C, 223-264.

Klatt, E.C. (2008). Histotechniques. The Internet Pathology Laboratory for Medical Education.

http://library.med.utah.edu/WebPath/HISTHTML/HISTOTCH/HISTOTCH.html

Kontiokari, T., Laitinen, J., Jarvi, I., Pokkam, T., Sunqvist, K. & Uhari, M. (2003). Dietary factors protecting women from urinary tract infections. Am. J. Clin. Nutr. *77,* 600- 604.

Kontiokari, T., Nutinen, M. & Uhari, M. (2004). Dietary factors affecting susceptibility to urinary tract infection. Pediatr. Nephrol. *19*, 378-383.

Krenn, L., Steitz, M., Schlicht, C., Kurth, H. & Gaedcke, F. (2007). Anthocyanin- and Proanthocyanidin-rich extracts of berries in food supplements –analysis with problems. Pharmazie *62,* 803-812.

Lin, L.U., Shu-wen, L.I.U., Jiang, S.-B. & Shu-Guang, W. U. (2004). Tannin inhibits HIV-1 entry by targeting gp41. Acta. Pharmacol. Sin. *25*, 213-218.

Lipson, S. M. (1992). Growth of human rotavirus by trypsin activation and centrifugation-enhanced shell vial culture. In: H. D. Isenberg (ed.). Clinical Microbiology Procedures Handbook: Amer. Soc. Microbiol., Washington, DC. Vol. *2*, pp. 8.16.1 – 8.16.5.

Lipson, S.M. & Kaplan, M.H. (1992). Atypical rotavirus genomic patterns identified by poly-acrylamide gel electrophoresis, J. Diarr. Dis. Res. *10*, 97-100.

Lipson, S. M., Leonardi, G.P., Salo, R.J., Schutzbank, T.E. & Kaplan, M.H. (1990). Occurrence of nonspecific reactions among stool specimens tested by the Abbott Test Pack^R enzyme immuno-assay. J. Clin. Microbiol. *28,* 1132-1134.

Lipson, S.M., Sethi, L., Cohen, P., Gordon, R.E., Tan, I.P., Burdowski, A. & Stotzky, G. 2007a. Antiviral effects on bacteriophage and rotavirus by cranberry juice. Phytomedicine. *14,* 23-30.

Lipson, S. M., Cohen, P., Zhou, J., Burdowski, A. & Stotzky, G. (2007b). Cranberry cocktail juice, cranberry concentrates, and proanthocyanidins reduce reovirus infectivity titers in African green monkey kidney epithelial cell cultures. Mol. Nutr. Food Res. *51*, 752-758.

Liu, R.H. (2004). Potential synergy of phytochemicals in cancer prevention: mechanism of action. J. Nutr. *134,* 3479S-3485S.

Liu, Y., Black, M.A., Caron, L. & Camesano, T.A. (2006). Role of cranberry juice on molecular scale surface characteristics and adhesion of *Escherichia coli.* Biotechnol. Bioeng. *93*, 297-305.

Malek, M.A., Curns, A.T., Holman, R.C., Fisher, T.K., Bresee, J.S., Glass, R.I., Steiner, C.A. & Parashar, U.D. (2006). Diarrhea- and rotavirus-associated hospitalizations among children less than 5 years of age: United States, 1997 and 2000. Pediatrics *117*, 1887-1892.

Mullen, W., Marks, S.C. & Crozier, A. (2007). Evaluation of phenolic compounds in commercial fruit juices and fruit drinks. J. Agr. Food Chem. *55*, 3148-3157.

Nair, M.P., Kandaswami, C., Mahajan, S., Nair, N.H., Chawda, R., Shanahan, T. & Schwartz, S.A. (2002a). Grape seed extract proanthocyanidins downregulate HIV-1 entry coreceptors, CCR2b, CCR3 and CCR5 gene expression by normal peripheral blood mononuclear cells. Biol. Res. 35, 421-431.

Nair, M. P., Mahajan, S., Chawda, R., Kandaswami, C., Shanahan, T. & Schwartz, S.A. (2002a). Grape seed extract activates Th1 cells *in vitro*. Clin. Diag. Lab. Immunol. *9*, 470-476.

Phuwapraisirisan, P., Sowanthip, P., Miles, D.H. & Tip-Pyang, S. (2006). Reactive radical scavenging and xanthine oxidase inhibition of proanthocyanidins from *Caralia brachiata*. Phytother. Res. *20,* 458-461.

Puupponen-Pimia, R., Nohynek,, L., Meier, C., Kahkonen, M., Heinonen, M., Hopia, A. & Oksman- Caldentey, K.-M. (2001). Antimicrobial properties of phenolic compounds from berries. J. Appl. Microbiol. *90,* 494-506.

Rrasad, D., Joshi, R.K., Pant, G., Rawat, M.S., Inoue, K., Shingu, T. & He, Z.D. (1998). An A-type proanthocyanidin from *Prunus armeniaca*. J. Nat. Prod. *61*, 1123-1125.

Santos-Buelga., C. & Scalbert, C. (2000). A Review: Proanthocyanidins and tannin-like compounds – nature, occurrence, dietary intake, and effects on nutrition and health. J. Sci. Food Agric. *80,* 1094-1117.

Scalbert, A (1991). Antimicrobial properties of tannins. Phytochemistry *30,* 3875-3883.

Shukitt-Hale, B., Carey, A., Simon, L., Mark, D. A. & Joseph, J.A.. (2006). Effects of Concord grape juice on cognitive and motor deficits in aging. Nutrition *22,* 295-302.

Weiss. E.I., Lev-Dor, R., Kashaman, Y., Goldhar, J., Sharon, N. & Ofek, I. (1998). Inhibitory interspecies coaggregation of plaque bacteria with a cranberry juice constituent. J. Am. Dent. Assoc. *129,* 1719-1723.

Weiss, E.I., Y. Houri-Haddad, Y., E. Greenbaum, E., N. Hochman, N., I. Ofek, I. & Zakay-Rones, Z. (2005). Cranberry juice constituents affect influenza virus adhesion and infectivity. Antiviral Res. 66, 9-12.

In: Fruit Juices: Properties, Consumption and Nutrition
Editor: Pauline G. Scardina
ISBN: 978-1-60741-505-3

Chapter 6

Characteristics of Chemical Components and Functional Properties of Chinese Quince (*Pseudocydonia Sinensis*) Fruit and Juice Extract

Yasunori Hamauzu
Shinshu University, Nagano, Japan

Abstract

The production of Chinese quince fruit is very few in the world, even in Japan. It is nevertheless a unique fruit, traditionally used in folk medicine. It cannot be eaten raw owing to strong astringency and large amounts of insoluble dietary fiber. Because of this fiber, it is difficult to extract juice from this fruit. However, it is rich in pectic substances, polyphenols, organic acids, and ascorbic acid. Juice extraction by applying sucrose osmotic pressure is time consuming but effective. Boiling is also a convenient and effective way of extracting the juice and bioactive constituents such as procyanidins and soluble pectins. Some phytochemicals have been identified as active ingredients responsible for the medicinal functions of the fruit or extract. Triterpenoid compounds and polyphenols are important phytochemicals with antibiotic, anti-inflammatory, anti-viral, and anti-ulcerative properties among others. However, many aspects remain to be studied, such as the change in functional compounds during processing, mechanisms of action of functional components, and verification of the effects of these components by clinical investigations.

1. Introduction

Chinese quince (*Pseudocydonia sinensis* (Thouin) C. K. Schneider) is believed to be a native of China (Zhejiang province) and is now widely planted in Japan, China, and Korea. It is a deciduous tree belonging to the family Rosaceae and grows 5 to 8 m tall. In 1906, C. K. Schneider classified Chinese quince as the only species in the genus *Pseudocydonia* [1]; however, many researchers continue to use the generic name *Chaenomeles*. Cuizhi & Spongberg [2] have described the morphological characteristics of Chinese quince under *Chaenomeles sinensis* along with four other species of the genus *Chaenomeles* (*C. speciosa, C. cathayensis, C. japonica,* and *C. thibetica*). Chinese quince is believed to have been imported from China to Japan around the Heian period (8th to 12th century). Since then, its trees have been planted around Shinto shrine precincts, temple grounds, and gardens. Horticultural cultivars are not yet well established and only a few commercial orchards exist (**Figure 1**). However, this fruit has always been popular in traditional culture as a medicinal fruit with antitussive and expectorant properties, among others. On one hand, the ripe fruit (**Figure 2**) has a yellowish smooth skin and emits a strong sweet fragrance, but on the other, it has woody hard flesh, strong astringency, and high acidity, rendering it inedible when raw. Therefore, it is consumed as a processed food product or used as an ingredient in folk or traditional Chinese medicine. Chinese quince fruit is prepared for consumption in a manner similar to that used for European quince (*Cydonia oblonga* P. Miller) fruit, and because of this, these two fruits have sometimes been confused.

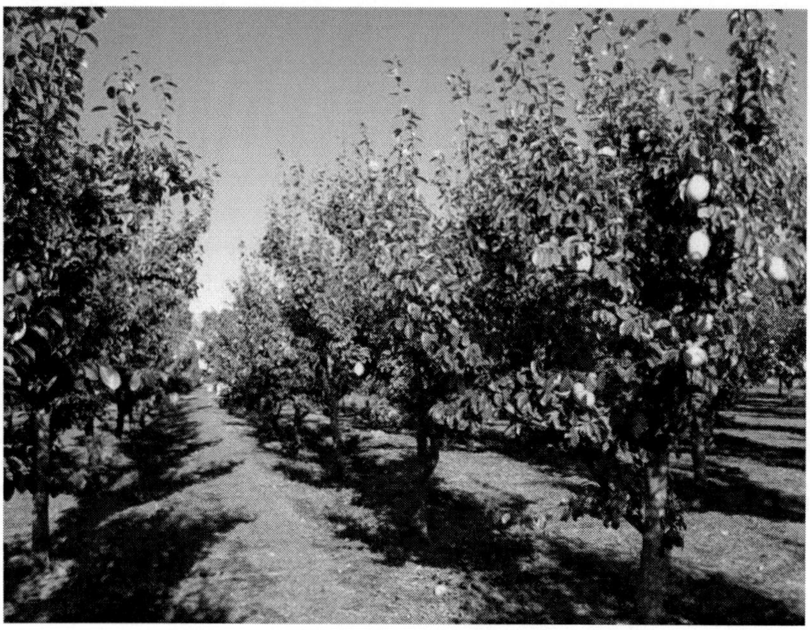

Figure 1. A Chinese quince (*Pseudocydonia sinensis*) orchard complete with trees and fruits

It is difficult to obtain large amounts of juice from Chinese quince fruit by standard procedures, and even after extraction, the juice cannot be consumed because of its strong acidity and astringency. Therefore, the juice is generally extracted by prolonged maceration

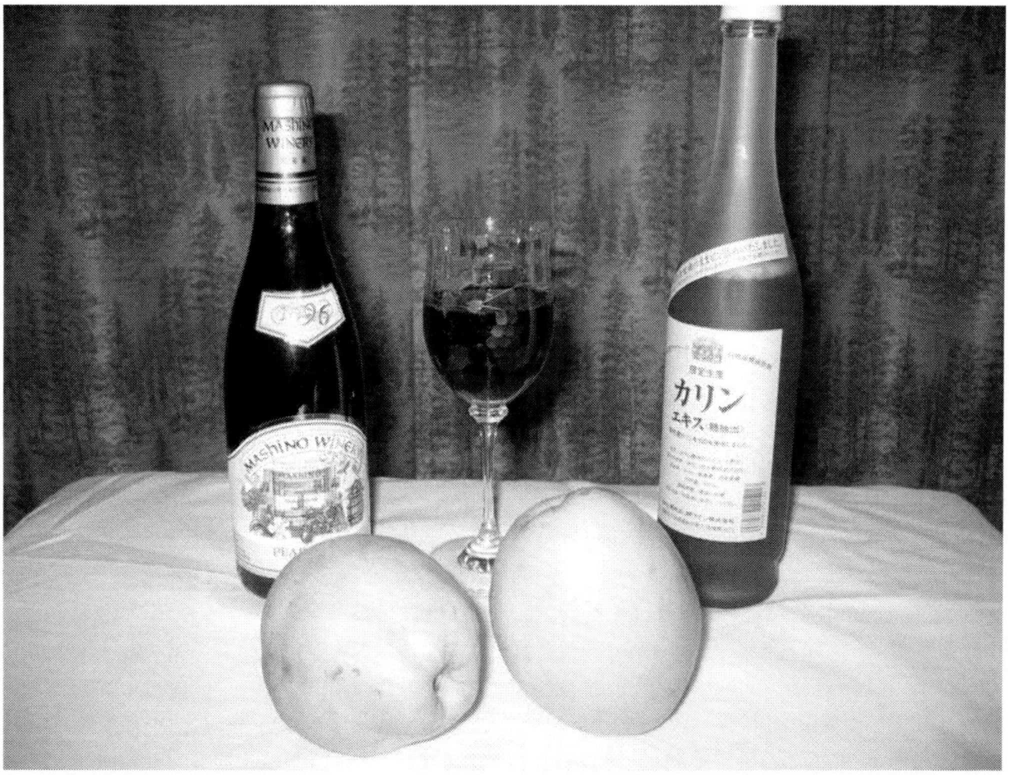

Figure 2. Ripe fruit, fruit liquor (left), and juice extract (right) of Chinese quince (*Pseudocydonia sinensis*)

of the flesh homogenate in sugar or by maceration of the fruit flesh slices in liquor with sugar added or by boiling the flesh pieces in water. Then, the extract obtained is ingested anticipating it to exert some medicinal effects. Consequently, the juice extract of Chinese quince fruit can be regarded as different from normal fruit juices; this fruit has nevertheless been savored by the common people since a long time ago. This chapter discusses the characteristics, utilities, and investigations of phytochemicals and the bioactivity of Chinese quince fruit and juice extract.

2. Utility Of Chinese Quince Fruit And Juice Extract

2.1. Characteristics of the Fruit and Ancient Medicinal Products

As described above, Chinese quince fruit is inedible when raw because of its hard flesh, strong astringency, and high acidity. In addition, it has numerous stone cells that are larger compared to those in normal (European) quince fruit, making the flesh unpleasant to eat. Therefore, Chinese quince fruit is usually consumed after processing to food products such as concentrated juice extracts, fruit liquor, jam, jelly, glutinous starch syrup, crystallized fruit, and throat lozenges. The dried fruit has also been used in folk medicine in the form of hot water extracts, for its antitussive and/or expectorant effects. Chinese quince fruit has been used for medicinal purposes since it was first imported from China to Japan. According to the "Wakansansaizue" encyclopedia, edited by a physician named Ryoan Terashima in 1712, the juice of Chinese quince was used for preparing "Karikou," an ointment or a paste prepared by mixing the juice with sugar and ginger extracts, and consumed as an antitussive and expectorant.

2.2. Juice Extract Obtained by Introducing Sucrose Osmotic Pressure

At present in Japan, the juice of Chinese quince fruit is often produced as a concentrated juice extract to be consumed after dilution. Unlike other fruits such as apple, it is difficult to separate the juice of Chinese quince fruit from the pulp using a blender. The pulp becomes mealy when the fruit is homogenized by the blender because the dietary fiber present in large amounts absorbs the juice such that almost no liquid remains. Merely squeezing the mealy homogenate is not an effective means of juice extraction; hence, large quantities of sugar are often added to create a sucrose osmotic gradient, and then the juice is extracted. That is, the crushed fruit obtained using a hammer crusher is added to a quantity of sugar approximately equal to 80% of the fruit weight and macerated for about three months, following which the mushy pulp is squeezed in a pressing machine to obtain the juice extract. The juice extract obtained contains approximately 60% sugar and can be consumed after dilution. This is the simplest method to produce concentrated juice extracts although the juice obtained is not exactly concentrated.

2.3. Effect of Clarification Step on Polyphenols in the Juice

In the food industry, processes such as enzyme deactivation by boiling (blanching); pureeing using a pulper finisher; and enzymatic degradation of dietary fiber using enzymes such as cellulase, pectinase, and hemicellulase are undertaken. An ultrafiltration (UF) membrane is sometimes used for juice clarification, but this treatment decreases the polyphenol concentration of Chinese quince juice extracts. A polyphenol concentration of 400 mg/100 mL (()-epicatechin equivalent) was obtained from cloudy juice extracts prepared by crushing the fruit with water, boiling, and pureeing. Subsequent clarification treatments such as the pulp removal using degradation enzymes followed by UF treatment (0.03 μm pore size) decreased the polyphenol concentration to 177 mg/100 mL. The reduction in polyphenol concentration due to UF treatment has also been observed in European quince juice. According to Ito & Toyomaki [3], a 430 mg/100 mL concentration of polyphenols in quince juice was decreased to 224 mg/100 mL by UF treatment (MWCO 500 k), and the effect was similar to that seen with Amberlite XAD-16 resin, a polymer adsorbent.

2.4. Extraction with Boiling

Extraction with boiling is an unusual method of juice production, but it has been used to prepare extracts from fruits that are hard to press. This traditional and convenient method extracts useful phytochemicals from the flesh through heat-induced degradation of cell wall components. In preparing traditional medicinal extracts, the dried fruit of Chinese quince is often used as a "decoction." This decoction is used in folk medicine as an antitussive and/or expectorant. Fruit jelly can be made from fresh fruit by boiling the extracts (or decoction). The jelly made from Chinese quince juice extracts has a bright red color similar to European traditional quince jellies such as "membrillo" and "marmelada."

2.5. Utility of Seeds

Seeds of Chinese quince secrete a viscous component when immersed in solvents such as water and aqueous ethanol. Therefore, commingling of seeds with juice extracts or extraction solvents is related to their solution property, especially in case of prolonged immersion. Because the viscous component of the seeds add thickness to the extract solution, some products such as fruit liquor or concentrated juice extracts of Chinese quinces have a thick consistency. This viscous component may be similar to that observed in the European quince seeds used as cosmetic ingredients. The component may also help relieve dysphagia. The yield of the viscous component from Chinese quince seeds is approximately 0.6% of the seed weight (after washing with 80% aqueous ethanol), which is slightly higher than that of European quince seeds (unpublished data). However, Chinese quince has an advantage in that it has a large number of seeds per fruit (approximately 150), five times more than that in European quince (30–40).

3. Characteristics Of Chemical Components In Chinese Quince Fruit And Juice Extract

3.1. Chemical Components of the Fruit

Few studies have reported the chemical components of Chinese quince fruit or juice extract. In Brazil, Chinese quince is called the "quince of Japan" and used as a rootstock in grafting for other quinces [4]. In addition to this, some characteristics of Chinese quince fruits such as their use in the preparation of "marmelada" have been also explored. Alvarenga et al. [5] reported the differences in physicochemical characteristics between Chinese quince 'Japonês' and European quince 'Portugal'. In their report, Chinese quince fruit contained moisture, 81.1%; total sugar, 8.5% (9.0% of total soluble solids); titratable acids, 1.4%; total pectins, 460 mg/100 gFW; soluble pectins, 54.4 mg/100 gFW (11.8% of total pectins); and total polyphenols, 1172 mg/100 gFW. Moreover, its total sugar, titratable acid, and total polyphenol content was higher than that of European quince, while its moisture, total pectin, and soluble pectin content was lower than that of European quince.

In our recent study (unpublished data), Chinese quince fruit contained moisture, 80%; total soluble solids, 17.3%; titratable acids, 1.2%; total pectins, 850 mg/100 gFW; soluble pectins, 53 mg/100 gFW (6% of total pectins); and total polyphenols, 1254 mg/100 gFW (**Table 1**). These results nearly agree with those of Alvarenga et al. [5]. However, the total soluble solids and total pectin (mainly insoluble pectin) content in our results was almost twice that reported by Alvarenga et al. [5]. Regarding the total soluble solids content, Manabe & Kadowaki [6] reported that Chinese quince fruit showed a large variation from 11% to 16%. The proportion of soluble pectin content to total pectin content in Chinese quince fruit is relatively small, a characteristic more often seen in root crops such as carrot, turnip, and radish than in fruits. Compared to European quince (cv. 'Smyrna'), the soluble pectin and total pectin content of Chinese quince fruit was lower and higher, respectively, indicating that the latter has larger amounts of insoluble pectic substances. To investigate the profile of dietary fiber in Chinese quince fruit, we prepared alcohol-insoluble solids (mainly contain cell wall polysaccharides) from the flesh, fractionated by sequential extraction with water, 1,2-cyclohexanediaminetetraacetic acid (CDTA), Na_2CO_3, 4% KOH, and 24% KOH.

Table 1. Some physicochemical properties of Chinese quince fruit

	Ref. [5]	Ref. [6]	Experimental
Physical characteristics of the fruit investigated			
Minor axis (cm)	6.96	NT	8.54
Major axis (cm)	8.14	NT	9.00
Fruit weight (g)	212	400–700	369
Chemical characteristics			
Moisture (%)	81.1	80.2–81.8	80.2
Starch (%)	2.68	1.8–2.1	NT
Total sugar (%)	8.53	NT	NT
Reducing sugar (%)	4.23	2.4–3.1	NT
Nonreducing sugar (%)	4.08	0.27–0.48	NT
Total pectin (mg/100 gFW)	460	NT	850
Soluble pectin (mg/100 gFW)	54.4	NT	53.1
%soluble pectin to total pectin	11.8	–	6.23
Total soluble solids (%)	9.00	11–16	17.3
Titratable acids (%)	1.44	1.5–2.0	1.23
Total polyphenols (mg/100 gFW)	1172	1200–2300	1254
Ascorbic acid (mg/100 gFW)	NT	85.6–96.0*	65.6**

NT, not tested. * Total ascorbic acid; **Ascorbic acid

Next we determined the pectic polysaccharide and hemicellulose content in each fraction. The results showed the fruit has large amounts of Na_2CO_3-soluble pectins and 24% KOH-soluble hemicellulose, indicating that pectic polysaccharides and hemicellulose develop a strong bond with the cell wall matrix to form a strong cell wall. Thus, large amounts of insoluble dietary fiber make the flesh hard, which leads to difficulty in obtaining juice by standard methods.

Chinese quince fruit also has large amounts of L-ascorbic acid. Manabe & Kadowaki [6] reported that the total ascorbic acid content of the fruit was 90 mg/100 gFW, with the highest value reaching 200 mg/100 gFW. In our study, the ascorbic acid content in the flesh ranged from 60 to 70 mg/100 gFW (average, 65.6 mg/100 gFW). Browning of Chinese quince juice is relatively slow, despite the high concentration of polyphenols. The high concentration of ascorbic acid might be related to this phenomenon.

As described above, Chinese quince fruit contains approximately 1.3% polyphenols. According to Manabe & Kadowaki [6], the highest value was 2.3%. In our recent study, polyphenol components comprised mainly polymeric procyanidins (composed of (+)-catechin and (−)-epicatechin) with monomeric catechins, other oligomeric procyanidins, and a relatively small amount of hydroxycinnamic derivatives [7]. Normal-phase HPLC analysis revealed that Chinese quince procyanidins exhibit varying degrees of polymerization from monomers to decamers and further (**Figures 3 and 4**). The HPLC condition was as follows: a 250 × 4.6 mm i.d. 5-μm Silica Luna column (Phenomenex Inc.) was used with the column temperature set at 40 °C. The mobile phase consisted of A, methanol/water/acetic acid (48:1:1, v/v/v), and B, dichloromethane/methanol/water/acetic acid (41:7:1:1, v/v/v). Elution was started with 100% B, followed by 100-82% B, 0-30 min; 82-70% B, 30-45 min; 70-10% B, 45-50 min; 10% B, 50-60 min; 10-100% B, 60-65 min. Separation was monitored using UV 280 nm. In our previous work, the mean degree of polymerization of procyanidins as analyzed by thioacidolysis was approximately 18 [7]. The degree of polymerization of procyanidins corresponds to the degree of bitterness and astringency. Although pure procyanidins are both bitter and astringent, the balance between these taste sensations depends on the molecular weight. Taste panel work has shown that tetrameric procyanidins are most bitter, while polymeric procyanidins are more astringent, on an equivalent weight basis [8,9]. Therefore, the strong astringency of Chinese quince fruit and juice extract is due to large amounts of highly polymeric procyanidins. In addition, Chinese quince fruit contains 3-caffeoylquinic acid (neochlorogenic acid), the concentration of which varies among different fruits and maturation stages.

3.2. Characteristics of Chemical Components of Juice Extract and Effect of Extraction

There exist no detailed reports on the chemical components or nutritional value of Chinese quince fruit juice. In our research, we determined polyphenol and soluble pectin concentrations of concentrated juice extracts, extracted by introducing sucrose osmotic pressure. The juice extracts contained 342 mg/100 mL of polyphenols and 1.3 mg/100 mL of soluble pectins (galacturonic acid equivalent), with a pH of 3.4 [10].

The characteristics of Chinese quince fruit or juice resemble those of *Chaenomeles* species along with which Chinese quince was previously classified. Ros et al. [11] investigated some chemical components of the juice from 21 genotypes of *C. japonica*, 1 of *C. cathayensis*, 1 of *C. speciosa*, and 1 of the hybrid *C.* × *superba* (a hybrid cross between *C.*

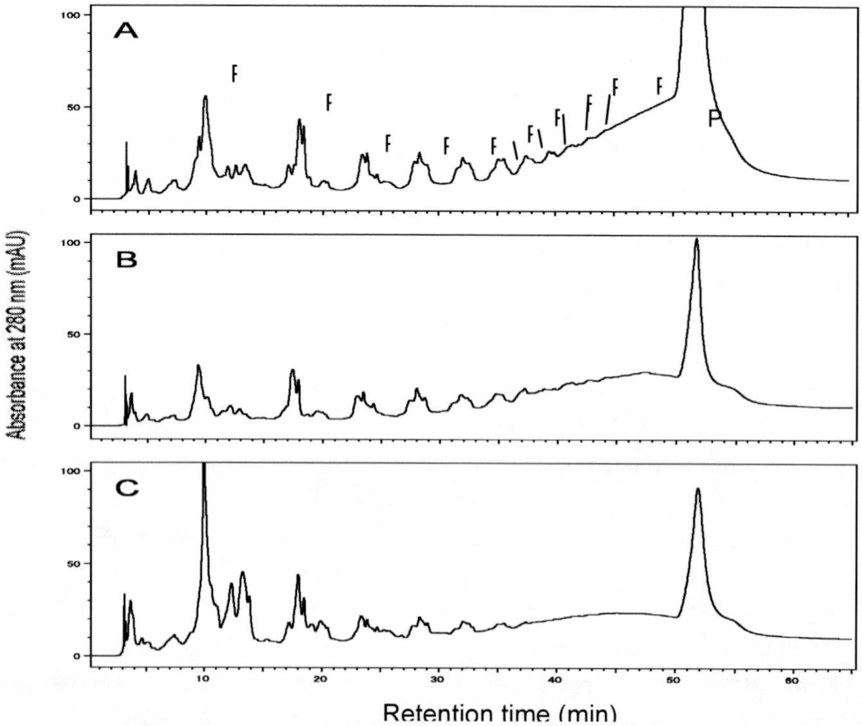

Figure 3. Normal-phase HPLC profile of Chinese quince polyphenols extracted by different procedures. A, 60% acetone extract (innate polyphenolic profile of the fruit); B, extract obtained with boiling; C, commercial juice extract prepared using the sucrose osmotic method. Labels P1–P10 indicate the degree of polymerization (DP) of procyanidins in the peaks. Polymeric procyanidins (PP) with DP >10 appeared as a single peak at the end of the chromatogram. *Peak P1 contains hydroxycinnamic derivatives.

speciosa and *C. japonica*), and showed that the proportion of juice to fruit ranged from 41 to 52% and the average values of the components of the juice were titratable acids (citric acid equivalent), 3.5%; total soluble solids, 7.1°Brix; vitamin C, 59 mg/100 mL; and polyphenols, 284 mg/100 mL. Soluble polysaccharides were not detected. The fruit and juice of *Chaenomeles* species and Chinese quince (*Pseudocydonia*) are comparable in terms of high ascorbic acid and polyphenol content.

Polyphenols have been regarded as bioactive constituents. Procyanidins, the main component of Chinese quince polyphenols, have recently been much focused on because of their strong antioxidant, anti-inflammatory, anti-tumor, anti-ulcerative, antibiotic, and anti-allergy effects in addition to enzymatic inhibitory activity. However, the concentration and composition of procyanidins in the juice and extracts are affected by the methods employed for extraction. Because of their high affinity to the cell wall matrix, highly polymerized procianidins are relatively hard to be released from the pulp and to enter the juice extracts. The proportion of highly polymerized procyanidins to total polyphenols in juice extracts obtained by the sucrose osmotic treatment or boiling the flesh for 60 min in water is lower than that in intact fruit (**Figure 3**). In addition, boiling causes changes in procyanidins during extraction since heat treatment has been reported to break down procyanidin polymers to oligomers under acidic conditions [12,13]. Bioavailability of oligomeric procyanidins has been reported to be higher than that of polymers [14]. The oligomers also have higher antioxidant activity [15] than polymeric procyanidins; therefore, extraction by heating may enhance the health benefits of Chinese quince extracts. This aspect is currently being studied in detail.

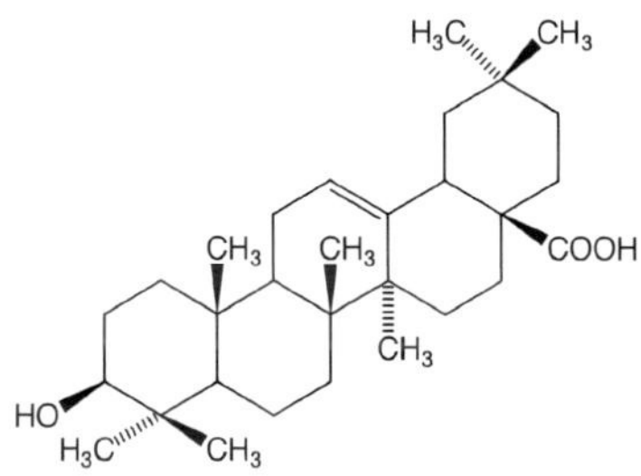

β-Sitosterol

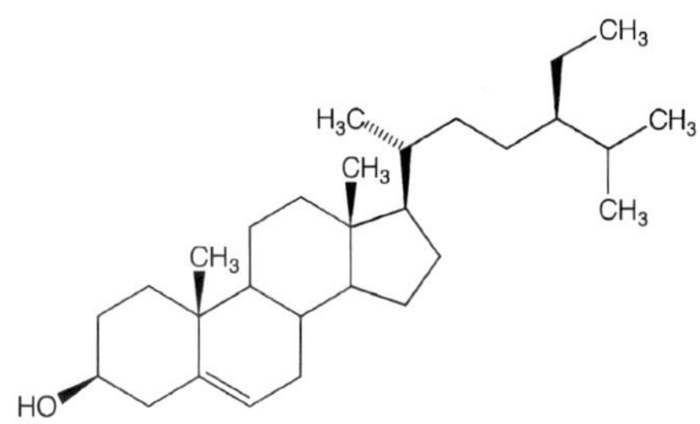

Oleanoric acid

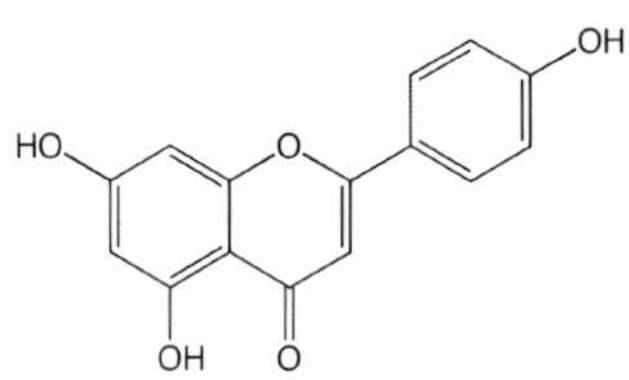

Apigenin

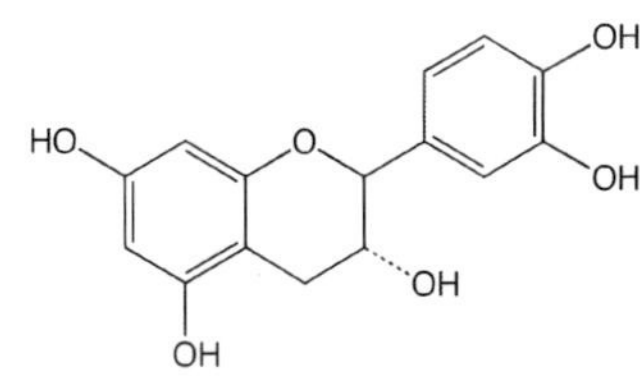

(–)-Epicatechin

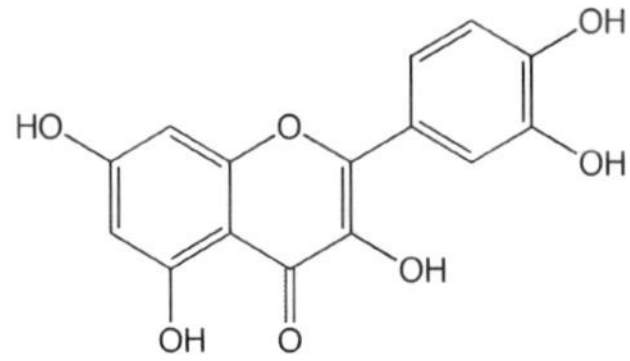

Quercetin

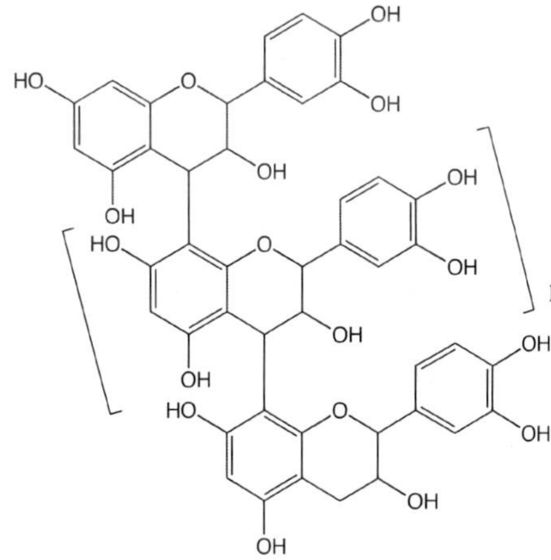

Procyanidins (n ≥ 0)

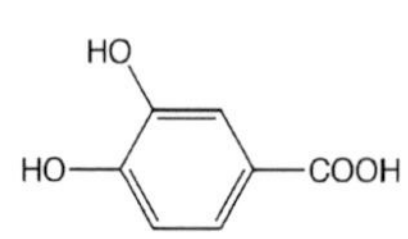

Protocatechuic acid

Figure 4. Typical phytochemicals identified in Chinese quince fruit

Pectic polysaccharides found in dietary fiber are regarded as an important functional component that exert hypoglycemic and cholesterol-lowering effects among numerous other pharmacological actions[16]. Pectic polysaccharides, especially soluble pectin, are contained in specified amounts in unclarified cloudy juices. However, the pectin concentration of Chinese quince juice may be limited because of the relatively low content of soluble pectin in the fruit. We compared the soluble pectin and polyphenol concentrations of Chinese quince juice extracts to those of cloudy apple juice and found that the soluble pectin concentration of Chinese quince juice extracts was one fourth that of cloudy apple juice, while the polyphenol content of Chinese quince juice extracts was four times higher [10]. Thus mild extraction techniques such as introduction of sucrose osmotic pressure do not increase the pectin concentration of Chinese quince juice extracts. However, extraction with boiling could increase the pectin concentration of these extracts because it causes solubilization of insoluble pectic polysaccharides in the cell wall. In our unpublished data, the amount of soluble pectin extracted by boiling was 5 to 7 times higher than the inherent amount in the fruit.

As discussed above, boiling is effective for extracting functional components such as oligomeric procyanidins and pectic polysaccharides. This concept is different from that used for making fresh juices. However, for medicinal characteristics, it is better to focus on the amount of functional ingredients in juice extracts. The boiling extraction process (or decoction) has been traditionally used for extracting medicinal ingredients from plants. Heat treatment such as boiling or decoction over a certain time period may cause decomposition of cell wall polysaccharides and/or polyphenols because the fruit contains large amounts of organic acids. Such decomposition results in increased amounts of functional constituents in the extracts. In addition, ethanolic extraction including the procedure of immersing in alcohol is another effective method for extracting medicinal components. However, since there are no reports on alcohol extraction from fresh Chinese quince fruit prepared with prolonged maceration, detailed investigations are necessary.

4. Functional Properties Of Chinese Quince Fruit And Juice Extract

4.1. Folklore and Scientific Research

Homemade medicines from Chinese quince fruit (including fruit liquor, decoction, syrup, and paste) are said to have antitussive, expectorant, antispasmodic, and antidiuretic actions. They are used for combating respiratory infections, intestinal dysregulation, and diuresis, and treating people with a weak constitution. At present, Chinese quince fruit is mainly used as a domestic antitussive and expectorant agent to treat coughs and colds. Various commercial products made from Chinese quince fruit (European quince fruit extracts are used in some cases in Japan) are also being advertised as being efficacious in treating throat conditions. However, to the best of our knowledge, there have been no reports clarifying the efficacy of Chinese quince fruit by clinical investigations, although there exist some reports based on *in vitro* and animal experiments.

4.2. Medicinal and Biological Functions

Some phytochemicals have been identified as active ingredients responsible for the medicinal function of Chinese quince fruit (**Figure 4**).

Anti-inflammatory activity

Osawa et al. [17,18] have identified some of the active components involved in the antitussive and expectorant actions of Chinese quince fruit extracts in an inflamed throat. According to their reports, triterpenes such as oleanolic acid, pomolic acid, 2-oxopomolic acid, and uvaol exerted strong antibiotic effects on *Streptococcus pyogenes*, the resident microbiota in the throat causing suppurative inflammation. Moreover, β-sitosterol and 2-oxopomolic acid exerted an inhibitory effect on streptolysin O, a hemolytic toxin produced by *S. pyogenes*. Polyphenolic compounds have also been shown to have anti-inflammatory effects. Osawa et al. [18] explored the active compounds involved in the inhibition of hyaluronidase and histamine release from rat mast cells, the indicators of inflammation. This indicates that higher molecular weight polyphenols (polymeric procyanidins) had a strong inhibitory effect on hyaluronidase and histamine release activities. In a small molecular weight fraction, protocatechuic acid was shown to be a strong active compound affecting histamine release. Polymeric procyanidins and protocatechuic acid are both strong antioxidants, and this antioxidant activity may contribute to producing the anti-inflammatory effect.

Anti-pruritic activity

Oku et al. [19] investigated the anti-pruritic effect of 35% ethanol extracts of the fruit on chemically induced scratching behavior in mice and identified quercetin, apigenin, and catechin derivatives as effective compounds. These compounds exhibited significant inhibitory effects on the pruritogenic agent compound 48/80 (COM)-induced scratching behavior. The active fraction from the 35% ethanol extracts and the active compounds (quercetin and apigenin) also inhibited serotonin-, platelet activating factor-, and prostaglandin E_2-induced scratching behavior, but did not inhibit histamine-induced scratching behavior or locomotive behavior. According to authors, Chinese quince fruit may be usable to treat allergic itching sensation.

Anti-ulcerative activity

Recently, we investigated the effect of Chinese quince juice extracts on ethanol-induced gastric ulcers in rats [10]. In control rats administered 1.5 mL of acidified ethanol (150 mM HCl:ethanol = 40:60, v/v), acute gastric ulcers were observed, while in rats given Chinese quince juice extracts (3 mL/rat) before administering acidified ethanol, almost no gastric ulcers were observed (**Figure 5**). We also investigated the effect of polyphenols and soluble pectin extracted from the fruit on gastric ulcer induction, and observed that polyphenols showed strong anti-ulcerative activity. Pectin obtained from the fruit also showed a certain preventive effect on ulcer induction (**Table 2**). However, in Chinese quince juice extracts, the main active components were polyphenols because of their concentration in the extracts (See section 3.2). We also compared the effect of administering cloudy apple juice and apple polyphenols, and observed that prior administration of cloudy apple juice or a lower dose of apple polyphenols showed a preventive effect on ulcer induction comparable to that of Chinese quince juice extracts. Interestingly, a high dose of apple polyphenols showed a promotive effect on ethanol-induced ulcers, indicating that a high intake of polyphenols might have an inverse effect. This result indicates a dangerous aspect of using purified phytochemicals as supplements. Polyphenols may have beneficial health effect, but the actual dose appropriate for humans remains unelucidated.

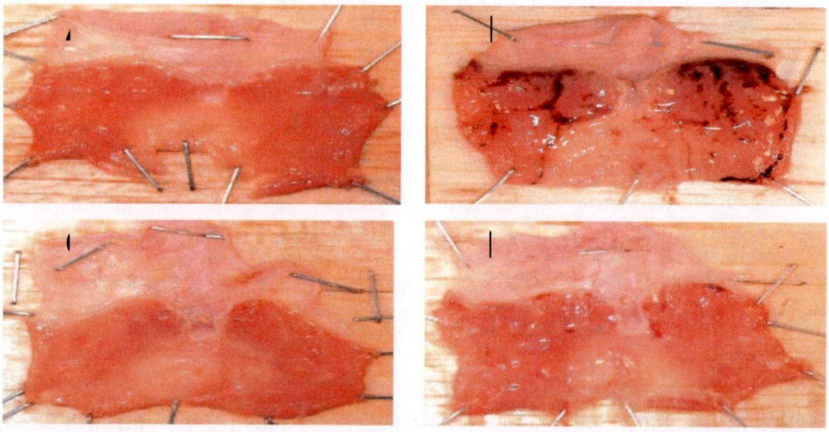

Figure 5. Photographs showing the inner surface of rat stomach (A) No treatment (normal stomach of rat); (B) Control (administered water before treatment with 60% ethanol containing 1.5 mM HCl); (C) Rat administered Chinese quince extract before the treatment; (D) Rat administered apple juice before the treatment. (Adapted from Ref. [10])

Table 2. Extent of gastric mucosal ulcer in rats administered water (control), polyphenols, or pectin from Chinese quince and apple fruits before treatment with 60% ethanol containing 1.5 mM HCl

	Polyphenol		Soluble pectin	
	Chinese quince	Apple	Chinese quince	Apple
Control (0 mg)	20.2 ± 2.4	20.2 ± 2.4	20.2 ± 2.4	20.2 ± 2.4
5 mg	3.3 ± 1.0	4.2 ± 1.5	8.3 ± 2.2	9.0 ± 2.3
10 mg	1.5 ± 1.1	6.4 ± 2.2	7.8 ± 3.9	7.6 ± 2.9
20 mg	0.7 ± 0.3	34.5 ± 3.9	NT	NT

Values (mean ± SE) represent the percentage of ulcerative area to total stomach surface area ($n = 5$). (Adapted from Ref. [10])

Anti-influenza virus activity

The anti-influenza virus activity of polyphenolic extracts has been investigated by Hamauzu et al. [7]. Influenza virus is known to interact with chicken erythrocytes to induce hemagglutination (HA), which reflects the ability of the influenza virus to adhere to the epithelial cells of the respiratory tract in a host as the first step of infection. Therefore, an inhibitory action of phytochemicals on the HA titer of the influenza virus represents inactivation of the virus in terms of its adhesive ability. We observed that Chinese quince polyphenols had a stronger anti-viral activity than European quince or apple polyphenols (**Figure 6**). At higher concentrations of polyphenols, European quince and apple fruit also showed anti-viral activity, but (−)-epicatechin and chlorogenic acid (5-caffeoylquinic acid) did not show any inhibitory action on HA at the same concentrations. This result indicates that a high proportion of polymeric procyanidins to the total polyphenol content may be an important factor for strong anti-viral activity. Chinese quince fruit juice or products rich in polymeric procyanidins appear to be effective in preventing influenza infection.

4.3. Future Trends

The health benefits of Chinese quince fruit and juice extracts have been partly clarified by *in vitro* experiments and animal trials that have focused on antibacterial, anti-hemolytic, anti-inflammatory, anti-pruritic, anti-viral, and anti-ulcerative activities. Triterpenes such as oleanolic acid, pomolic acid, 2-oxopomolic acid, and uvaol; β-sitosterol; and polyphenols such as protocatechuic acid, procyanidins, and flavonoids have been identified as active compounds. However, details of the health benefits of Chinese quince fruit used in folk medicine have not been explained by the research conducted until date. An unknown compound relating to the health effect might be found. Moreover, the processing procedure or extraction method may have a great influence on the concentration and/or composition of active compounds. Therefore, research on the control of active compounds during processing, clinical trials of products for evidence-based health claims, and clarification of the mechanisms involved are needed.

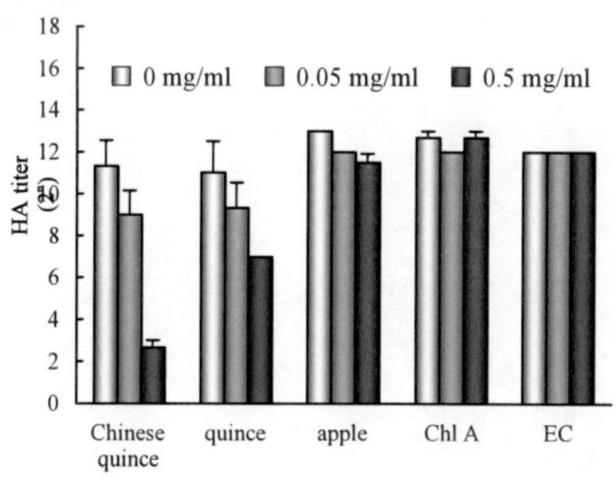

Figure 6. Hemagglutination (HA) activity of influenza virus treated with polyphenols from different fruits and with different phenolic standards. Chl A, chlorogenic acid; EC, (–)-epicatechin. Bars indicate SE ($n = 3$).

5. Red Coloration Of Chinese Quince Juice And Other Products

5.1. Red Coloration and Utility

Red coloration is a characteristic of Chinese quince juice extracts and other products. Chinese quince fruit liquor and juice extracts stored for a long time or decocted syrup subjected to heating for several hours turn red or reddish-brown in color. A similar phenomenon has been observed in products obtained from European quince (e.g., Spanish "membrillo," French "cotignac d'Orleans," and Portuguese "marmelada"). In the middle of the 16th century, Michel Nostradamus introduced this phenomenon in his book "Traité des Fardemens et Confitures (Treatise on Cosmetics and Conserves)." According to this book, in the chapter entitled "To make a quince jelly of superb beauty, goodness, flavour and excellence fit to set before a King," the quince jelly produced is described as having a beautiful red color in the phrase "for the colour will be as diaphanous as an oriental ruby." In his recipe, the quince juice was collected from boiled flesh by squeezing through a thick piece of linen cloth, following which it was decocted with sugar. Chinese quince fruit can also be used for preparing a similar fruit jelly that has "superb beauty." (**Figure 7**)

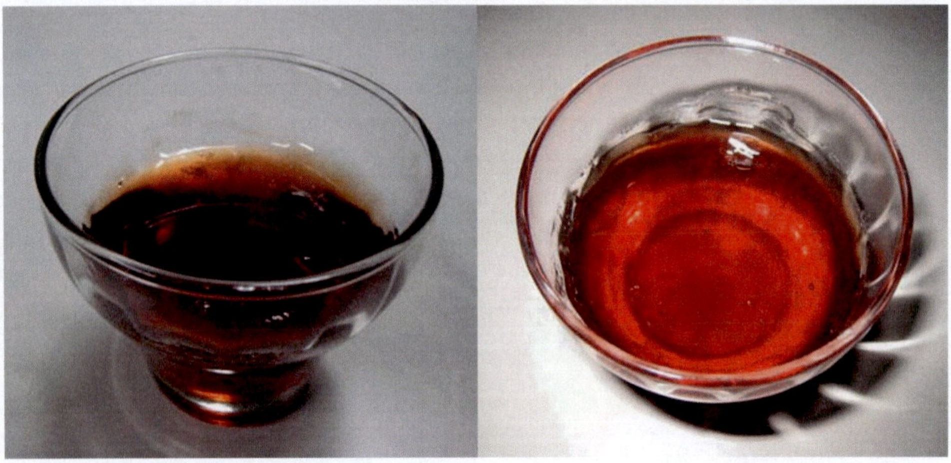

Figure 7. Red colored fruit jelly made from Chinese quince juice. The juice was collected from boiled flesh and then decocted with sugar for a long time (2–3 hours).

5.2. Involvement of Procyanidins in Coloration

On investigating the red coloration in Chinese quince fruit products, we found that the color change which occurs during heat processing is due to changes in procyanidins, the main polyphenols in the fruit. Degradation and/or denaturation of high polymeric procyanidins are the predominant cause, and the changes are accelerated in the presence of organic acids [13]. Although details of the changes and their effects on health-related functions are under investigation, these changes seem to involve the degradation of high polymeric procyanidins to low polymer such as monomeric catechins and cyanidin, and the formation of novel substances containing re-polymerized flavanol derivatives exhibiting absorption in the visible light range. With these changes in procyanidins, the anti-viral activity decreased slightly but retained moderate activity, while the antioxidant activity of polyphenols increased. Thus, if denatured red polyphenols gain some biological activity, the red color change in Chinese quince polyphenols during processing may increase the food functions with respect to not only appearance but also health benefits.

6. Conclusion

Of late, the importance of "food and health" has been gaining increased public interest in many developed countries. Because Chinese quince fruit or juice extract have been used in traditional Chinese or folk medicine, using this fruit as a functional food product is a worthwhile endeavor. As shown above, Chinese quince fruit has various medicinal and functional compounds. The concentration and composition of these active compounds in fruit products may be greatly affected by the processing conditions, including those encountered during juice extraction, preparation, and cooking. Consideration should also be given to the influence of the maturation stage and post-harvest handling conditions. However, few studies have dealt with these aspects. Processing conditions that enable full utilization of the functional characteristics of Chinese quince fruit or juice phytochemicals, such as their antibiotic, anti-inflammatory, anti-viral, and anti-ulcerative activities, remain to be studied. Further research should be conducted through clinical trials to determine the efficacy of fruit products and clarify their mechanisms of action.

References

[1] Schneider, C. K. (1906) Species varietatesque Pomacearum novae. *Repertorium novarum specierum regni vegetabilis*, *3*, 177–183.

[2] Cuizhi, G. & Spongberg, S. A. (2003) Chaenomeles. *Flora of China*, *9*, 171–173.

[3] Ito, H. & Toyomaki, K. (1994) Preparation of the marumero juice (in Japanese with English summary). *Science of Cookery*, *27*, 265–270.

[4] Pio, R.; Chagas, E. A.; Campo Dall'Orto, F. A.; Barbosa, W.; Alvarenga, Â. A. & Abrahão, E. (2005) Marmeleiro 'Japonês': nova opção de porta-enxerto para marmelos (in Portuguese). *O Agronômico, Campinas*, *57*, 15–16.

[5] Alvarenga, Â. A.; Abrahão, E.; de Souza, M.; de Carvalho, V. D.; Lopes, P. S. N. & Gonçalvas, C. A. A. (1994) Physical and chemical caracterization of Japonese quince (*Chaenomeles sinensis* Koehne)(in Portuguese with English summary). *Ciência e Prática*, *Lavras*, *18*, 178–180.

[6] Manabe, T. & Kadowaki, R. (1998) Some physico-chemical properties for non edibility of Chinese quince (*Chaenomeles sinensis* Koehne) (in Japanese with English summary). *The Bulletin of Hiroshima Prefectural University*, *9*, 103–109.

[7] Hamauzu, Y.; Yasui, H.; Inno, T.; Kume, C. & Omanyuda, M. (2005) Phenolic profile, antioxidant property, and anti-influenza viral activity of Chinese quince (*Pseudocydonia sinensis* Schneid.), quince (*Cydonia oblonga* Mill.), and apple (*Malus domestica* Mill.) fruits. *Journal of Agricultural and Food* Chemistry, *53*, 928–934.

[8] Lea, A. G. H. & Arnold, G. M. (1978) The phenolics of ciders: Bitterness and astringency. *Journal of the Science of Food and Agriculture*, *29*, 478–483.

[9] Spanos, G. A. & Wrolstad, R. E. (1992) Phenolics of apple, pear, and white grape juices and their changes with processing and storage–A review. *Journal of Agricultural and Food* Chemistry, *40*, 1478–1487.

[10] Hamauzu, Y.; Irie, M.; Kondo, M. & Fujita, T. (2008) Antiulcerative properties of crude polyphenols and juice of apple, and Chinese quince extracts. *Food Chemistry*, *108*, 488–495.

[11] Ros, J. M.; Laencina, J.; Hellín, P.; Jordán, M. J.; Vila, R. & Rumpunen, K. (2004) Characterization of juice in fruits of different *Chaenomeles* species. *Lebensmittel-Wissenschaft und-Technologie*, *33*, 124–131.

[12] Spencer, J. P. E.; Chaudry, F.; Pannala, A. S.; Srai, S. K.; Debnam, E. & Rice-Evans, C. (2000) Decomposition of cocoa procyanidins in the gastric milieu. *Biochemical and Biophysical Research Communications*, *272*, 236–241.

[13] Hamauzu, Y.; Kume, C.; Yasui, H. & Fujita, T. (2007) Reddish coloration of Chinese quince (*Pseudocydonia sinensis*) procyanidins during heat treatment and effect on antioxidant and antiinfluenza viral activities. *Journal of Agricultural and Food* Chemistry, *55*, 1221–1226.

[14] Spencer, J. P. E.; Schroeter, H.; Rechner, A. R. & Rice-Evans, C. (2001) Bioavailability of flavan-3-ols and procyanidins: Gastrointestinal tract influences and their relevance to bioactive forms *in vivo*. *Antioxidants & Redox Signaling*, *3*, 1023–1039.

[15] Lu, Y. & Foo, L. Y. (2000) Antioxidant and radical scavenging activities of polyphenols from apple pomace. *Food Chemistry*, *68*, 81–85.

[16] Wang, Q.; Pagán, J. & Shi, J. (2002) Pectin from fruits. In J. Shi, G. Mazza, & M. Le Maguer (Eds.). *Functional Foods* (Vol. 2, pp. 263–309). Boca Raton: CRC Press.

[17] Osawa, K.; Yasuda, H.; Morita, H.; Takeya, K. & Itokawa, H. (1997) Antibacterial and antihemolytic activity of triterpenes and β-sitosterol isolated from Chinese quince (*Chaenomeles sinensis*) (in Japanese with English summary). *Natural Medicines*, *51*, 365–367.

[18] Osawa, K.; Miyazaki, K.; Imai, H.; Arakawa, T.; Yasuda, H. & Takeya, K. (1999) Inhibitory effects of Chinese quince (*Chaenomeles sinensis*) on hyaluronidase and histamine release from rat mast cells (in Japanese with English summary). *Natural Medicines*, *53*, 188–193.

[19] Oku, H.; Ueda, Y.; Ishiguro, K. (2003) Antipruritic effects of the fruits of *Chaenomeles sinensis*. *Biological and Pharmaceutical. Bulletin*, *26*, 1031–1034.

In: Fruit Juices: Properties, Consumption and Nutrition
Editor: Pauline G. Scardina
ISBN: 978-1-60741-505-3

Chapter 7

Effect of Temperature, Pressure and Concentration on the Viscosity of Fruit Juices: Experimental and Modeling*

A. I. Abdulagatov,[2] M. A. Magerramov,[1] I. M. Abdulagatov[2*] and N. D. Azizov[3]

[1]Azerbaijan State Economic University, Az 1001 Baku, 31 Istiglaliayt Str., Azerbaijan
[2]Institute of Physics of the Dagestan Scientific Center of the Russian Academy of Sciences, 367003 Makhachkala, Shamilya Str. 39-A, Dagestan, Russia
[3]Azerbaijan State Oil Academy, Baku, 370601, Azerbaijan

Abstract

Viscosity of four fruit (pomegranate, pear, tangerine and lemon) juices have been measured at temperatures from 292 to 403 K and at pressures from 0.1 to 10 MPa for the concentrations from 11 to 45 °Brix. The best and complete comprehensive compilations all of the available viscosity data for liquid foods at the present time are provided. The effect of temperature, pressure, and concentration on the viscosity fruit juices were studied. The measured values of the viscosity were used to calculate the temperature, $(\partial \ln \eta / \partial T)_x$, and concentration, $(\partial \ln \eta / \partial x)_T$, coefficients for the fruit juices. Various theoretical models (polynomials, power, exponential, logarithmic, and their various combinations) for the viscosity of fruit juices were stringently tested with

---

* A version of this chapter was also published in *Progress in Food Engineering Research and Development*, edited by Jerrod M. Cantor published by Nova Science Publishers, Inc. It was submitted for appropriate modifications in an effort to encourage wider dissemination of research.

* Present address: Physical and Chemical Properties Division, National Institute of Standards and Technology, 325 Broadway, Boulder, Colorado 80305, USA. †To whom correspondence should be addressed. ilmutdin@boulder.nist.gov, Fax: (303) 497-5224, Tel: (303) 497-4027

new accurate measurements on pomegranate, pear, tangerine and lemon juices. The applicability, accuracy and predictive capability of the various models were studied. New models were developed to accurately represent the combined effect of temperature and concentration on the viscosity of the fruit juices. Models which represent the viscosity of fruit juices relative to pure water viscosity was considered. The empirical extension of the various theoretically based models for the viscosity of aqueous solutions to the fruit juices is considered. It was found that theoretically based models originally developed for the viscosity of aqueous system can be adopted with success for fruit juices. The average absolute deviation (AAD) between measured and calculated values from these models for the viscosity of fruit juices was within 0.8 % to 2 %.

The values of the Arrhenius equation parameters (flow activation energy, E_a, and η_0) were calculated for the measured viscosities of pomegranate, pear, tangerine, and lemon juices as a function of concentration. The new viscosity models for the fruit juices are recommended for the future scientific and engineering used.

Keywords: Arrhenius equation; pomegranate, pear, tangerine, lemon juices; viscometer; viscosity

1. Introduction

Modeling, optimization and automation of food processes is difficult due to complexity of the raw materials and product involved, which affect thermophysical properties such as density, heat capacity, viscosity, thermal conductivity, and thermal diffusivity. The thermophysical properties of fruit juices exhibit substantial changes with temperature, pressure, and concentration during processing (storage, transport, marketing and consumption, chilled, change temperature, tank farm change concentration, evaporator change concentration), see for example, Moressi & Spinosi [1] and Crandall et al. [2]. For this reason the thermophysical properties (density, heat capacity, viscosity, thermal conductivity, and thermal diffusivity) should be studied as a function of temperature, pressure, and concentration. Last 20 years the high-temperature and high-pressure technologies (high-temperature and high-pressure treatment in food preservation and pasteurization) was expanded to food industry. The preservation temperature is about 60 to 90 °C. Many fluid foods are subjected to high temperatures (above 90 °C) and high pressure (up to 350 MPa) during pasteurization and thermal processing [3-9] (high pressure food processing technologies and other industrial operations) . High pressure presents unique advantages over conventional thermal treatments including, application at low temperature, which improves the retention of food quality. Almost all previous thermophysical properties measurements for liquid foods were performed at atmospheric pressure, although high pressure food processing technologies requires accurate knowledge of thermophysical properties at moderate (3-10 MPa) and high pressures (up to 350 MPa). Therfeore, viscosity (flow properties) and other thermophysical properties of liquid foods at high temperatures and high pressures are need in these processing conditions. Very few measurements are available in the literatures at high temperatures. A literature survey revealed that there are no viscosity and other thermophysical data for liquid foods under prerssure, except our recent density, viscosity, and thermal conductivity measurements for fruit juices (Magerramov [10] and Magerramov et al. [11-15]). Little is known about the effect of temperature, pressure, and concentration on the thermophysical properties of liquid foods.

Knowledge of the viscosity is of primary importance to the fruit juice industry. For example, viscosity is an important property of juices in the prediction of heat – and mass-transfer coefficients and in the design of heat- and mass-transfer equipment for fruit juice industry. The accurate viscosity data and their variation with operating conditions (over wide temperature and concentration regions) are need also for a various research and engineering applications in any branches of the food industry, such as developing food processes and processing equipment (detailed design and evaluate food processing equipment such as pumps, heat exchangers, evaporators, equipment sizing, filters and mixers, engineering calculations on evaporation rates, pumping and pipe requirements), control of products, quality evaluation and an understanding of the structure of food and raw agricultural materials. Viscosity changes are determinant factors in operations such as concentration by evaporation and reverse osmosis, pumping, homogenization and blending.

Variations in the viscosity of fruit juices affect the energy usage in a fruit processing plant (Crandall et al. [2]). The type of evaporator, direction of feed, and heat transfer rate are all affected by viscosity. High shear rates are utilized in modern evaporators to reduce the viscosity, increase the heat-transfer rate, and thus safe energy. If the viscosity of the concentrate exceeds a threshold value then the output products concentration must be reduced or the concentrate will "burn on" the inside of the evaporator (Crandall et al. [2]). This would cause a loss of energy and product. Viscosity can become an important factor during the concentration juices, especially in the production of high density concentrates, due to the inefficiency of the operation when the product becomes highly viscous. Viscosity of fruit juices changes with content of soluble and suspended solids. Pectin and sugar concentration are the main factors in changes of viscosity.

For engineering utility, reliable methods for estimation of the viscosity and other thermophysical properties of fruit juices over wide ranges of concentration, temperature, and pressure would be extremely valuable. To understand and control those processes which used liquid foods, it is necessary to accurately know their thermodynamic (density, heat capacity, vapor pressure, activity coefficient) and transport (viscosity, thermal conductivity, and diffusivity) properties. However, the lack of reliable data for fruit juices over wide temperature, pressure, and concentration ranges makes it necessary to estimate the missing properties by empirical and semi-empirical prediction methods. Therefore, a new accurate experimental data for viscosity of fruit juices at high temperatures and high pressures needed also to improve and extend the range of validity of available estimation and correlation methods which will be capable of reproducing the experimental viscosity data within their uncertainty and develop new more reliable prediction techniques. Unfortunately, the thermophysical properties of liquid food products cannot be accurately predicted theoretically, due to their complicated physical and chemical structure. Therefore, the thermophysical properties measurements of liquid foods are also research interest. The available theoretical models for liquids cannot describe complex real system as they met in practice. Better prediction models can be developed based on reliable experimental information on thermophysical properties liquid foods. Thus, there is great practical and theoretical interest in the study of the effect of temperature, pressure, and concentration on the thermophysical properties fruit juices at equipment operating conditions. The main objectives of this study are: (a) review of the often used techniques for the viscosity measurements for liquids; (b) present for the readers the comprehensive review all of the available experimental viscosity data for liquid foods (viscosity data compilation); (c) experimental and theoretical study of the effect of temperature, pressure, and concentration on the viscosity behavior of fruit juices; (d) examine the accuracy and predictive capability various empirical, semi empirical, and predictive models for the viscosity of liquid foods; (e) develop accurate models for the combined effect of the temperature and concentration on the viscosity of fruit juices; (f) provide for the readers the recommendations of the best viscosity models for fruit juices for the future scientific and engineering used. Available experimental thermophysical properties (density, heat capacity, viscosity, thermal conductivity, and thermal diffusivity) data for liquid foods have been reviewed previously by various authors [16-32]. We also provided a new accurate experimental viscosity data for four fruit (tangerine, lemon, pomegranate, and pear) juices at high temperatures (up to 120 °C), at pressures up to 10 MPa and at concentrations up to 45 °Brix using a capillary-flow techniques, which have been previously used for the accurate measurements on other fluids [33-37] at high temperatures and high pressures. The present results considerably expand the temperature, pressure, and concentration ranges in which viscosity data for these fruit juices are available.

1.1. Material Descriptions

Experimental samples 11.0, 15.2, 15.0, and 17.0 °Brix of pomegranate, pear, tangerine, and peach juices used in this study were obtained from fresh full-ripe fruits from a plant in Baku, Azerbaijan. The natural juices were obtained by squeezing the full-ripe fruits with a laboratory screw press, eliminating the suspended solids by filtering and clarifying. Concentrated juices with various soluble solids contents were obtained from the original concentrate using a rotary glass vacuum evaporator (SPT-200, Zeamil-Horyzont, Poland) at temperature below 60 °C. The evaporation chamber was rotated at a constant rotational speed in water bath at 40°C. The soluble solids content as °Brix was measured using a universal laboratory refractometer (RLU-1, Russia) at room temperature (20 °C). In order to adjust the concentration of the juice, the concentrated juice was diluted with distilled water. The samples were stored in glass vessel at 2-4 °C (8 hours) until used for the density measurements. Microelements (potassium, calcium, magnesium, and phosphates) were determined using an atomic absorption spectrophotometer (C-115-M1, Russia). The glucose and fructose contents were determined by the method of Bertrand. The total sugar was calculated by summation of individual sugars. The pH was measured using a digital pH-meter (Kent EIL 7020, UK) at 20 °C. Total acidity was determined by potentiometric titration with NaOH 0.1 N until pH 8, monitored with pH-meter. Physical and chemical characteristics of pomegranate, pear, tangerine, and lemon juices are given in Table 1.

2. Viscosity Measurements

The viscosity of a liquid is known to determine the relationship between the gradients of pressure and corresponding flow. However, this flow enters hydrodynamic equation which contains nonlinear terms. The response of the system to the presence of finite pressure gradient is so intricate that it is difficult to take this gradient into account in experiment. For example, the pressure gradient induces secondary flows and energy dissipation in addition to laminar flow. This difficult is challenge researcher to develop special techniques for measuring of viscosity which would diminish the effect to a minimum.

Table 1. Physico-chemical characteristics of fruit juices

Pear juice		**Pomegranate juice**	
Soluble solids	15.2 °Brix	Soluble solids	11°Brix
Pectin	0.25 %	Citric acid	1 %
Total sugar	8.70 %	Limon acid	1 %
Glucose	1.43 %	Glucose	6 %
Fructose	6.91 %	Sucrose	-
Sucrose	0.36 %	Acidity	-
Amino acid nitrogen	0.141 %	Fructose	7 %
Tannic acid	0.0171	Potassium*	1100
Cellulose	0.90	Chlorides*	500
pH	4.15	Magnesium*	-
Potassium	48 mg l^{-1}	Phosphates*	300
Calcium	12 mg l^{-1}	Other minerals	5
Magnesium	3 mg l^{-1}	-	-
Phosphate	13 mg l^{-1}	-	-
Ash	0.3	-	-
Lemon juice		**Tangerine juice**	
Soluble solids	17 °Brix	Soluble solids	15 °Brix
Total sugar	3.0 %	Total sugar	5.4 %
Sucrose	-	Glucose	1.1 %
Glucose	-	Fructose	3.8 %
Fructose	2.9 %	Sucrose	0.4 %
Pectin	-	Acidity	-
Potassium*	30	Potassium*	33 mg
Calcium*	6	Calcium*	6 mg
Magnesium*	5	Magnesium*	6 mg
pH	2.4	pH	3.5

* mg in 100 g juice.

For fluids that obey Newton's Law, the dynamic viscosity of a fluid is a measure of its tendency to dissipate energy when it is disturbed from equilibrium by a velocity field v. The dynamic viscosity, η, is thus defined by the relationship

$$\sigma_{ij} = -P\delta_{ij} + \eta\left(\frac{\partial v_i}{\partial x_j} + \frac{\partial v_j}{\partial x_i} - \frac{2}{3}\delta_{ij}\frac{\partial v_k}{\partial x_k}\right). \tag{1}$$

In this equation, σ_{ij} are the instantaneous stresses, P, the pressure and δ_{ij} is the Kronecker symbol. The viscosity depends on the thermodynamic state, (T, P, x) or (T, ρ, x), of the fluid and fluid mixture (where T is the temperature, ρ the density, and x the concentration).

2.1. Experimental Techniques

The definition of the dynamic viscosity given by Eq. (1) presumes the ability to measure local shear stresses. Since however, it is impossible to measure local shear stresses, and viscometers undoubtedly do not have a constant shear rate, methods of measurement of the viscosity must be based on the determination of some integral effect of the stresses amenable to precise measurement in a known flow field. Inevitably, the imposition of a shear field generates small pressure differences, and dissipation causes local temperature gradients, both of which change slightly the reference thermodynamic state to which a measurement is assigned, from the initial, unperturbed, equilibrium state. The reference state for the measurement will be obtained by averaging so it is important that the system is disturbed as little as possible from equilibrium during measurement.

Techniques frequently employed to measure the viscosity of liquids are: 1. capillary flow; 2. oscillating discs; 3. oscillating cups; 4. falling body; 5. rotating cylinders; 6. torsional crystal oscillator; and 7. vibrating wire. In Table 2 all available measurements, to our knowledge, of the viscosity of fruit juices are presented. It can be seen that almost all data were derived by a capillary-flow technique and coaxial cylinder, while only very few datasets were obtained by the falling-body technique and rotational viscometer.

Table 2. Summary of experimental viscosity data for liquid foods

Liquid food	Authors	Concentration	Temperature (°C)	Method
Cranberry	Peleg and Noble [185]	12 °Brix	5-25	CC
Passion fruit	Vitali et al. [186]	15.6-33.4 °Brix	20-50	CC
Passion fruit, peanapple, banana, guava, papaya	Garciá et al. [187]	12.6-26.5 °Brix	22-40	CV
Apple	Geller et al. [214]	12-60 °Brix	20	CC
Apple, grape,	Saravacos [160]	19-70 °Brix	27	CV
Apple, grape, orange,	Saravacos [38]	10.5-75° Brix	20-70	CC
Apple, grape	Rao [112]	15-75° Brix	-5-41	RV
Orange	Barros [109]	54.99-68.83	30	-

		°Brix		
Orange	Steverson [163]	-	30	-
Orange	Moresi and Spinosi [162]	9.6-65 °Brix	25-50	FSV
Orange, grapefruit	Ezell [167]	23-67	30	RV
Orange	Vitali and Rao [113]	65 °Brix	-19-30	CC
Orange	Hernandez et al. [169]	12.2-66.5 ° Brix	5-75	CV
Orange	Mizrahi and Berk [164]	11-60 °Brix	30-70	CV
Orange	Mizrahi and Berk [165]	60-65 °Brix	30-80	CC
Orange	Dubois and Murdock [170]	42, 58.5 °Brix	-1.1-23.3	-
Orange, peanapple	Varshney and Kumbhar [168]	7-36 °Brix	30-45	CC
Orange	Crandall et al. [2]	12.8-65 °Brix	-10-25	CC
Liquid food	Authors	Concentration	Temperature (°C)	Method
Orange	Berk [171]	60 °Brix	-	CV
Orange	Ibarz et al. [101]	30.7-63.5 °Brix	5-70	CC
Orange (concentrate)	Mizrahi and Firstenberg [166]	1.5-11°Brix	30	CC
Orange	Rouse et al. [39]	57.3-65.1 °Brix	25.6	CV
Orange	Rouse et al. [172]	45 °Brix	25.6	CV
Orange	Ingram [173]	63-69.5°Brix	15-45	-
Grape	Bayindirli [95]	19-35 °Brix	20-80	CV
Grape	Moresi and Spinosi [174]	0-73.1 °Brix	20-50	RV
Grape musts	Lopez et al. [188]	990-1100 $kg \cdot m^{-3}$	14-22	RV, CC
Raspberry	Ibarz and Pagán [104]	15-30°Brix	5-60	CC
Peach	Ibarz et al. [105]	40-69°Brix	5-60	CC
Loquat	Ibarz et al. [102]	40-72°Brix	5-65	CC
Sloe	Ibarz et al. [103]	25-58.5°Brix	5-65	CC
Blackcurrant	Ibarz et al. [106]	35-64.5 °Brix	5-60	CC
Sea buckthorn	Oomah et al. [189]	48°Brix	25-80	SR
Pear, apple, grape, lime, plum, tomato, pineapple, watermelon, babaco, orange, lemon, tangerine	Alvarado and Romero [92]	8.4-70 °Brix	10-80	CV
Pear	Ibarz et al. [108]	40-71 °Brix	5-60	CC
Apple	Gochiyaev [159]	15-57 °Brix	23-65	CV
Apple	Constenla et al. [98]	12-68.5 °Brix	20-80	CC
Apple	Bayindirli [93]	14-39 °Brix	20-80	CV
Apple	Rao et al. [110]	51-70 °Brix	23-43	CC
Apple, pear	Ibarz et al. [107]	70, 71 °Brix	5-60	CC
Apple	Schwartz and Costell [161]	-	-	-
Celery	Lau et al. [190]	0-30 %	-9.1-25	ROV

Table 2. Continued

Liquid food	Authors	Concentration	Temperature (°C)	Method
Tomato	Fito et al. [176]	5-28 °Brix	15-70	RV
Tomato	Foda and McCollum [177]	-	35-95	RV
Tomato	Molwane and Gunjal [180]	6-18 °Brix	30-80	CC
Tomato	Krapivin and Fedotkin [181]	8-35 °Brix	25-70	CV
Tomato	Harper and El-Sahrigi [179]	5.8 - °Brix	32-82	CC
Tomato	Luh et al. [182]	6.67	20	RV
Tomato	Saravacos et al. [178]	9-32 °Brix	25	CV
Tomato	Alviar et al. [217]	11.78-35.74 °Brix	23	SR
Tamarind	Manohar et al. [191]	7-62 °Brix	25-70	CC
Liquorice extract	Maskan [192]	3-50 °Brix	10-60	RV
Malus floribunda	Cepeda and Villaran [97]	17-70 °Brix	25	RV
"Baneshan" and "Neelum" Mangoes	Gunjal and Waghmare [193]	20 °Brix	40-80	SV
Watermelon	Sogi [194]	23.59-42 °Brix	5-50	RV
Gilaboru	Altan et al. [158]	35-59.7 °Brix	5-60	SR
Strawberry	Juszczak and Fortuna [99]	50-67.1 °Brix	10-60	CC
Strawberry	Simpson [195]		22.8	CV
Cherry	Juszczak and Fortuna [100]	50-63.8 °Brix	10-60	CC
Cherry	Giner et al. [183]	22-74 °Brix	5-70	CC
Sour cherry	Bayindirli and Özsan [94]	13.8-26.1 °Brix	20-70	CV
Banana	Khalil et al. [175]	20-79.7 °Brix	30-70	CC
Pomegranate	Kaya and Sözer [114]	45.3-71 °Brix	5-60	SR
Pomegranate	Altan and Maskan [184]	17.5-75 °Brix	10-55	SR
Pomegranate, pear	Magerramov et al. [14]	11-40 °Brix	19-130	CV
Pomegranate	Bayindirli et al. [96]	0.5, 1.0, 1.5, 2.0 g/L gelatin		CV
Tangerine, lemon	Magerramov et al. [15]	15-40 °Brix 17-45 °Brix	30-119 30-119	CV
Guava	Vitali and Rao [196]	9.8-16 °Brix	25-60	CV
Guava	Brekke and Myers [197]	7.2-40.8°Brix	24	CV
Corn sirup	Erickson et al. [128]	20-85 D.S.	15.6-82.2	FSV
Corn sirup, silicone oil	McCarthy and Seymour [218]	-	-	CM
Mango	Manohar et al. [198]	16-30 °Brix	30-70	CC
Mango	Rao et al. [111]	11-26 °Brix	25-62	CC

concentrates				
Mango	Singh and Eipeson [199]	15-66 °Brix	15-85	RV
Mulberry	Kaya [115]	46-72 °Brix	10-60	SR
Apricot	Watson [200]	22 °Brix	4.4-25	CC
Pear purees	Harper and Lebermann [201]	18-46 °Brix	32-82	CC
Guar gum and locust bean gum solution	Elfak et al. [202]	20 wt % Glucose, 40 wt % water; 20 wt % sucrose, 40 wt % water;	25	RV
Silicon and mineral oils	Aution and Houska [216]	-	20, 30	RV
Cassava starch pastes	Odigboh and Mohsenin [213]	2-8 wt %	50-95	RV

* CV-capillary viscometer; FSV-falling sphere viscometer; CC-coaxial cylinders; SR-stress rheometer; RV-rotational viscometer; ROV-routine viscometer; SV – synchrolectric viscometer; CM-consistometer.

In this section a brief analysis of these methods is presented. The theoretical basis of the methods, and the working equations employed are presented, together with a brief description of the experimental apparatus and the measurements procedure of each technique. For a more thorough discussion of the various techniques employed for the viscosity measurements of liquids and liquid foods, the reader is referred to the works [18,19,25,26,29,41].

2.1.1. Capillary-flow technique

As seen in Table 2, capillary viscometers are the most extensively used instruments for the measurement of viscosity of fruit juice. They have the advantage of simplicity of construction and operation.

2.1.1.1. Theoretical

The principle of the capillary viscometer is based on the Hagen-Poiseuille equation of fluid dynamics (first formulated by Hagenbach [42] in 1860) and its alteration for practical viscometry by Barr [43] in order to include the so-called kinetic-energy correction and the end correction. The resulting equation expresses the viscosity of a fluid flowing through a thin capillary, in terms of the capillary radius, R, the pressure drop along the tube, ΔP, the volumetric flow rate, Q, and the length of the tube, L, as

$$\eta = \frac{\pi R^4 \Delta P}{8Q(L+nR)} - \frac{m\rho Q}{8\pi(L+nR)} \tag{2}$$

where n is the end-correction factor and m is the kinetic-energy correction factor with $L >> R$. The above equation is derived on the assumptions that, (a) the capillary is straight with a uniform circular cross section; (b) the fluid is incompressible and Newtonian and (c) the flow is laminar and there is no slip at the capillary wall - to avoid turbulence (Reynolds number, Re, over 2000), viscometers are designed to operate where the Reynolds number is well bellow 300. The correction factors n and m reflect the fact that in a practical viscometer two chambers must be placed at either end of the capillary in order to measure the pressure drop. Thus, for example, the parabolic velocity distribution characteristic of most of the flow can only be realized some distance downstream from the inlet of the capillary.

In the range of Reynolds numbers between 0.5 and 100, the theoretical values of the correction factors m and n are represented as $m = m_0 + 8n/Re$ with $m_0 = 1.17 \pm 0.03$ and $n = 0.69 \pm 0.04$ [44]. The values of m and n can also be determined experimentally. Other corrections - capillary shape and slip, non-uniform cross-sections, elliptical cross-section, coiled capillaries, wall roughness, fluid properties effects, compressibility, non-Newtonian [45], and surface tension correction can be found in the respective literature [41,45].

2.1.1.2. Experimental

Figure 1 shows a schematic diagram of a typical capillary viscometer (Abdulagatov and Azizov [46]). A very similar capillary viscometer, differing only in the actual capillary dimensions, was developed by other authors (see [47-51]). The working capillary-1 with ID of 0.3 mm and length of 216 mm is made from stainless steel. The capillary-1 is soldered to the extension tube-6. The fluid under study flows to a cold zone through the extension tube-6. Capillary-1 with extension tube-6 located in the high temperature and high pressure autoclave-4. The extension tube-6 is connected to a movable cylinder-9, which in turn is connected to the fixed cylinder-11 by means of the flexible tube-10. Both cylinders (9 and 11) are supplied with identical expanded bottles, employed to stabilize the fluid efflux through the capillary. The input and output sections of the capillary have conical extensions. All parts of the experimental installation in contact with the sample are made out of stainless steel.

The capillary tube-1 is filled with the fluid and when the movable cylinder is moved vertically at constant speed, the fluid flows through the capillary. To create and also measure accurately the pressure, the autoclave is connected to a dead-weight pressure gauge by means of separating vessel-13. Mercury is used as the separating liquid.

2.1.1.3. Working Equation and Uncertainty

In the capillary viscometer shown in Figure 1, if we denote by t the time required for a volume of fluid V to flow through the capillary, and take into consideration the variation of the geometrical size of the capillary, and that of mercury and sample densities, then Eq. (2) becomes

$$\eta = \frac{\pi R^4 \Delta P t}{8(L + nR)V}(1 + \alpha \Delta T)^3 - \frac{m \rho V}{8\pi(L + nR)t}, \tag{3}$$

where, α is the linear expansion coefficient of the capillary material, ΔT the temperature difference between experimental temperature and room temperature. The pressure drop, ΔP, is determined from the relation

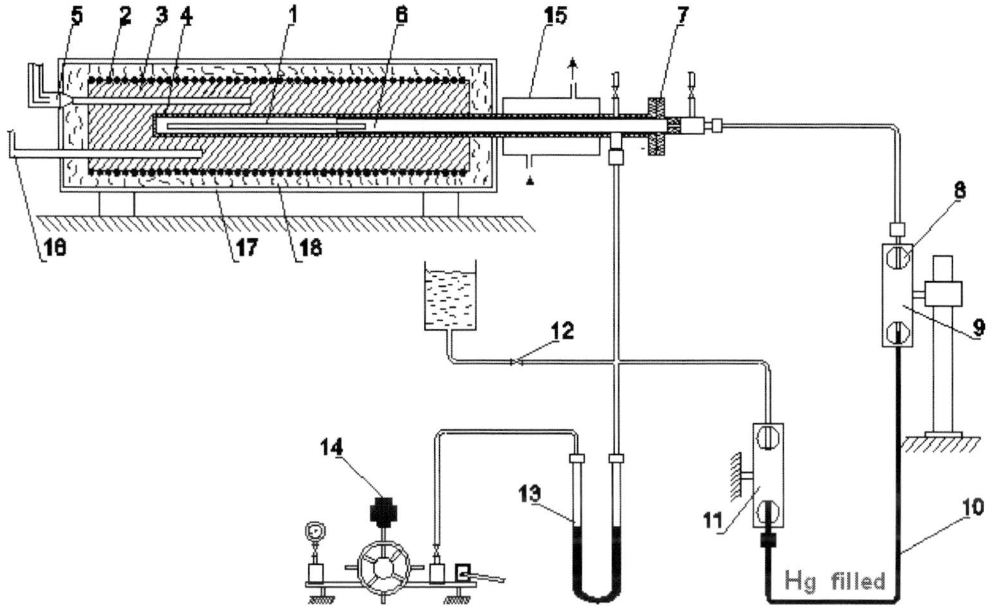

Figure 1. Schematic diagram of the experimental apparatus employed for the measurement of viscosity of aqueous solutions at high temperatures and high pressures by the capillary method (Abdulagatov and Azizov [46]). Working capillary-1; two electrical heaters-2; solid (substantial) red copper block-3; high pressure autoclave-4; thermocouple-5; extension tube-6; flange-7; viewing windows-8; movable cylinder-9; flexible connecting tube-10; unmovable (fixed) cylinder-11; valve-12; separating vessel-13; dead-weight pressure gauge (MP-600)-14; PRT-15.

$$\Delta P = g\,\Delta H(\rho_{\mathrm{Hg}} - \rho), \tag{4}$$

where, ΔH, is the average mercury level drop in the movable and fixed cylinders at the beginning and ending of the measurements, ρ_{Hg}, is the density of mercury at room temperature and experimental pressure, and ρ is the density of the fluid under study. Mercury level in the cylinders was measured with a cathetometer. Equation (3) can be simplified to

$$\eta = c_1 t - \frac{c_2}{t}. \tag{5}$$

where constants c_1 and c_2 can be obtained from Eq. (3).

In Eq. (3) the viscosity obtained is proportional to the fourth power of the capillary radius. Hence a very accurate value of the radius is required. The inner surface of the capillary walls is perfectly polished with powders of successively smaller grain size (1 to 40 nm). The average capillary radius is measured using a weighing technique or/and by calibration (relative method, see Abdulagatov and Azizov [46]) from the viscosity of a standard fluid (pure water) with well-known viscosity values (IAPWS formulation, Kestin et al. [52]). The correction for capillary radius, due to the meniscus curvature (surface forces in a capillary), is made. Typical values (obtained by Abdulagatov and Azizov [46]) of the capillary radius determined with both weighing and by the calibration techniques are 0.15091 mm and 0.15048 mm, respectively, resulting in a value for R^4 of (51.27 ± 0.59)x10^{-5} mm^4. The length, L, of the capillary is measured with a microscope with an uncertainty of ±0.005 mm. Typically the final value of the capillary length (obtained by Abdulagatov and Azizov [46]), is 540.324 ± 0.005 mm. Flow time measurements are usually made electronically and the uncertainty in this value is never more than 0.1s (0.5 %).

To assess the uncertainty of the technique, the uncertainty of each quantity that enters into Eq. (3) must also be taken into consideration. After a very careful analysis of the uncertainty of these quantities (Abdulagatov and Azizov [46]), it is estimated that the combined relative uncertainty in measuring the viscosity (up to the highest temperature of 575 K) is 1.5 %. The uncertainty in the pressure measurements is 0.05 %.

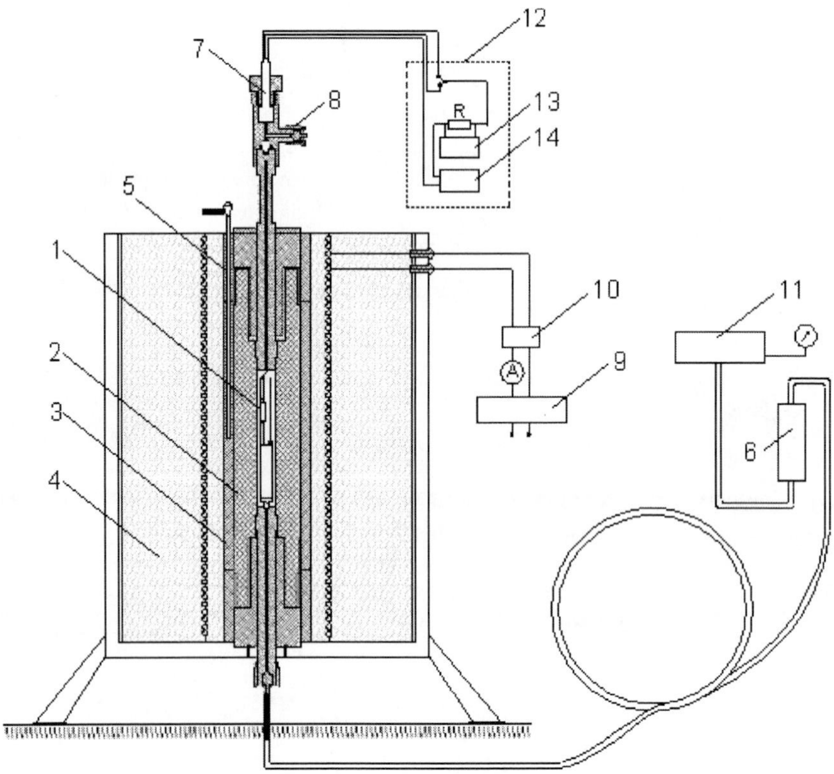

Figure 2a. High temperature and high pressure capillary viscometric system (Semenyuk *et al.* [49]). Titanium viscometer-1; high-pressure autoclave-2; copper block-3; cylindrical electro-heater-4; PRT-5; separating vessel-6; high-pressure electro-input unit-7; removal (withdrawal)-8; electronic voltage stabilizer (П71M)-9; auto-transformer-10; dead-weight pressure gauge (MP-2500)-11; indicated circuit-12; electronic oscillograph-13; audio-frequency oscillator-14.

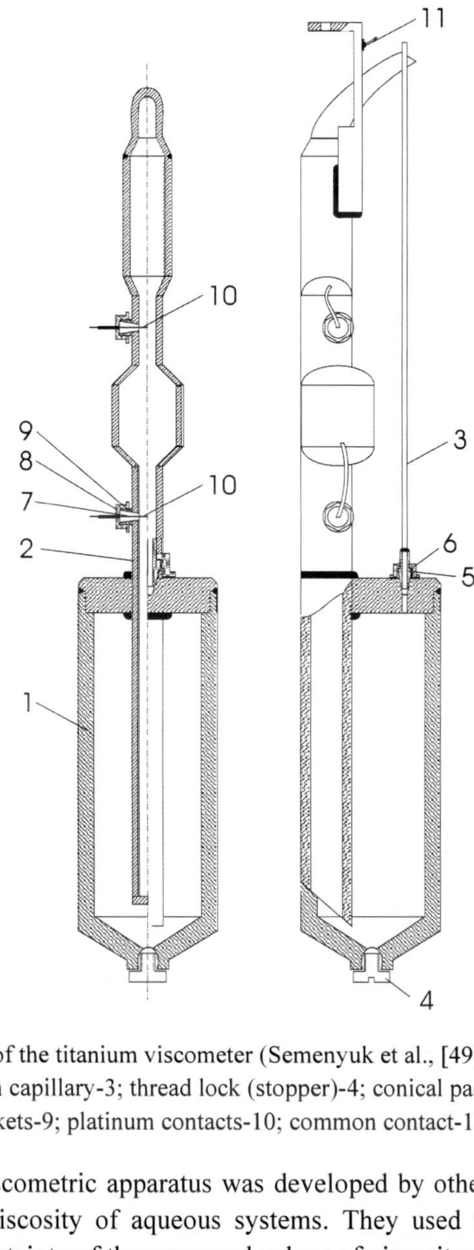

Figure 2b. Construction of the titanium viscometer (Semenyuk et al., [49]). Cylindrical bulb-1; shaped (figured) tube-2; titanium capillary-3; thread lock (stopper)-4; conical packing-5; adapter nuts-6 and 8; insulators-7; conical pockets-9; platinum contacts-10; common contact-11.

A very similar viscometric apparatus was developed by other authors in the works [47-51] to measure the viscosity of aqueous systems. They used nickel, glass, and platinum viscometers. The uncertainty of the measured values of viscosity quoted is 1.5 % for the glass viscometer and 1.0 to 1.5 % for the nickel viscometer. The internal radius and length of the metallic capillary was 0.15 mm and 13.5 cm, respectively. The viscometric apparatus used by Semenyuk et al. [49] schematically shown in Figure 2a,b. Figure 2b shows the details of the construction of titanium viscometer.

Recently we developed new apparatus (glass capillary viscometer) to measure the viscosity of liquid substances. This apparatus was use to measure the viscosity of fruit juices (Magerramov et al. [14,15]). The apparatus used to the viscosity measurements is schematically shown in Figure 3a,b. Details of the apparatus and procedure were described elsewhere [14,15,33-37]. The apparatus for the viscosity measurement consisted of (see

Figure 3a) a high pressure vessel -1, hydraulic press -2, pinching vessel-3, and glass viscometer -4. Main part of the apparatus is glass viscometer-4 which was located in the high temperature and high pressure autoclave with conical packing-5. The high pressure vessel-1 was made from stainless steel (1X18H9T). In order to equalization and maintain homogeneous temperature during the measurements the steel vessel was covered on the cooper block- 8. The high pressure viscometric vessel was supplied with two semi-axis -7 to maintain on the frame and for the rotation around the horizontal axis. The grooves were milled and drilled the well in the copper block for the resistance thermometer and controlling differential chromel–copel thermocouples. One of the semi-axis of the high pressure vessel was supplied with stopper mechanism to fix of the vessel strict vertical position by reading control pointer and scale, maintained on the end of second semi-axis -7. The high pressure autoclave was immersed in a thermostat-6 which was made from the two semispherical iron sheets. The gap between the sheets was filled with asbestos isolator. Two electrical heaters were wound around the surface of the copper block. To create and measure of the pressure, the autoclave was connected with a dead-weight pressure gauge (MP-600) by means of separating vessel. The temperature of the juices was measured with a PRT-10 (platinum résistance thermometer, 10 Ω) using potentiometer circuit. The high-pressure electro-output units were used to connect the viscometer with time of fluid flowing measuring circuit. The high-pressure electro-output unit consists of pinching cone with lock nut, pinching holder -9 and connecting tube. High pressure vessel was immersed in thermostat -6 and maintained on the supports of frame and can rotate around horizontal axis-7. Viscometer was made from refractory glass "supremacs". A construction of the capillary viscometer is shown in Figure 3b. The viscometer consists of a lower bulb. The connecting tube with oval shape is located inside the lower bulb. The lower end of the connecting tube is 2-3 mm above the bottom of the bulb. The upper end of the connecting tube goes to measuring and preliminary bulb. The capillary was welded to the side of the preliminary bulb parallel to the vertical axis of the viscometer. For the centering of the viscometer in the high pressure vessel the lower bulb supplied with shoulders and with funnel for the mercury filling. In order to contact with mercury the platinum wires were seal to 3 contacts– two on the inlet of the measuring bulb and other one on the lower bulb. The platinum contacts of the viscometer were welded to insulated nichrome wires which were connected to the outs of the pressure vessel by an electrically insulated feed-through. The viscometer was suspended to packing cone in the high-pressure vessel by using tag. The tag was supplied with four branches to supporting electro-output units of the viscometer.

Operating Procedure

Initially at vertical position mercury is in the lower bulb. When the high-pressure viscometric vessel is turned by an angle of 90° the viscometer is in a horizontal position and the mercury spills over the whole viscometer volume. When the viscometer returns to its initial vertical position, the level of mercury will be higher than the upper contact. Due to the difference of the mercury levels in the viscometer, flow of the fluid through the capillary takes place. While lowering, the mercury successively disconnects at the inlet and the outlet of the measuring bulb and the flow time is fixed.

The time of fluid flowing through the capillary τ was measured automatically by a frequency-meter with an uncertainty of 0.01 s. The upper contact of the viscometer was connected to brand "start" and the middle to brand "stop". The measurement of the flow time was repeated 5-6 times for each temperature and pressure in order to confirm the reproducibility of the results. The flow time for the investigated juices was about 45 s at high temperatures (120-130 °C) and 1000 s at low temperatures (at room temperature).

The viscosity was obtained from the measured quantities (r_0^4, H_0, h_0, L_0, l_0, V_{10}, τ, ρ_{Hg}, ρ_{Hg0}, T, P, ρ, and m): geometric sizes of the viscometer; radius and the length of the capillary; the volumes of the measuring and preliminary vessels, the difference of the mercury levels, and total length of the mercury column in the beginning and the end of the flow. The geometrical size of the viscometer was determined using the method (mercury – weighing method) described in (Abdulagatov and Rasulov [37]). The viscometer constants were determined using microscope (MIR) and cathetometer. The radius was determined by weighing and relative methods. The dimensions and geometric characteristics of the viscometer are: V_{1H}=1.675×10^{-6} m^3; V_{2H}=1.430×10^{-6} m^3; r_0=12.58×10^{-5} m; l_0=5.942×10^{-2} m; L_0=9.572×10^{-2} m; H_0=5.154×10^{-2} m; h_0=5.052×10^{-2} m.

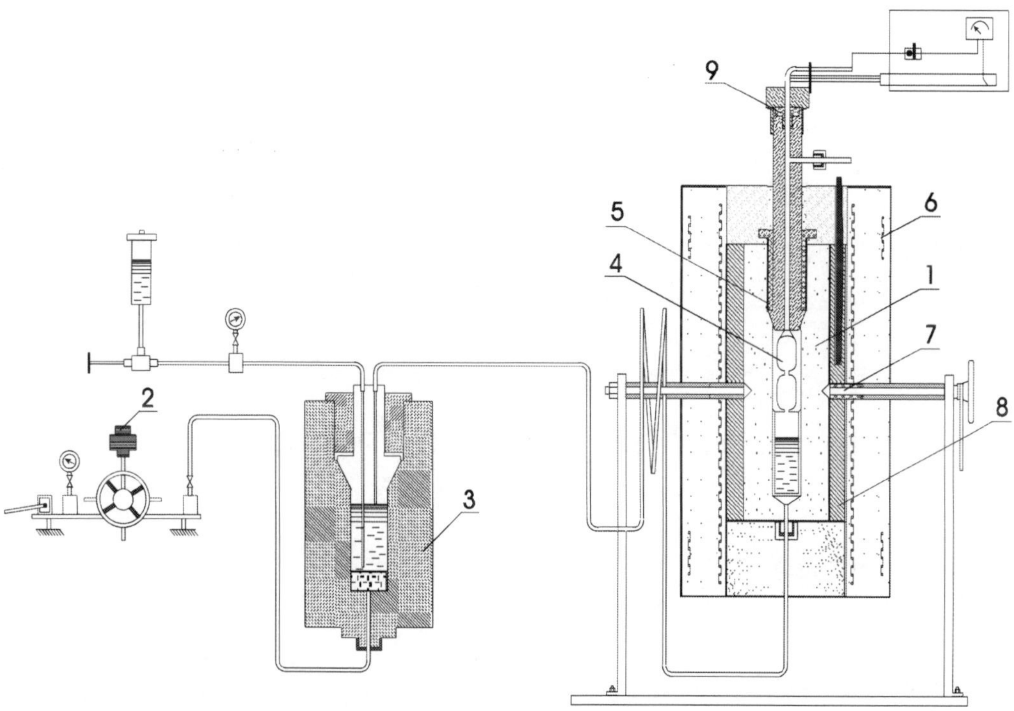

Figure 3a. Schematic diagram of the experimental apparatus for viscosity measurements at high temperatures and high pressures (Magerramov et al. [14,15]). 1 – high-pressure vessel; 2- hydraulic press; 3- pinching vessel; 4-glass viscometer; 5-conical packing; 6- thermostat; semi-axis-7; 8-copper block; 9-packing cartridge.

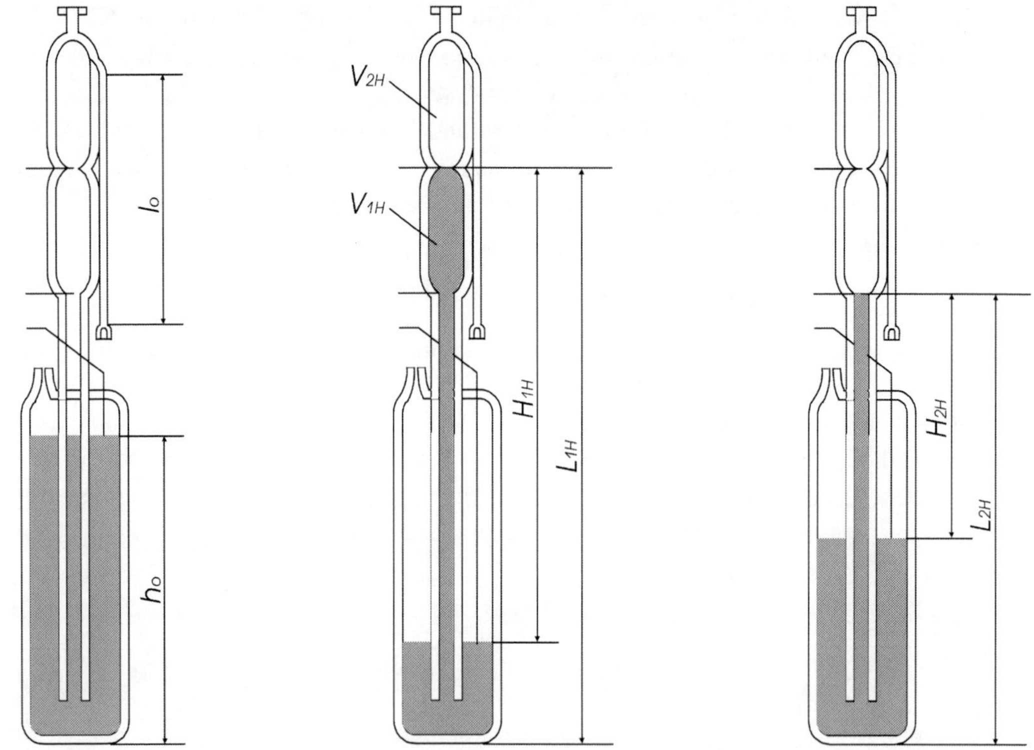

Figure 3b. Construction and geometric characteristics of the high-pressure capillary viscometer (Magerramov et al. [14,15]). V_{1H} and V_{2H} are volumes of the measuring and preliminary bulbs, respectively; H_{1H} and H_{2H} are the mercury level drop at the beginning and the end of the flow; L_{1H} and L_{2H} are the height of the mercury column at the beginning and at the end of the flow, respectively; h_0 is the height of the mercury in the lower bulb; l_0 is the capillary length.

Working Equation

The measurements of the viscosity is based on Poiseuille's law which relates viscosity η to the rate $v = V/\tau$ of fluid flow through a capillary tube

$$\eta = \frac{\pi r^4 \Delta P \tau}{8Vl}, \tag{6}$$

where ΔP is the pressure drop ($\Delta P = P_{in} - P_{out}$, where P_{in} is the inlet pressure, P_{out} is the outlet pressure), r is the inner radius of the capillary, V is the volume of the fluid flowing through the capillary for the time τ , l is the capillary tube length, τ is the time of flow. After corrections (which take into account the acceleration of a fluid at the inlet and outlet; corrections for the effect of thermal expansion of the mercury and glass; corrections for the changing of the mercury level in the viscometer with temperature and pressure) the variation of the geometrical sizes of the capillary, mercury and sample densities at the experimental conditions were varied with temperature and pressure; the final working equation for the viscosity can be written as

$$\eta = A\left(C_t - a\frac{\rho_{Hg0}}{\rho_{Hg}}\right)(\rho_{Hg} - \rho)\tau - B_t\frac{\rho}{\tau}, \tag{7}$$

where the viscometer constants are

$$A = \frac{\pi g r_0^4 H_0}{8V_{10}l_0},\ B_t = \frac{mV_{10}}{8\pi l_0}(1 + 2\alpha\Delta t),\ C_t = \left(1 + \frac{h_0 + 3\alpha\Delta t L_0}{H_0}\right),\ \text{and } a = \frac{h_0}{H_0}, \tag{8}$$

where V_{10} is the measuring volume, ρ_{Hg} is the density of mercury at the experimental conditions (at experimental T and P); ρ is the density of the liquid under study at the experimental conditions, ρ_{Hg0} is the density of mercury at room temperature; H_0 is the average mercury level drop; L_0 is the average height of the column at the flowing process; h_0 is the height of the column in the lower vessel at the initial position; $\alpha = 4.31\times10^{-6}$ K^{-1} is the linear expansion coefficient of the capillary material; r_0 is the capillary radius; l_0 is the length of capillary; Δt is the temperature difference between experimental temperature and room temperature; m=1.12 is a constant introduced to take account of the shape of the capillary ends (correction factor).

The values of the parameters (viscometer constants) A, B_t, and C_t in Eq. (8) can be also determined by means of a calibration procedure from the viscosity of a reference fluid (for example, pure water IAPWS standard data, Kestin et al. [52]) with well-known viscosity values. In the present study the values of parameters A and B_t were determined by calibration (5.895×10^{-10} m^2 s^{-2} and 1.2498×10^{-6} m^2, respectively) on pure water and by the geometric characteristics of the apparatus (5.849×10^{-10} m^2 and 1.2571×10^{-6} m^2, respectively). The values of the parameters a and C_t calculated with geometric characteristics are 0.97497 and 1.9808, respectively. The change in the capillary radius (r_0), length of capillary (l_0), and in the measuring volume (V_{10}), therefore, and in the values of viscometer constants A due to pressure, was considered negligible due to the low volume compressibility of the capillary material (stainless steel 1X18H9T). The effect of pressure on geometrical characteristics of the cell is also negligibly small in the pressure range of the experiments since the entire viscometric capillary was under pressure.

Uncertainty of the Measurements

The uncertainty analysis was based upon the ISO Uncertainty Guide (IOS 4787 [53]) and Coleman & Steele [54]). The uncertainties reported in this paper are expanded uncertainties at 95 % confidence level with a coverage factor of k=2. The accuracy of the viscosity measurements strongly depends on the uncertainty of each individual measurement involved in the overall determination. In this method the measurement of the following basic quantities are needed: r_0^4, H_0, h_0, L_0, l_0, V_{10}, τ, ρ_{Hg}, ρ_{Hg0}, T, P, ρ, and m. The accuracy of the viscosity measurements was assessed by analyzing the sensitivity of Eq. (7) to the experimental uncertainties of the measured quantities from which the viscosity is determined. The uncertainties all of the measured quantities are given in Table 3. The expanded total uncertainty ($\delta\eta/\eta$) with a coverage factor of k =2 at 95 % confidence for the viscosity measurement in this method is

$$\frac{\delta\eta}{\eta} = \frac{1}{\eta}\sqrt{\left(\frac{\partial\eta}{\partial R^4}\right)^2 S_{R^4}^2 + \left(\frac{\partial\eta}{\partial \Delta H_0}\right)^2 S_{\Delta H_0}^2 + \cdots + \left(\frac{\partial\eta}{\partial x}\right)^2 S_X^2}\,, \tag{9}$$

where $S_{R^4}^2$, $S_{\Delta H_0}^2$, ..., and S_X^2 are the root-mean-square deviations of R^4, ΔH_0, ..., and m, respectively. The systematic uncertainties of the viscosity measurements can be estimated from the equation

$$Q_\eta = \frac{1}{2}\left[\left(\frac{\partial^2\eta}{(\partial R^4)^2}\right)S_{R^4}^2 + \left(\frac{\partial^2\eta}{\partial(\Delta H_0)^2}\right)S_{\Delta H_0}^2 + \cdots + \left(\frac{\partial^2\eta}{\partial x^2}\right)S_X^2\right]. \tag{10}$$

Table 3. The uncertainty of the measured quantities

No.	Measured quantities	Uncertainty
1	Height of the mercury column in the viscometer, L_0, *m*	9.572×10^{-2}
2	Level of the mercury in the lower vessel, h_0, *m*	5.248×10^{-2}
3	Mercury level drop at the beginning of flow, H_0, *m*	5.154×10^{-2}
4	Measuring volume, V_{10}, m^3	1.675×10^{-6}
5	Length of the capillary, l_0, *m*	5.942×10^{-2}
6	Thermal expansion coefficient of the viscometer, α, K^{-1}	4.31×10^{-7}
7	Uncertainty in capillary radius determination, *m*	2.16×10^{-7}
8	Uncertainty in capillary length determination, *m*	5.5×10^{-8}
9	Uncertainty in measuring volume of viscometer, m^3	1.65×10^{-10}
10	Uncertainty in height of the mercury column, *m*	5.0×10^{-2}
11	Uncertainty in temperature measurements, *K*	2.5×10^{-2}
12	Uncertainty in fluid flowing time measurement, *s*	1.0×10^{-2}
13	Relative uncertainty in liquid density measurements,	2.0×10^{-4}
14	Relative uncertainty in pressure measurements	6.0×10^{-5}
15	Relative systematic root-mean-square uncertainty in viscosity measurement	1.6 %
16	Random root-mean-square uncertainty in viscosity measurement	0.1 %
17	Total root-mean-square uncertainty in viscosity measurement	1.7 %

The uncertainty all of the measured quantities was determined as $S = \sqrt{\sum_{i=2}^{n} (x_i - \bar{x})^2 / n(n-1)}$, where x_i is the measuring quantity; $\bar{x}$ is the mean value; n is the number of measurements. Based on the detailed analysis of all sources of uncertainties likely to affect the determination of viscosity with the present apparatus, the combined maximum relative uncertainty $\delta\eta/\eta$ in measuring the viscosity was 1.5 %. The relative systematic uncertainties Q_η/η was 0.001 %.

2.1.2. Oscillating-disk Technique

Oscillating-disk viscometers consist of an axially symmetric disk placed between two fixed parallel plates and suspended from a torsion wire, so that it performs oscillations in the fluid about its axis of symmetry. Such a viscometer has been used by several researchers as an instrument for viscosity measurements (see, for example [55-62]). The theoretical and experimental problems of this technique have been discussed in detail elsewhere [61,63-67].

2.1.2.1. Theoretical

The theoretical aspects of the technique are described in the works [65-67]. The characteristic equation which relates the motion of an oscillating body to that of the fluid is [67]

$$(s + \Delta_0)^2 + 1 + D(s) = 0, \tag{11}$$

where Δ_0 is the logarithmic decrement in a vacuum. Here, $D(s)$ is the torque on the body, calculated from solutions for the fluid flow close to the oscillating body. It is therefore the torque $D(s)$ that is characteristic of the particular type of oscillating viscometer employed.

Apart from roots that are associated with the initial oscillatory behavior of the body, the roots associated with the long-time behavior can be written in the form

$$s = \pm(i - \Delta)/\theta \tag{12}$$

where i is the imaginary unit and $\theta = T/T_0$. Here, T is the period of oscillation in the fluid and the subscript zero denotes the same quantity in vacuo. The function $D(s)$ can be expressed as

$$D(s) = \frac{s\,M(s)}{I\omega_0^2\,[s\alpha(s) - \alpha_0]}, \tag{13}$$

where $M(s)$ is the Laplace transform of the torque function $M(\tau)$ (torque exerted by the fluid on the body), $\tau = \omega_0 t$ is a dimensionless time, $\omega_0 = 2\pi T_0$ is the angular frequency of oscillation in a vacuum, I is the moment of inertia of the oscillating system. The symbol, α_0, denotes the initial angular displacement, while $\alpha(s)$ is the Laplace transform of the angular displacement $\alpha(\tau)$ of an axially symmetric body, defined as

$$\alpha(\tau) = \frac{\alpha_0}{2\pi i} \int_C \left\{ \frac{1}{s} - \frac{1 + \Delta_0^2}{s\left[(s + \Delta_0)^2 + 1 + D(s)\right]} \right\} e^{s\tau} ds \tag{14}$$

or

$$\alpha(\tau) = \alpha_0 e^{-\Delta\theta\tau} \cos(\theta\tau) . \tag{15}$$

During an experiment, the logarithmic decrement Δ and the period *T*, are determined from the motion of the body. The form of the torque functions *D*(s) for various oscillating-body viscometers are discussed in the literature [66, 68-71].

Before proceeding to examine different forms of the function *D*(s), it is important to introduce a natural length scale that appears in oscillatory systems in general, namely the boundary-layer thickness, *δ*, defined as

$$\delta = \left(\frac{\eta}{\rho\,\omega_0} \right)^{1/2} . \tag{16}$$

As it will be shown in the following paragraphs, this natural length scale is important in the selection of the dimensions of oscillating-disk viscometers.

In the particular case of viscometers consisting of a disk of thickness d and radius *R*, oscillating between two fixed horizontal plates, and provided $\delta >> 2b+d$ (where *b* is the separation between the disk and one of the fixed horizontal plates), the solution for *D*(s), is [61]

$$D(s) = \frac{\pi\rho\, R^4 \delta}{I} s^{3/2} \left[\coth\left(\frac{b}{\delta} s^{1/2} \right) + \frac{(C_{\mathrm{N}} - 1)\,\delta}{b} s^{1/2} \right], \tag{17}$$

where C_N is calculated from the viscometer geometry [72].

For the oscillating-disk viscometers consisting of a thick disk oscillating in an infinite fluid (i.e. a free thick disk), and provided that $\delta << d/2$ and $R >> \delta$, the analytical solution for $D(s)$ is [61]

$$D(s) = \frac{\pi\rho\, R^4 \delta}{I} s^{3/2} \left[1 + \frac{2d}{R} \frac{K_2(\xi_0 s^{1/2})}{K_1(\xi_0 s^{1/2})} + \varepsilon(s) \right], \tag{18}$$

where K_1 and K_2 are the modified Bessel functions of order 1 and 2, and $\xi_0 = R/\delta$. The edge-effects $\varepsilon(s)$ for this type of geometry are given by

$$\varepsilon(s) = \frac{16}{3\pi}\left[\frac{4\pi}{3\sqrt{3}} - 1\right]\frac{1}{\xi_0 s^{1/2}} + \frac{17}{9}\frac{1}{\xi_0^2 s} + \ldots \tag{19}$$

The solutions represented by Eqs. (16) and (19) are valid for oscillations of small amplitude.

For all disks the general torque function can be expressed (Nieuwoudt et al. [69]) in the form of

$$D_k(s) = \frac{\rho}{\overline{\rho}} s^{3/2}\left[A_k \xi_0^{-1} + B_k s^{-1/2}\xi_0^{-2} + C_k s^{-1}\xi_0^{-3} + D_k s^{-3/2}\xi_0^{-4} + Q_k(s)\right], \tag{20}$$

where k denotes the type of configuration and $\overline{\rho}$ is the effective density of the oscillating body. The term A_k arises from the torque on the flat and cylindrical sides of the disk, while the high-order terms contain the effects of the sharp edges at the rims of the disk. The values of the coefficients A_k, B_k, C_k and D_k appearing in Eq. (20) for various oscillating-body viscometers, can be found in literature [41].

2.1.2.2. Experimental

During the last fifty years, many designs of oscillating-disk viscometers, operating in a relative or in an absolute way, have been reported and their theory has been developed in the works [56,60,61,63-67,73-75]. However, due to design limitations, absolute measurements of the viscosity of aqueous solutions with an oscillating-disk viscometer are almost impossible. Kestin and coworkers [56,58,61] employed relative methods, based upon the development of previous formulations [64-67] in order to measure the viscosity of aqueous solutions at temperatures up to 200 °C and pressures up to 30 MPa. Calibration of the viscometer involves measurement of the viscosity of distilled water, whose viscosity is well known, in order to determine the dependence of the edge-correction factor C upon the boundary-layer thickness δ. Calibration was performed over the temperature range from 25 to 150 °C, which corresponds to a boundary-layer range from 0.73 to 1.53 mm.

The oscillating-disc viscometer used by Kestin et al. [56,57,60], Grimes et al. [74], and Kestin and Shankland [75] to measure the viscosity for aqueous solutions at high temperatures and high pressures, is schematically shown in Figure 4.

The viscosity body is divided into a solid lower part -3 and hollow upper part- 7 forming the viscometer cavity, effectively sealed against an internal pressure in excess of 30 MPa. The oscillating-disk -5 is suspended between two Hastelloy fixed plates -4 and -6 by means of a stress relieved 92 Pt thin strand -9. The upper end of the wire is gripped at the top of the suspension cartridge. The top suspension assembly -11 is designed to permit controlled adjustments in the elevation of the disk as well as in the angular orientation of the oscillating system. Two side windows at the lower part of the instrument provide access to the disk and the fixed plates.

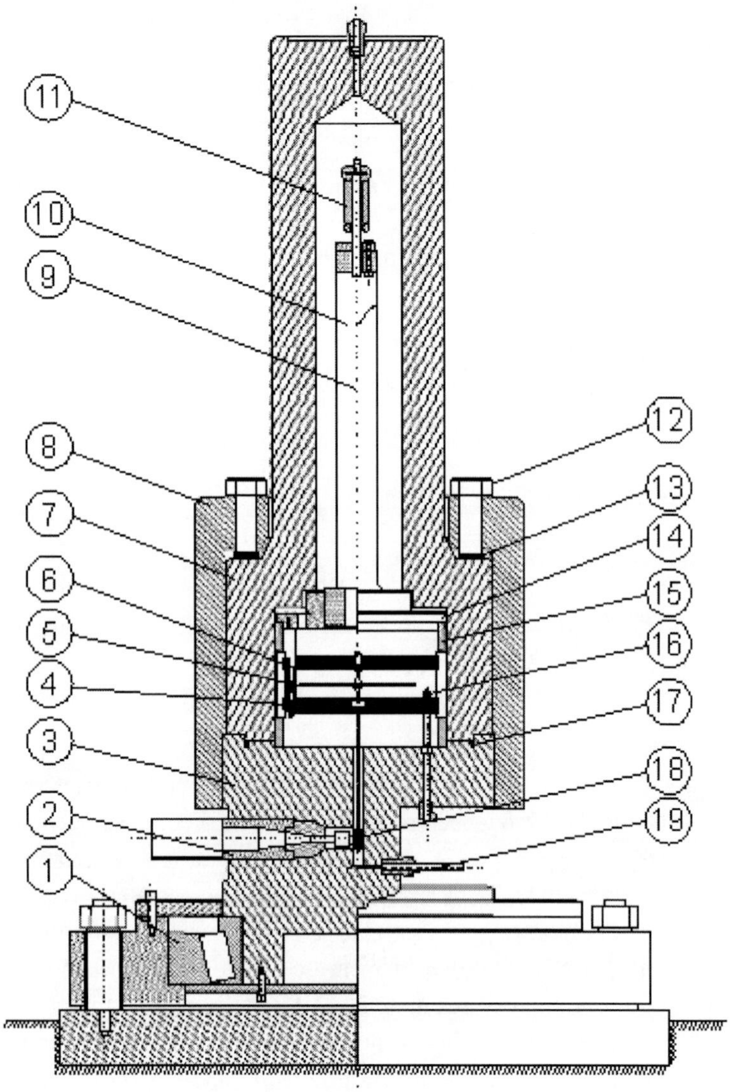

Figure 4. Cross-section view of the viscometer by Kestin *et al.* [56]. Bearing for rotating viscometer-1; window-2; solid lower part of the viscometer-3; fixed plates-4,6; disk-5; hollow upper part of the viscometer-7; buttress-threaded stainless steel cap-8; Pt/W thin strand-9; alumina column-10; suspension assembly-11; ten bolts-12; pressure ring-13; suspension mounting plate-14; thick-walled cylinder-15; thermocouple-16; O-ring seal-17; mirror-18; filling connection-19.

2.1.2.3. Working Equation and Uncertainty

As already mentioned, the value of the viscosity (obtained in a relative way), is derived from measurements of the logarithmic decrement Δ and the period of oscillation T. The working equation for the viscometer reduces to [56,58]

$$\frac{2}{\theta}\left(\frac{\Delta}{\theta}-\Delta_0\right)-C\frac{\pi\rho R^4\delta}{I}\left[H_1K_2+H_2K_1+\frac{2d}{R}\left(H_1+\frac{3\delta}{2R\theta}\right)\right]=0, \tag{21}$$

where, θ is the ratio of the period of oscillation in the liquid to that in vacuum, R is the radius of the disk, I its moment of inertia, and δ is a measure of the boundary layer thickness (Eq. (16), $\delta=\sqrt{\eta/(\rho\,\omega_0)}$). Parameter C is an edge-correction factor depended on the dimensionless boundary-layer thickness (δ/b), determined by calibration. Finally, the functions $H_{1,2}$ and $K_{1,2}$ are defined by

$$H_{1,2}=\left(1\pm1.5\Delta-0.375\Delta^2\right)/\sqrt{2}\theta^{3/2}, \tag{22}$$

and $K_1=\dfrac{\sin Y}{\cosh X-\cos Y}$, $K_2=\dfrac{\sinh X}{\cosh X-\cos Y}$, (23)

with $X,Y=\dfrac{2}{\sqrt{2\theta}}\left[1\pm0.5\Delta+0.125\Delta^2\right]\dfrac{b}{\delta}$. (24)

Eq. (21) is first employed in combination with viscosity measurements of a liquid of “known” viscosity, in order to obtain the edge-correction factor $C(\delta)$. Consequently having obtained this factor, it is applied to measure the viscosity of other liquids from measured values of Δ and θ.

The precision of the viscometer depends both upon the accuracy of the mathematical model describing its operation and on the precision of each individual measurement involved in the overall determination. In this method the measurement of the following basic quantities are needed: temperature T, pressure P, a series of the times, and the period of oscillation.

The temperature inside the viscometer is usually measured by means of a Pt/Pt-Rh thermocouple with an uncertainty of 0.05 K. The uncertainty in pressure measurements is 50 kPa. The time intervals were measured with the aid of digital timers and a photo-electric circuit. The accuracy of the time interval measurements is 1 ms; this translates into a logarithmic decrement, known to within 0.1 % and a period that is known to within 0.001 %. On the basis of these values the estimated uncertainty of the viscosity measurements does not exceed 0.4 %. Kestin et al. [60] numerically evaluated the sensitivity of the viscometer working equation to uncertainties in density. They found that at room temperatures, the viscosity is insensitive to any uncertainty in density, while at 200 °C, the relative uncertainty in density is amplified by a factor of approximately 2 in viscosity.

2.1.3. Falling-body Technique

This method is usually employed to measure the viscosity of liquids and high-dense gases. This method is characterized by high uncertainty (3-4 %), but has some advantages for measurements at high pressures. The theoretical and experimental problems of this technique have been discussed by Kawata et al. [76].

2.1.3.1. Theoretical

The method is based on Stoke's law, according to which, the force, W, exerted by the liquid on a sphere of radius, r, falling in an infinite homogeneous liquid at a constant velocity v, is related to viscosity η of the liquid via the equation $W = 6\pi \eta r v$. This relation is valid for very small Reynolds numbers, Re. At greater Reynolds numbers, this relation should be corrected for the effect of walls. Stoke's law assumes that the following conditions are satisfied, during the free-fall under gravity of a sphere through the liquid of interest (Wakeham et al. eds. [41]): (a) the motion of the sphere is sufficiently slow; (b) the liquid is of infinite extent; (c) there is no slip between the liquid and the surface of the sphere; (d) the sphere is rigid; (e) the liquid is incompressible; and (f) the liquid is Newtonian.

For falling bodies of various shapes (a cylinder, a cylinder with semispherical ends, or an arrow-like body), the viscosity is determined by measuring the time t of fall through a fixed distance at a constant velocity as

$$\eta = C\left(\rho_b - \rho_l\right)t, \tag{25}$$

where C is the instrument's constant (function of the dimensions and the design of the apparatus), ρ_b is the density of the falling body, and ρ_l is the density of the liquid studied. The value of the instrument's constant, C, is usually determined by a calibrating procedure, from the viscosity of a standard fluid (usually pure water) with well-known viscosity values (IAPWS formulation, Kestin et al., [52]).

For a free-fall of a sphere of radius r through a distance h, in a liquid enclosed in a tube of radius R, the viscosity equation is derived as

$$\eta = \frac{2r^2 g}{9h}(\rho_b - \rho_l)t f_w. \tag{26}$$

In the above equation f_W is the correction factor for the wall effect. The correction factor f_W has been studied theoretically and experimentally [76-79]. Faxen [77] expressed the factor f_W as a function of the Reynolds number, Re, and the ratio (r/R)

$$f_w = 1 - 2.104(r/R) + 2.09(r/R)^3 - 0.95(r/R)^5. \tag{27}$$

Stoke's law is applicable provided the Reynolds number, Re, is much less than unity. Oseen [80] derived the following working equation for a sphere moving with a velocity v, which is applicable for a wide range of Re number

$$\eta = \frac{2r^2 g}{9v(1+3Re/16)}(\rho_b - \rho_l) \text{ for } Re = \frac{2Rv\rho_l}{\eta} < 1 \tag{28}$$

There are several modifications of the Stoke's law for a wide range of Re numbers (see, for example, [79-83]). Other corrections to the working equation of this technique, such as the effect of the fall-tube ends, the fall-tube dimensions, and the selection of spherical material, are well documented in literature [84-86].

For a cylinder of mass m, radius r_l and length L_b, falling under the influence of gravity a distance h along the axis of a tube of radius r_2, the viscosity of the liquid can be expressed as

$$\eta = \frac{(\rho_b - \rho_l)}{A\rho_b} t \tag{29}$$

where $$A = \frac{2\pi L_b h}{mg\left[\ln(r_2/r_1) - [(r_2^2 - r_1^2)/(r_2^2 + r_1^2)]\right]}. \tag{30}$$

In practice the value of the instrument's constant A is determined by a calibration procedure employing fluids of well-known viscosity (pure water, for example). This method was used to measure the viscosity of water, alcohols, and their mixtures [87,88].

2.1.3.2. Experimental

Melikov [89-91] employed the falling-body technique to measure the viscosity of aqueous solutions at temperatures up to 300 °C and pressures up to 30 MPa. The main part of the apparatus is a viscometric tube - the fall-tube - (see Figure 5a-c), with 40 mm OD, 10.33 mm ID, and a length of 500 mm, made out of stainless steel. The working section of the viscometric tube is 400 mm (see Figure 5b). The inner surface of the tube walls is perfectly polished with powders of successively smaller grain size (1 to 40 nm). On the outside surface of the fall-tube (50 mm from the ends), the two inductance coils (electromagnetic transducers) are mounted, connected to potentiometers. When the falling-body passes the inlet and outlet of the fall-tube, an induced signal triggers the appropriate timing circuitry. The cylindrical falling body with a diameter of 10.214 mm and a density $\rho_b = 6.290$ g·cm^{-3}, is made out of magnetic steel. The viscometer is located in a liquid thermostat with 7 heaters and can be rotated upside down in order to let the ball return to its starting position.

To perform accurate viscosity measurements with the falling-body technique, various corrections (fall-tube dimensions, effect of fall-tube ends, terminal velocity, falling-body shape, position of the fall-tube) ought still to be considered (Wakeham et al. eds. [41]).

2.1.3.3. Uncertainty

The uncertainty of the viscosity values is directly connected to the uncertainty associated with several other factors, including the measurement of the dimensions, mass and density of the falling body, the radius of the fall tube, the distance traveled and time taken, the density of the falling body and that of the liquid. These uncertainties are connected through the corresponding working equation. In particular the radius of the falling body and that of the tube are of primary importance as they strongly affect the viscosity. For the instrument described here (Melikov [89-91]), the uncertainty in the radius of the falling cylinder and the tube is 0.001% in both cases. Density of falling body and liquid were measured with an uncertainty of 0.002% and 0.0052% respectively. The temperature and the pressure were measured with an uncertainty of 0.1 K and 0.005 MPa. Hence, the resulting total uncertainty in the viscosity measurements was about 3.3 %. It should also be pointed out that as a test of the operation of his instrument, Melikov [89-91] measured the viscosity of pure water at pressures between 0.1 and 40 MPa and over the temperature range from 298 to 573 K. His values agreed with the IAPWS formulation values (Kestin et al. [52]) within 1.5 %.

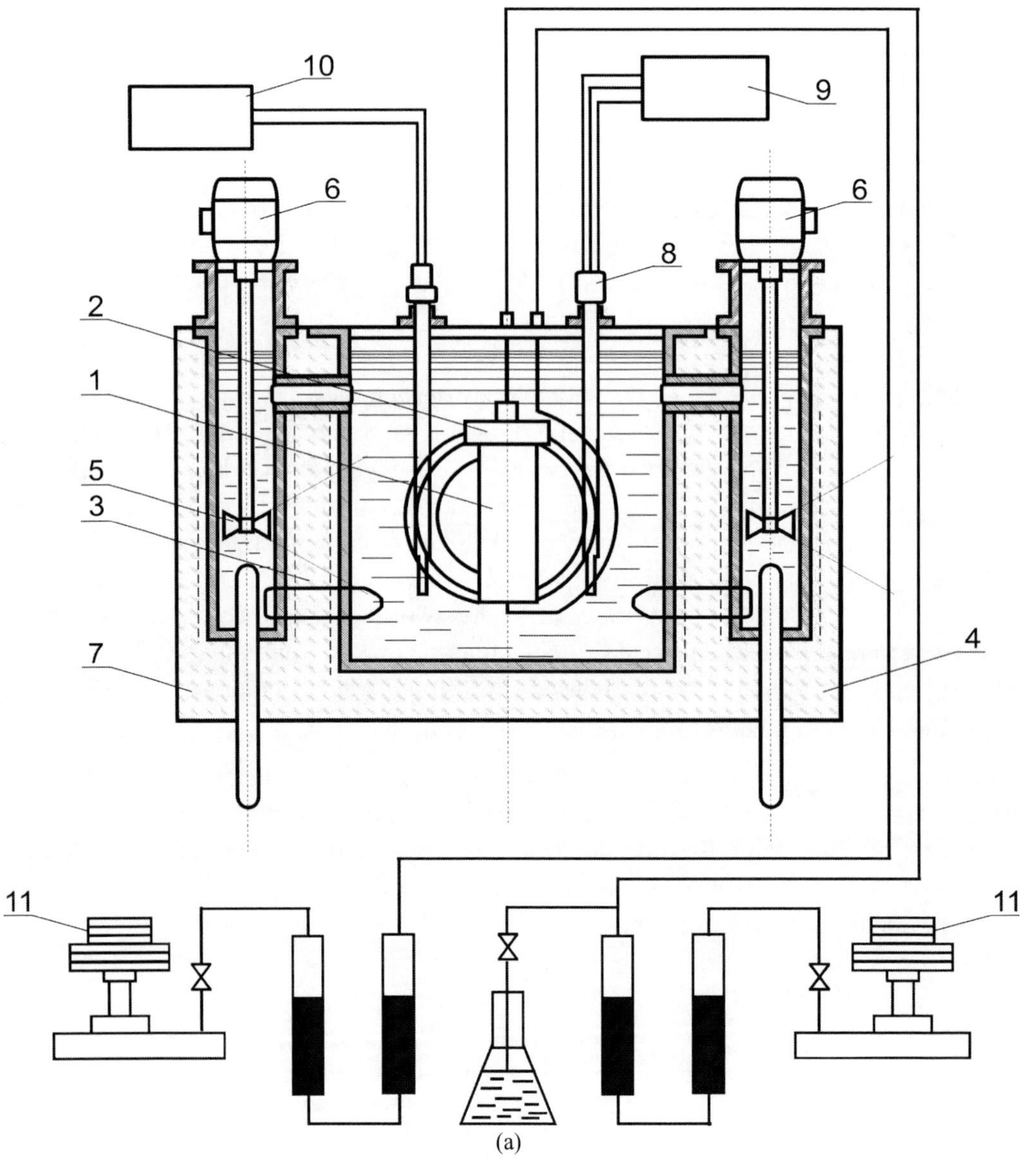

(a)

Figure 5. (Continued)

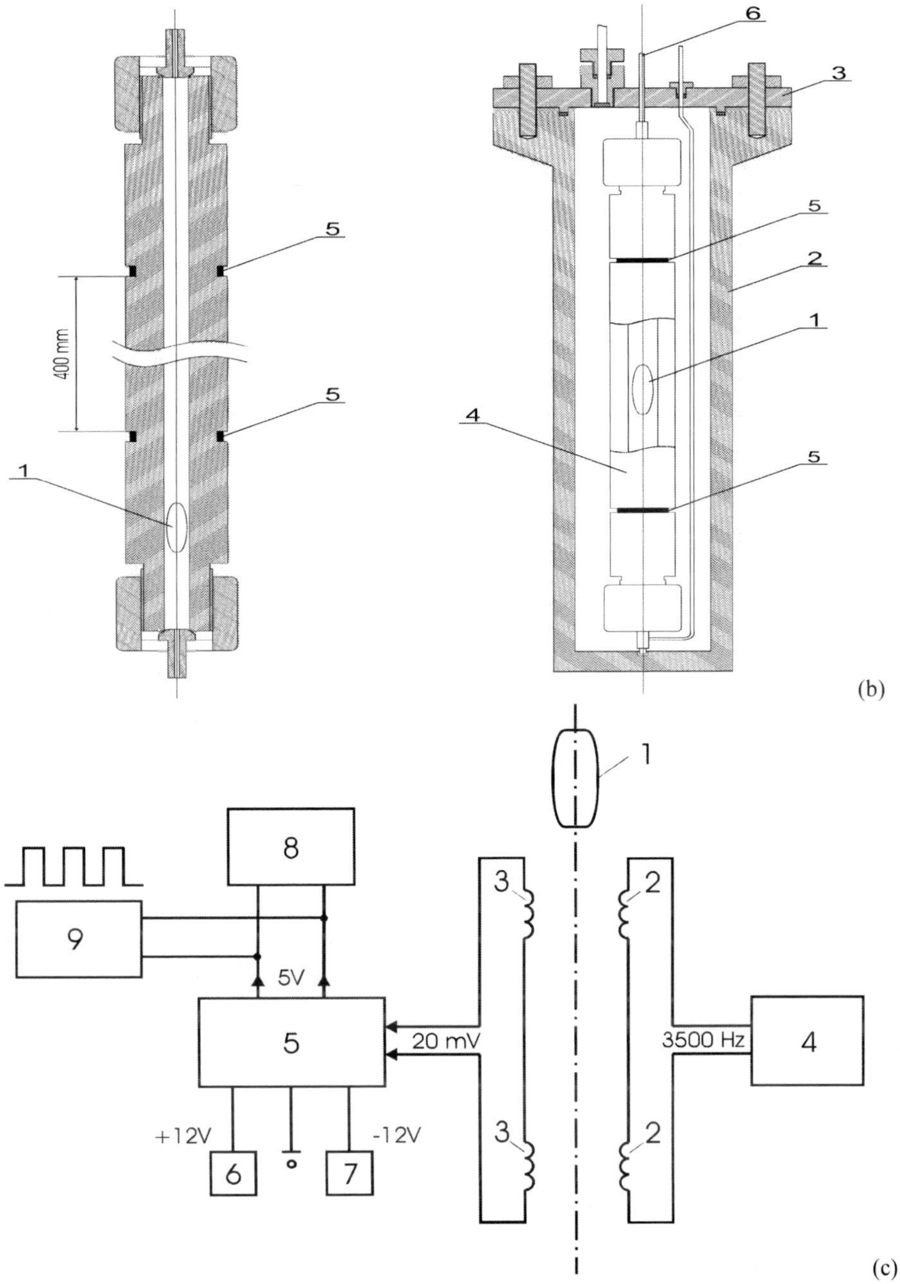

Figure 5a-c. Schematic diagram of a falling-body viscometer (Melikov [89]). Experimental apparatus (5a), fall-tube construction (5b), and fall-time measure unit (5c). (a): 1-high-pressure autoclave; 2-cover of the high-pressure vessel; 3-rotary encoder; 4-liquid thermostat; 5-mixer; 6-circulating pump; 7-thermostating liquid; 8-PRT-10; 9-patentiometer (P363/1); 10-high precise temperature regulator (HPTR-3); 11-manometer, (b): 1- falling-body; 2-high pressure autoclave; 3- cover of the high-pressure vessel; 4- fall-tube; 5- inductance coils (electromagnetic transducers); 6-filling tube, (c): 1- falling-body; 2-primary winding of the transducer; 3-secondary winding of the transducer; 4- generator of the signals; 5-amplifier; 6,7-direct current power supply unit; 8- frequency meter; 9-oscillograph.

3. Discussion of Available Experimental Viscosity Data for Fruit Juices

In Table 2, a summary of all viscosity measurements, to our knowledge, is presented for liquid foods. In the same table, for every fruit juice, the authors, the concentration and the temperature ranges, and the experimental method employed are shown. The tables provide (to our knowledge) the largest and most useful collection of viscosity data at the present time for the liquid foods. As one can see from this Table 2, most available experimental viscosity data sets for liquid foods basically cover a low temperature range (below 60 °C) and limited concentration range. All previous viscosity measurements for liquid foods were performed at atmospheric pressure. Very restricted (about 25 datasets) measurements are available in the literatures at high temperatures (see Table 2) and no data reported at high pressures, except the data reported by the present authors (Magerramov et al. [14,15]) for four fruit (pomegranate, pear, lemon, and tangerine) juices. Majority of viscosity measurements of fruit juices have been made using the concentric cylinder (Haake Rotovisco RV 12), capillary tube, falling sphere, rotational viscometers, and controlled stress rheometer (RheStress RS1) techniques. Most authors used the measured viscosity data to calculate the values of parameters (flow activation energy E_a and η_0) in the Arrhenius viscosity equation. The effect of temperature and concentration on viscosity of fruit juices was study using the various type models (Arrhenius-type equation, polynomial, exponential type, power law and their various combinations).

Figures 6 to 10 shows the typical dependence of the viscosity of fruit juices on temperature, pressure, and concentration. The following four sections 4.1 to 4.4 will provide a brief outline of the available schemes describing the temperature, the pressure and the concentration dependence of the viscosity of liquids and fruit juices. These schemes will be employed to the viscosity of fruit juices in order to perform examine the predictive capability and accuracy of the models and their applicability to the viscosity of fruit juices.

Below we briefly analyzed the reported viscosity datasets for fruit juices. The viscosity measurements for four fruit (pomegranate, pear, tangerine, and lemon) juices have been performed in the temperature range from 292 to 403 K at pressures up to 10 MPa by using the method described above (section 2.1.1.2). The concentration range was between 11 and 45 °Brix. All experimental viscosity data were obtained as a function of temperature for the several fixed concentrations at three isobars (0.1, 5, and 10 MPa). The experimental temperature, viscosity, pressure, and concentration values for the pomegranate, pear, tangerine, and lemon juices are presented in Appendix. The comparison of the data with the values reported by other authors is shown in Figures 11 to 14.

The comparison of the datasets given in Table 2 for various fruit juices was difficult because the viscosity and other thermophysical properties of fruit juices are depend on various factors such as composition and soluble solids content due to: fruit type, generic characteristics, variety, ripening, place in the plant, size, plant nutritive level, agricultural practices, weather. This could explain the published data discrepancy (see below) for fruit juices. Below we briefly discussed the various datasets for some fruit juices.

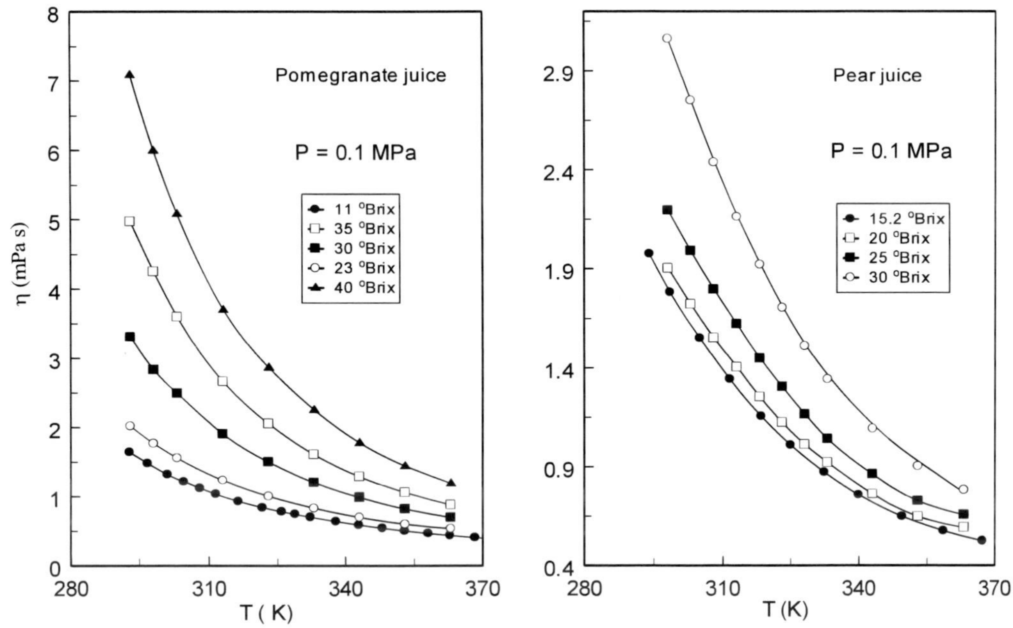

Figure 6. Measured values of viscosity η of pomegranate and pear juices as a function of temperature T along the various constant concentrations. Symbols – experimental values (Magerramov et al. [14]), solid lines calculated with correlation model (Eq.32).

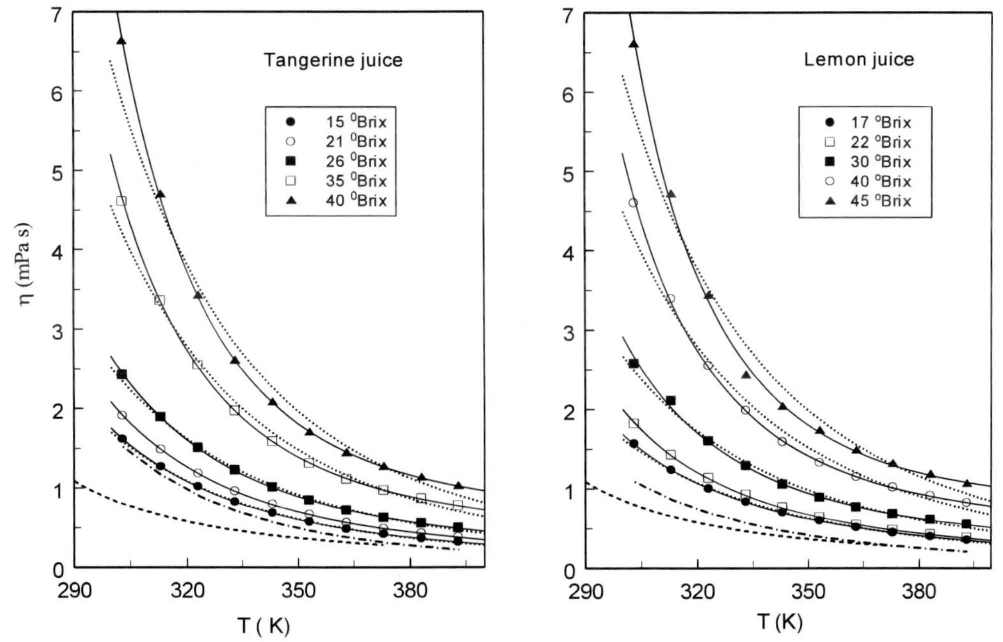

Figure 7. Measured values of viscosity η of tangerine and lemon juices as a function of temperature T along the various constant concentrations. (------), pure water calculated with IAPWS formulation (Kestin et al. [52]); (———), calculated with Eq. (32); (-·· - · - - -), Alvarado and Romero [92] for x=9.4 °Brix (tangerine juice) and x=8.4 °Brix (for lemon juice).

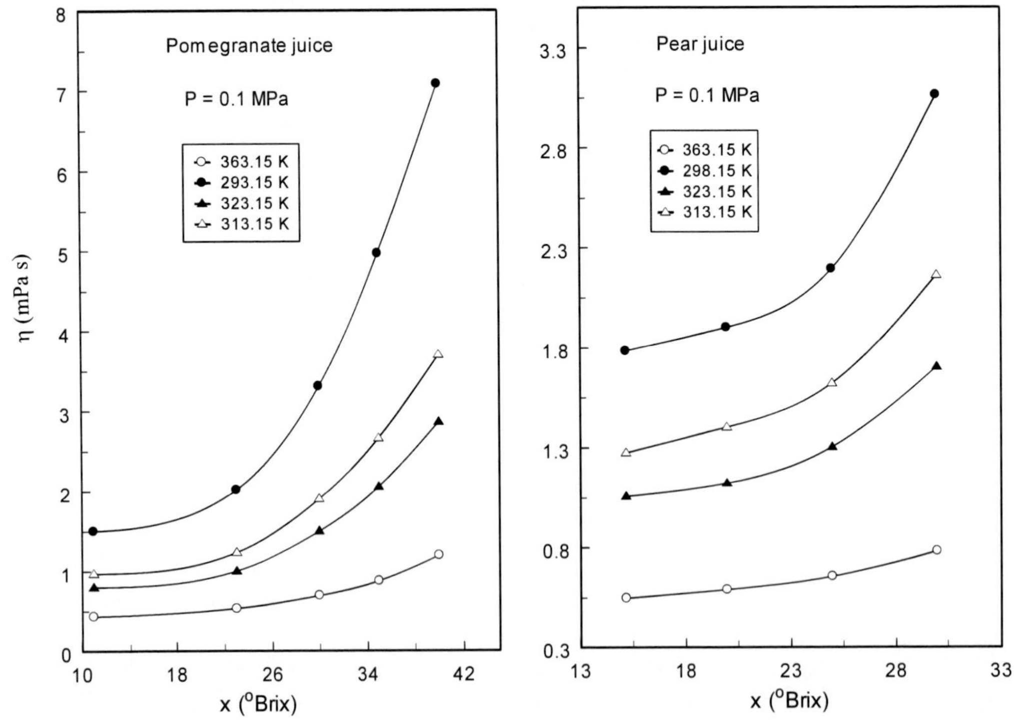

Figure 8. Measured values of viscosity η of pomegranate and pear juices as a function of concentration along the various selected isotherms (Magerramov et al. [14]).

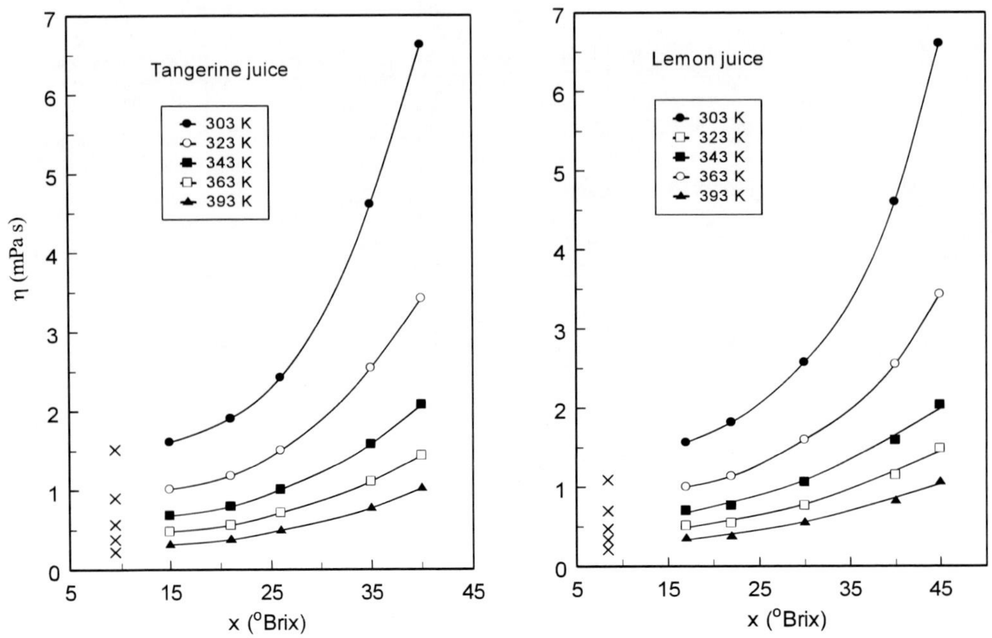

Figure 9. Measured values of viscosity η of tangerine and lemon juices as a function of concentration along the various selected isotherms (Magerramov et al. [15]). ×, Alvarado and Romero [92].

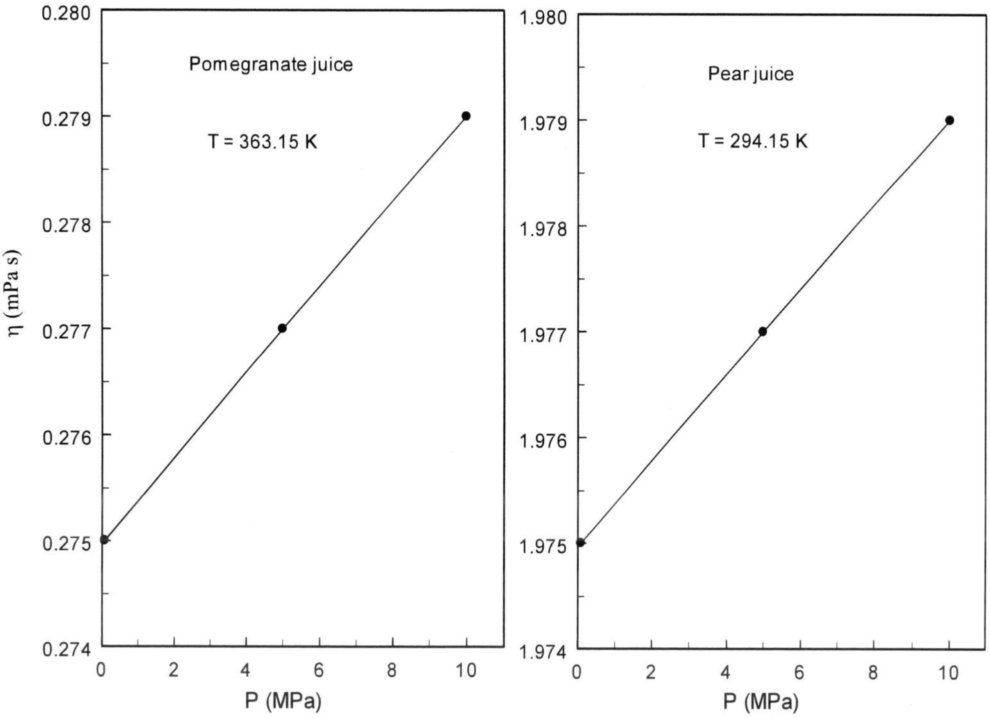

Figure 10. Viscosity of pomegranate and pear juices as a function of pressure along two selected isotherms 294.15 and 363.15 K (Magerramov et al. [14]).

Apple Juice

Nine datasets [38,93,98,107,110,112,159,160,161] were found in the literature for apple juice. Different techniques (capillary tube, coaxial cylinder, rotational viscometers) were used to measure the viscosity of apple juices. These data cover the temperature range from -5 to 80 °C and concentrations from 11 to 75 °Brix. Figure 15 demonstrate the comparison between the experimental data by Ibraz et al. [107] and the data reported by Alvarado and Romero [92] and the values calculated with the model by Bayindirli [93] and Rao [110]. At low concentrations (up to 40-45 °Brix) the agreement between the various datasets is satisfactory (dscrapances within 5-10 %), while at high concentrations (above 50°Brix) the deviations are very large. Probably this is due to difference in physical and chemical characteristics of the juices. Unfortunately some authors is not provide detailed information about physical and chemical characteristics of the studied sample of fruit juices. This is making difficult to estimate the reliability of the various reported datasets for the viscosity of fruit juices.

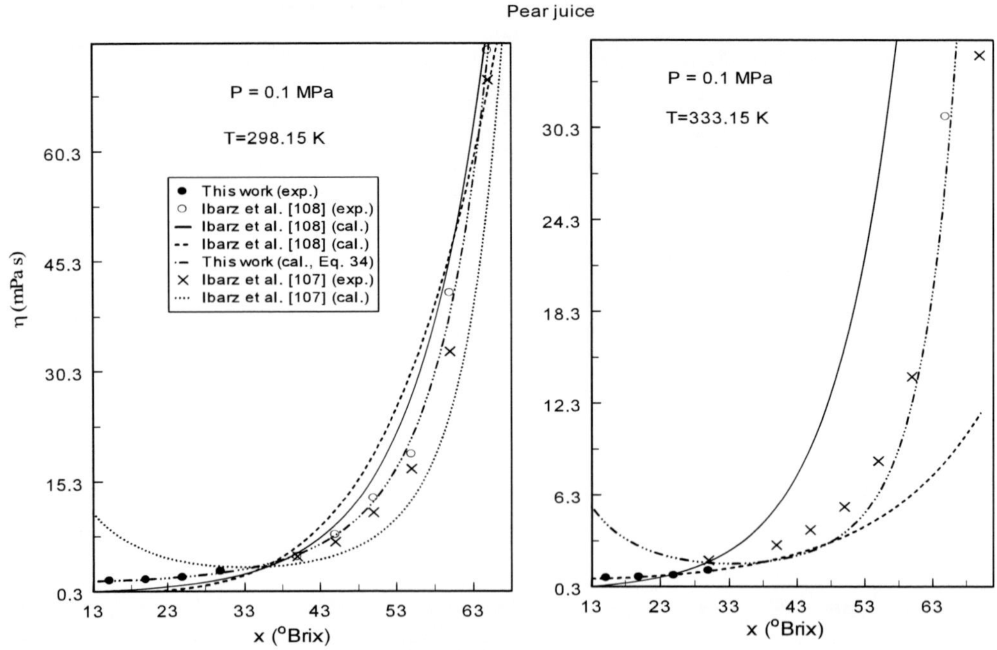

Figure 11. Comparisons of the concentration dependence of the measured and calculated values of the viscosities of pear juice using various models at fixed temperatures of 298.15 and 333.15 K and at atmospheric pressure.

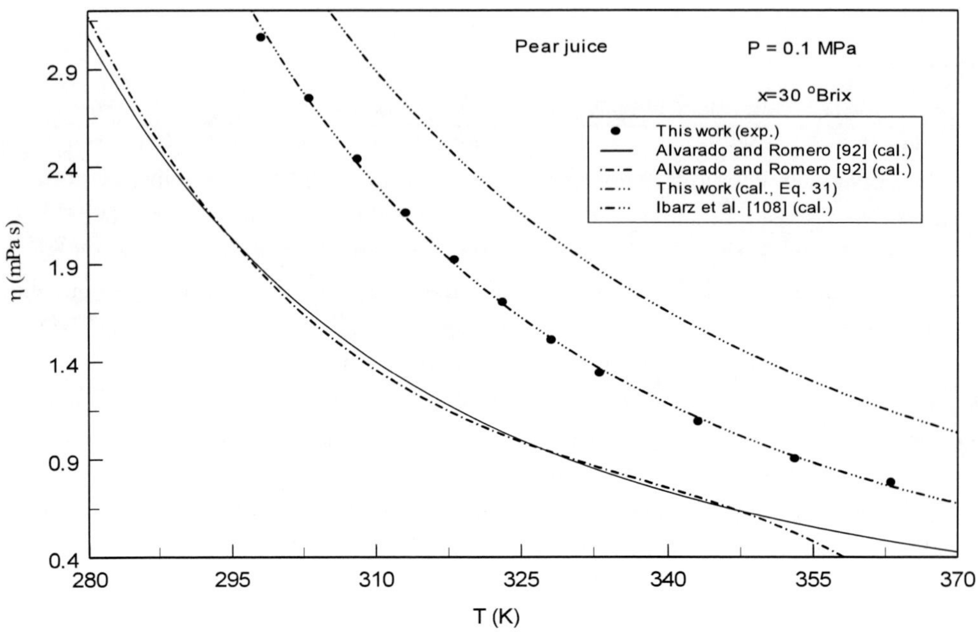

Figure 12. Comparisons of the temperature dependence of the measured and calculated values of the viscosities of pear juice using various models at fixed concentration of 30 °Brix and at atmospheric pressure.

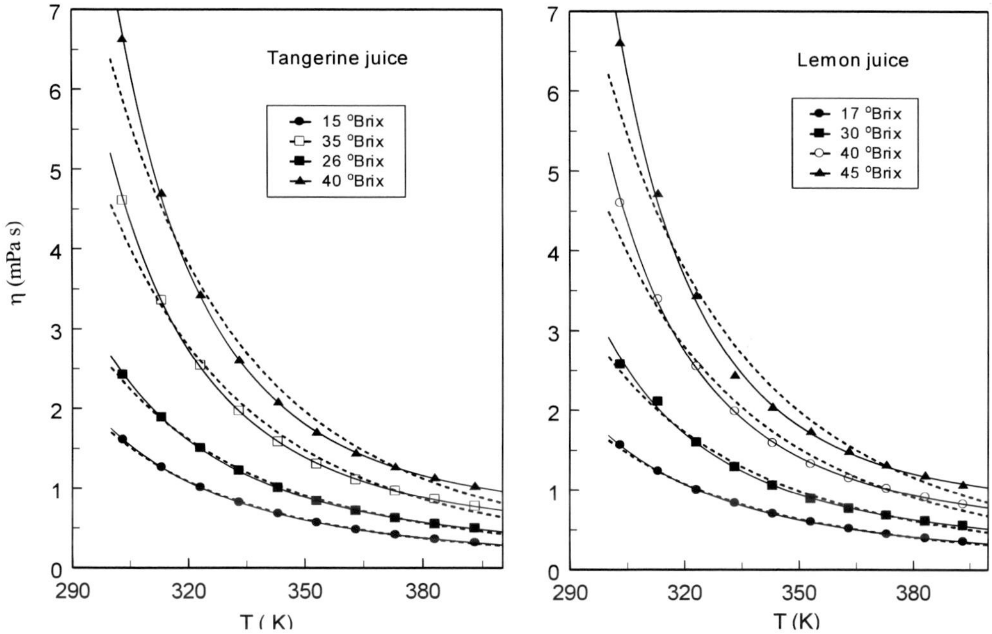

Figure 13. Comparisons of the temperature dependence of the measured (Magerramov et al. [15]) and calculated values of the viscosities of tangerine and lemon juices using various models at fixed concentrations. (------), calculated with original Arrhenius Eq. (31); (———), calculated with extended Arrhenius Eq. (32).

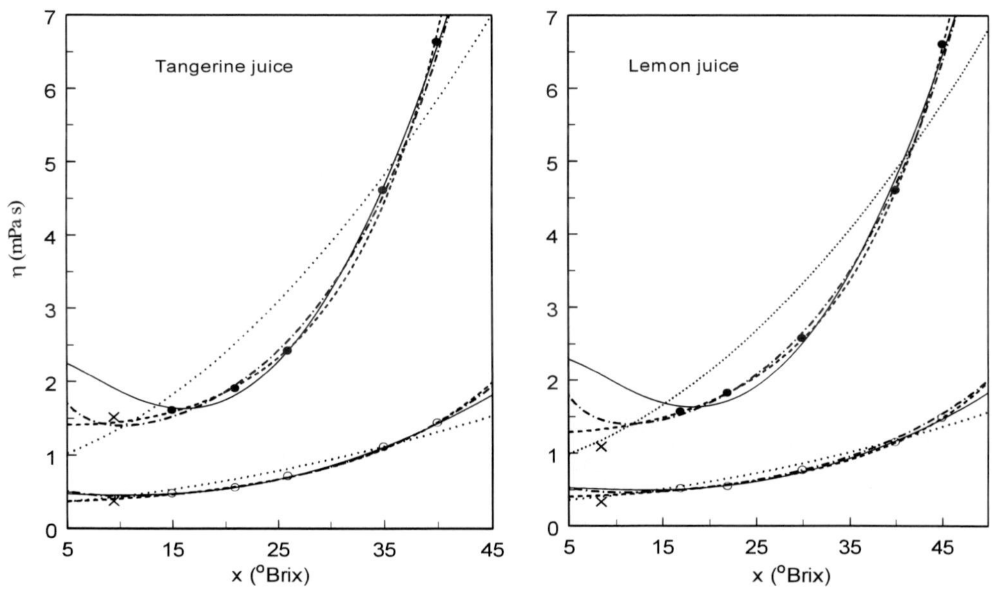

Figure 14. Comparisons of the concentration dependence of the measured and calculated values of the viscosities of tangerine and lemon juices by using the various models at two selected temperatures (303.15 and 363.15) K. ●, this work (303.15 K); ○, this work (363.15 K); ×, Alvarado and Romero [92]. (———), Eq. (37); (--------), Eq. (34); (-· - · - · -), Eq. (35); (·········), Eq. (40).

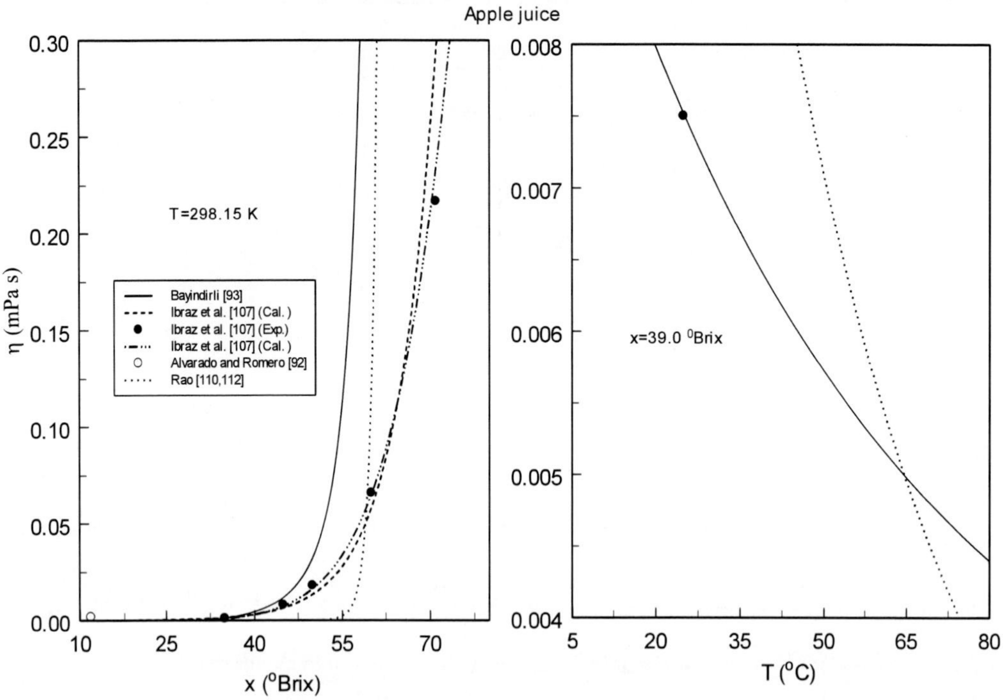

Figure 15. Experimental and calculated values of viscosity of apple juices as a function of concentration (left) and temperature (right) reported by various authors.

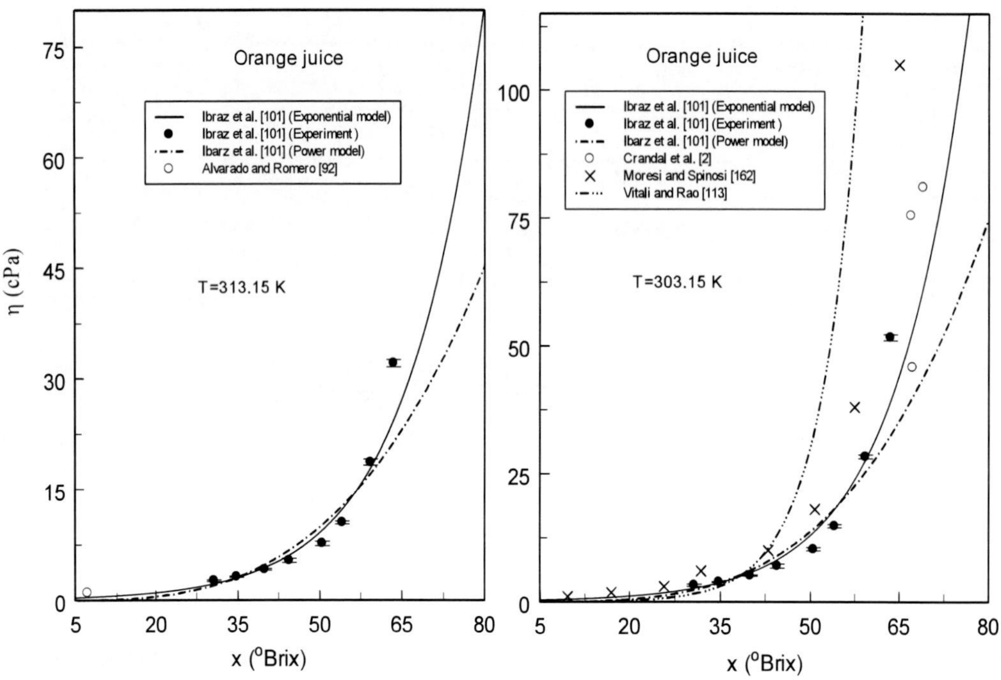

Figure 16. Measured and calculated with various models values of the viscosity of orange juices at two selected temperatures.

Orange Juice

Seventeen datasets [2,39,101,109,113,162-173] were reported by various authors in the literature. These data cover the temperature range from -19 to 80 °C and the concentration from 7 to 69.5 °Brix. Majority of the reported data were derived by using the coaxial cylinders and capillary viscometers. The direct comparison between the various reported viscosity data for orange juice and the values calculated with various viscosity models at selected isotherm of 303.15 K is presented in Figure 16. As one can see, the consistence between various datasets is satisfactory. Good agreement is found at low concentrations, while at high concentration the scattering various datasets is large.

Grape Juice

Six datasets are available in the literature for the grape juice [38,110,112, 160,174,175]. Three different techniques, capillary tube, coaxial cylinders, and rotational viscometer, were used to perform the measurements. Measurements were made over the wide temperature range from -5 to 80 °C at concentrations between 0 and 75 °Brix. Figure 17 provide the comparison between the values of the viscosity of grape juice calculated with the models reported by Bayindirli [95] and Constenla et al. [98] at selected isotherm of 293.15 K and fixed concentration of 13.9 °Brix. The agreement is only qualitatively. The discrepancy is probably due to difference in the chemical composition of the grape juice sample.

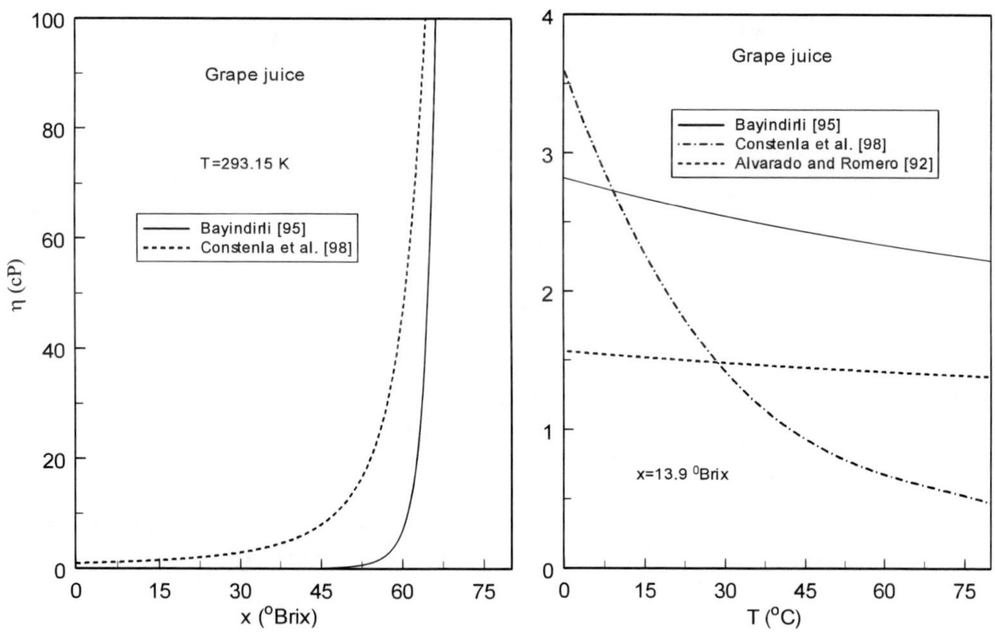

Figure 17. Viscosity of grape juice as a function of concentration (left) and temperature (right) calculated with various models reported in the literature.

Cherry Juice

Only two datasets are available for cherry juice Juszczak and Fortuna [100] and Giner et al. [183]. Both datasets were derived by using the coaxial cylinders technique. The data cover the range from 5 to 70 °C and concentrations from 22 to 74 °Brix. The uncertainty of the reported viscosity data by Genier et al. [183] vary within 0.08 to 190 mPa·s (or 2.77 to 5.9 %) depending on temperature and concentration. Figure 18 demonstrate the comparison between the both datasets for cherry juice in the $\eta - T$ and $\eta - x$ projections for the selected isotherms and concentrations. As one can see, the agreement is acceptable because the uncertainty of the values of viscosity calculated with Juszczak and Fortuna [100] model within 11-12 %. No physical and chemical characteristics of juice are presented in the work by Juszczak and Fortuna [100]. Both authors used the same viscosity model (see below section 4.4 Eqs. 44 and 47) to represent own experimental viscosity data. As one can see from Figure 18, these models fails to represent the experimental data at low temperatures and high concentrations.

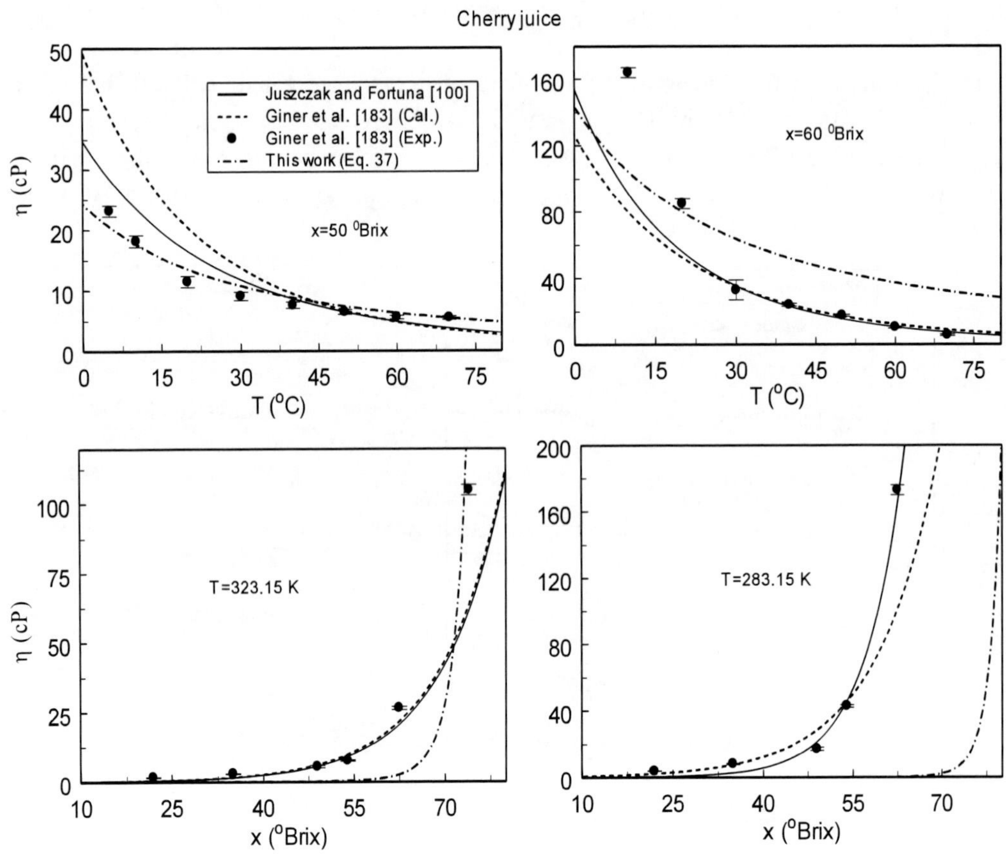

Figure 18. Experimental and calculated values of the viscosity of cherry juice as a function of temperature and concentration reported by various author in the literature.

Pear Juice

Four datasets were found for pear juice [15,92,107,108]. Two different (coaxial cylinders and capillary tube) techniques were employed to measure the viscosity of pear juice at temperatures from 5 to 130 °C and at concentrations between 8 and 71°Brix. The measurements by Magerramov et al. [15] were performed under pressure. The detailed comparison various data sources and prediction model for pear juices is presented in section 4 (see Figures 11 and 12).

Watermelon

Two datasets were reported in the literature for watermelon juice by Alvarado and Romero [92] and Sogi [194]. Measurements by Alvarado and Romero [92] were performed as a function of temperature along the only one concentration of 7.2 °Brix, while Sogi [194] made the measurements at temperatures from 5 to 50 °C and at concentrations from 23 to 42 °Brix. These data were derived by using the capillary tube [92] and rotational [194] viscometers. The comparison between the models reported by Sogi [237] and Alveredo and Romero [92] for watermelon is presented in Figure 19. As one can see the agreement is acceptable.

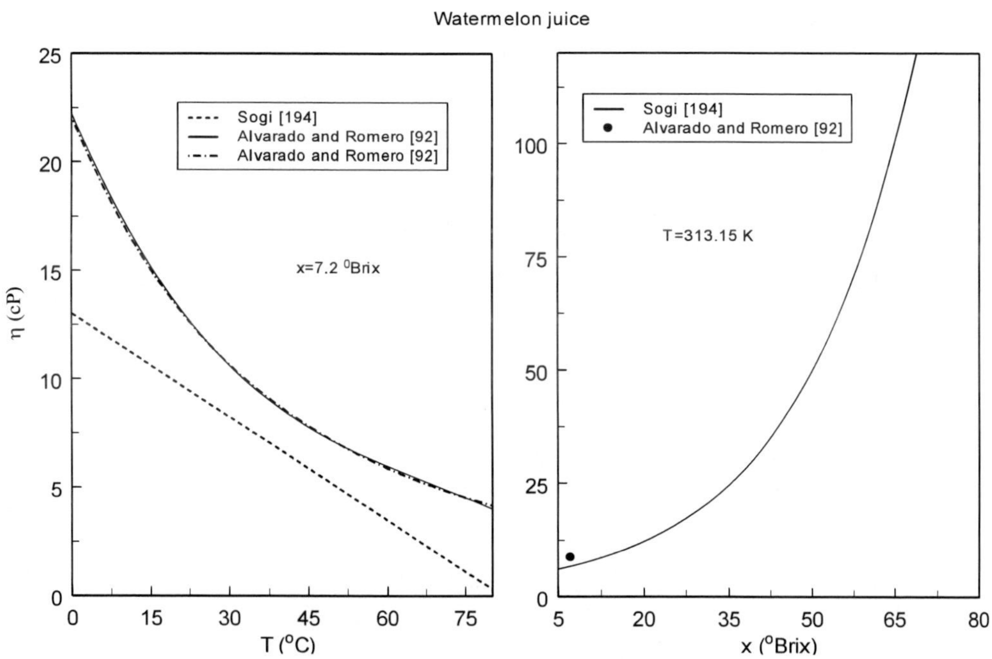

Figure 19. Temperature and concentration dependences of the viscosity of watermelon juice calculated with various models.

Pineapple Juice

Viscosity data for this juice reported by Alvarado and Romero [92], Garciá et al. [187], and Varshney and Kumbhar [168]. The reported data are cover the temperature range from 22 to 45 °C and concentrations range was between 7 and 36 °Brix. Measurements were performed with coaxial cylinder [168] and capillary viscometers [92,187]. The viscosity data for pineapple juices by Garciá et al. [187] and Varshney and Kumbhar [168] together with values calculated from correlation by Alvarado and Romero [92] at selected concentration of 13.9 °Brix are presented in Figure 20. The comparison of the viscosity results reported by various authors is difficult because of temperature and concentration differences between the measurements. Therefore, some time to comparison the various datasets reported by other authors in the literature, we used an interpolating procedure (analytical method). As Figure 20 shows, the agreement between various datasets and prediction models is reasonable.

Pomegranate Juice

The viscosity of pomegranate juice was measured by several authors [15,114,184,185]. The measured range of temperature is from 5 to 130 °C. The concentration ranged from 11 to 75 °Brix. The capillary tube and stress rheometer were used to measure the viscosity. The lack of the enough information provided by the authors in the publications is precluded the comparison reported viscosity data for pomegranate juices. Figures 6,8, and 10 provide the experimental temperature, concentration, and pressure dependences of the viscosity of pomegranate juices together with values calculated from Eq. (32).

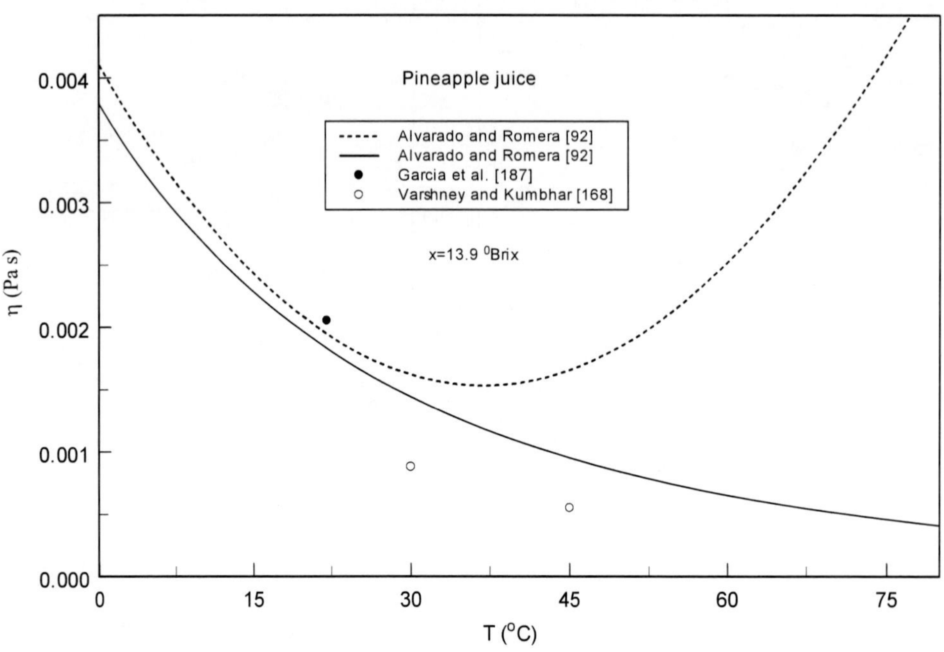

Figure 20. Effect of temperature on the viscosity of pineapple juice at selected concentration.

Mango Juice

Three datasets were reported in the literature by Manohar et al. [198], Rao et al. [111], and Singh and Eipeson [199] for mango juices. Measurements were made with coaxial cylinder and rotational viscometers in the temperature range from 15 to 85 °C and at concentrations between 11 and 66 °Brix. The measured values of viscosity for mango juices were used by Singh and Eipeson [199] to calculate the Arrhenius equation parameters as a function of concentration in the range from 15 to 66 °Brix. The concentration dependence of the Arrhenius equation parameters was presented as exponential function.

Lemon and Tangerine Juices

Only two datasets were found for lemon and tangerine juices (Alvarado and Romero [92] and Magarremov et al. [15]). These data cover the range of temperature from 10 to 119 °C and concentrations between 8.4 and 45 °Brix. Measurements were made with capillary viscometer. The measurements by Magarremov et al. [15] were performed under pressure (up to 10 MPa). Alvarado and Romero [92] reported temperature dependence of the viscosity for lemon and tangerine juices only at one concentration of 8.4 and 9.4 °Brix, respectively. The details of the comparison various datasets and prediction models for lemon and tangerine juices is presented in section 4 (Figures 7 and 14).

Strawberry Juice

Two datasets were found also for strawberry juices (Juszczak and Fortuna [99] and Simpson [195]). Measurements were performed using the capillary tube and coaxial cylinders techniques in the temperature range from 10 to 60 °C and at concentration from 50 to 67.1 °Brix. The measured values of the viscosity by Juszczak and Fortuna [99] were used to calculate the parameters of the combined models (see section 4.4. Eqs. 44 and 47).

Guava Juice

Three datasets were found in the literature for this guava juices reported by Vitali and Rao [196], Garciá et al. [187], and Brekke and Myers [197]. All data were derived by using the capillary tube viscometer. The temperature and concentration ranges were between 22 and 60 °C and 7.2 to 40.8 °Brix, respectively.

Banana Juice

The viscosity of banana juices was measured by Garciá et al. [187] and Khalil et al. [175]. These data cover the temperature range from 22 to 70 °C and concentrations between 13 and 80 °Brix. Measurements were made with coaxial cylinder and capillary viscometers.

Tomato Juice

Seven datasets were found for this juice [176-182]. These data cover the temperature range from 10 to 95 °C and concentrations from 5 to 32 °Brix. Three different techniques (capillary tube, coaxial cylinder, and rotational viscometer) were used to measure the viscosity of the juice.

Cranberry, Raspberry, Peach, Blackcurrant, Celery, Mulberry, and Apricot, Papaya, Grapefruit Juices

For these juices only one reported viscosity dataset was found in the literature. These data were derived by using the coaxial cylinder [104-106,185,200], capillary tube [187], and rotational [167,194]. The comparison between the reported data is not possible due to lack the enough information provided by the authors.

4. Modeling. Prediction and Correlation Techniques

Various models were used in the literature to describe the temperature, concentration, and pressure dependences and their combined effect on the viscosity of liquid foods and aqueous solutions. Most frequently used by various authors models for the viscosity liquid foods and aqueous solutions are summarized in Table 4. Below we briefly reviewed the most often used models to describe the effect of temperature and concentration and their combined effect on the viscosity of fluids and fluid mixtures. We examined the accuracy of the models and their applicability for the fruit juices.

Table 4. Summary of the models used for the correlation of the viscosity of fruit juices and aqueous solutions

Functional Form of the Models	Reference
Temperature dependency models at x=constant	
$\eta(T)=\eta_\infty exp(E_a/RT)$	Juszczak and Fortuna [99,100], Ibraz et al. [102-107], Kaya and Sözer [114], Altan and Maskan [184], Khalil et al. [175], Rao and Anantheswaran [40]
$log\,\eta = a+\dfrac{b}{T-c}$	Rao [19], Soesanto and Williams, [203]
$\eta=\eta_0\exp\left(\dfrac{b}{T}+\dfrac{c}{T^2}\right)$	Magerramov et al. [14,15]

$log\,\eta = a_0 + a_1 T + a_2 T^2$	Rao [204]
$\eta = a_0 + a_1 T + a_2 T^2 + a_3 T^3$	Alvarado and Romero [92]
Concentration dependency models at *T*=constant	
$\eta(T) = \eta_1 x^n$, $\eta(T) = \eta_1\, exp(bx)$	Ibraz et al. [102-107], Juszczak and Fortuna [99, 100], Sogi [194], Altan and Maskan [184], Khalil et al. [175], Singh and Eipeson [199]
$\eta = \eta_3 a_W{}^n$, $\eta(T) = \eta_4\, exp(ba_W)$, a_W -water activity	Ibraz et al. [102-107]
$log\,\eta = 1.1x/(100 - 0.856x)$	Mizrahi [205]
$\eta_S = \eta_{wis} \exp[f(x)]$, $f(m) = a_1 x + a_2 x^2 + \cdots$	Leyendekkers and Hunter [129,130], Leyendekkers [131], Ibarz et al. [108]
$\eta = \dfrac{\eta_0 \exp(xE)}{1 + xV}$,	Goldsack and Franchetto [132,133], Chirife [128] Chirife and Buera [134]
$\eta/\eta_0 = 1 + A\sqrt{x} + Bx$, $\eta/\eta_0 = 1 + A\sqrt{x} + Bx + Dx^2$, $\eta/\eta_0 = 1 + A\sqrt{x} + Bx + Dx^2 + Fx^{2.5}$	Jones and Talley [206], Kaminsky [144-147], Desnoyers and Perron [149], Desnoyers et al. [148], Feakins and Lawrence [150], Robertson and Tyrrell [151], Abdulagatov et al. [127,141-143,152], Abdulagatov and Azizov [140,122-126]
$\eta/\eta_0 = 1 + d_1 x + d_2 x^2 + d_3 x^3$	Kestin and Shankland [61,75], Grimes et al. [74]
$\eta/\eta_0 = 1 + 2.5\phi + 10.05\phi^2 = 1 + 2.5V_k x + 10.05V_k^2 x^2$	Thomas [153], Charm [207]
$\eta/\eta_0 = 1 + 2.5\overline{V}x + k_1\overline{V}^2 x^2 + k_2\overline{V}^3 x^3 + k_3\overline{V}^4 x^4$	Sahu and Behera [157]
Temperature and concentration dependency models at *P*=constant (Combined models for the viscosity of fruit juices)	
$\eta(T) = \eta_3\, exp(E_a/RT + bx)$, $\eta(T) = \eta_4 x^n\, exp(E_a/RT)$	Juszczak and Fortuna [99,100], Alvarado and Romero [92], Altan and Maskan [184], Khalil et al. [175]

Table 4. Continued

Functional Form of the Models	Reference
$\eta(T)=\eta_3\, exp(E_a/RT+ba_W)$, $\eta(T)=\eta_3(a_W)^n\, exp(E_a/RT)$	Ibarz et al. [102-107]
$\eta=a_0(9/5t+32)^{0.9982}(b_0+b_1x+b_2x^2)$	Balint [208]
$\eta=exp(a+b/T+cx)$	Altan et al. [158]
$\eta=\eta_0\exp\left(\frac{(a+b/T)x}{100-(c+dT)x}\right)$	Bayindirli [93-96,209]
$\eta=K_2\exp\left(\frac{E_a}{RT}+K_3x+K_4x^2\right)$	Ibraz et al. [108]
$\eta(T)=\eta_0\, exp(b/T)$, $\ln\eta_0=\sum_{i=0}^{4}a_ix^i$, $b=\sum_{i=0}^{4}b_ix^i$	Magerramov et al. [14,15]
$\eta/\eta_0=1+A\sqrt{x}+Bx+Dx^2$, $A(t)=\sum_{i=0}^{3}A_it^i$, $B(t)=\sum_{i=0}^{3}B_it^i$, $D(t)=\sum_{i=0}^{3}D_it^i$	Magerramov et al. [14,15]
$log\eta=a_0+a_1T+a_2T^2+(b_0+b_1T+b_2T^2)x+(c_0+c_1T+c_2T^2)x^2$	Fernéndez-Martin [210]
$log_{10}\eta=a_0N-a_1(30-T)(a_2+a_3N^{1.25})/(91+T)$, $N=x(1900-18x)$	Peacock [211]
$\eta/\eta_0=1+d_1x+d_2x^2+d_3x^3$, $d_i=\sum_{j=0}^{3}d_{ij}t^j$	Kestin and Shankland [61,75], Grimes et al. [74]
Models which represent the viscosity of juice relative to pure water viscosity (see also Table 11)	
$\eta_r=1+ax/(1+bx^{1/2})+dx$, $\eta_r=\eta/\eta_0$ is the relative viscosity	Elfak et al. [212]

* $log\frac{\eta_0(\theta)}{\eta(20\,°C)}=\frac{\theta}{116-\theta}\{1.2378-1.303\times10^{-3}\theta+3.06\times10^{-6}\theta^2+2.55\times10^{-8}\theta^3\}$,
where θ=20– T/°C, is the viscosity of pure water; The estimated uncertainty of equation is better than ±0.1% (Kestin *et al.* [73])

4.1. Temperature Dependence of the Viscosity of Fruit Juices

The experimental temperature dependences of the viscosity of fruit (pomegranate, pear, tangerine, and lemon) juices along the selected constant concentrations are presented in the Figures 6 and 7 as an example of the typical temperature effect on the viscosity of fruit juices. The viscosity of fruit juices considerably decreases with temperature. For example, as one can see from Figure 6 (left) (see also Table 1 in Appendix), at constant pressures (from 0.1 to 10 MPa) between temperatures (293 and 403) K the viscosity of pomegranate juice is significantly (by a factor of 4 to 7) affected by temperature at high concentrations (above 30 °Brix). However, at low concentrations (below 23 °Brix), the temperature is little (by a factor of 1 to 2) influences viscosity. The effect of temperature on viscosity of fruit juice is different for distinct temperature range. The viscosity of juices is considerably affected by temperature below 360 K. At high temperatures (above 360 K) the rate of the viscosity decreasing with temperature is small. For example, at constant concentrations (from 15 to 40 °Brix) between temperatures (303 and 360) K the viscosity of tangerine and lemon juices changes by factor of 4.5, while at high temperatures (above 360 K) the viscosity changes by factor of 1.5 only. The temperature effect on viscosity strongly depends also on the concentration of juice. At low concentrations (below 30 °Brix) the rate of viscosity changes is small (changes by factor 4), while at high concentrations the rapid changes (by factor 6) of viscosity with temperature is observed (see Figures 6 and 7). To quantitatively estimate the effect of temperature on the viscosity of juices the temperature coefficient of viscosity, $(\partial \ln\eta / \partial T)_x$ was calculated from the measured values of viscosity for tangerine and lemon juices. The temperature coefficient of viscosity for tangerine juice is changes within (0.007 to 0.04) K^{-1} depending on concentration and temperature. At low temperatures the rate of temperature changes of the viscosity, $(\partial\eta / \partial T)_x$, of tangerine juice changes within (0.025 to 0.040) K^{-1}. The highest rate up to 0.04 K^{-1} was found in the low temperature range and high concentrations.

Table 4 provides the list of the various models which were used in the literature to describe the temperature dependence of the viscosity of liquid foods and aqueous solutions. The empirical equation of Arrhenius is valid for temperature dependence of the viscosity of liquid foods [14,15,18,19,29,33,40,92-98,99-108,110,111,112,113-115,116,117]

$$\eta = \eta_0 \exp\left(\frac{b}{T}\right), \tag{31}$$

where η_0 (values of viscosity at high temperatures, $T \to \infty$) and $b = E_a/R$ (E_a is the flow activation energy) are function of concentration. This relation also often used to represent experimental viscosity data for pure fluid and fluid mixtures (for example, aqueous solutions, see [118-127]). However, Eq. (31) failed to represent experimental viscosity data at high temperatures and high concentrations. One more term is required to accurate describe the experimental viscosity data at high temperatures

$$\eta = \eta_0 \exp\left(\frac{b}{T} + \frac{c}{T^2}\right). \tag{32}$$

Equation (31) was theoretically rigorous substantiated by the Eyring's absolute rate theory for concentrated aqueous electrolyte solutions (Glasstone et al. [118]) in the form

$$\eta = \frac{hN}{V}\exp\left(\frac{\Delta G^+}{RT}\right) \text{ or } \eta = A\exp\left(\frac{\Delta H^+}{RT}\right), \tag{33}$$

where ΔG^+ and ΔH^+ are the free enthalpy of activation and enthalpy of activation, h is Planck's constant, N Avogadro's constant, and R the gas constant, V is the molar volume.

Table 5. The Arrhenius Eqs. (31) and (32) parameters ($\ln\eta_0$, $b = E_a / R$, and c) for tangerine and lemon juices as a function of concentration

Equation (31)

	Tangerine juice			**Lemon juice**	
x (°Brix)	$\ln\eta_0$ (mPa s)	$b = E_a / R$ (K)	x (°Brix)	$\ln\eta_0$ (mPa s)	$b = E_a / R$ (K)
15	-6.68899	2165.783	17	-6.10088	1975.496
21	-6.51205	2159.819	22	-6.35765	2097.062
26	-6.17033	2127.509	30	-5.98611	2089.936
35	-6.36895	2365.660	40	-6.09457	2279.163
40	-6.39998	2476.157	45	-6.15909	2395.723
	Pomegranate juice (0.1 MPa)			**Pear juice (0.1 MPa)**	
x (°Brix)	$\ln\eta_0$ (mPa s)	$b = E_a / R$ (K)	x (°Brix)	$\ln\eta_0$ (mPa s)	$b = E_a / R$ (K)
11	0.8590	1898.44	15.2	0.7299	2014.76
23	0.5901	2049.47	20.0	0.7238	2037.26
30	-0.0457	2382.97	25.0	0.6444	2106.70
35	-0.5544	2650.71	30.0	0.1817	2343.95
40	-0.4099	2711.51	40.0	-0.4099	2711.51
	Pomegranate juice (5 MPa)			**Pear juice (5 MPa)**	
11.0	1.0956	1817.28	15.2	0.9075	1958.77
	Pomegranate juice (10 MPa)			**Pear juice (10 MPa)**	
11.0	0.9505	1871.97	15.2	1.3376	1826.50

Equation (32)

	Tangerine juice				**Lemon juice**		
x (°Brix)	$\ln\eta_0$	b	$c\times10^{-5}$	x (°Brix)	$\ln\eta_0$	b	$c\times10^{-5}$
15	-4.5578	693.639	2.5247863	17	-3.4798	164.955	3.1051494

Tangerine juice				Lemon juice			
x (°Brix)	$\ln\eta_0$	b	$c\times10^{-5}$	x (°Brix)	$\ln\eta_0$	b	$c\times10^{-5}$
21	-3.1557	-158.638	3.9762453	22	-2.0487	-879.422	5.1047882
26	-2.0514	-717.649	4.8795601	30	0.5156	-2401.194	7.7024672
35	3.2081	-4249.82	11.345803	40	4.8281	-5265.764	12.939851
40	6.2801	-6282.718	15.021821	45	8.6979	-7866.905	17.600817

The measured values of the viscosity of pomegranate, pear, tangerine, and lemon juices were expressed by the Arrhenius relationship (31) and by Eq. (32). The values of the Arrhenius parameters for pomegranate, pear, tangerine, and lemon juices calculated with the measured viscosity data at atmospheric pressure and at pressures of 5 and 10 MPa as a function of concentration are given in Table 5. This equation represents experimental values of viscosity for fruit juices within 0.65 % in the temperature range from 292 to 363 K. The experimental viscosity data for pear juice as a function of temperature are shown in Figure 12 at selected concentration of 30 °Brix together with the values calculated from Eq. (31) and various correlation models reported by other authors [92,108]. As one can see from Table 5, the values of activation energy for the flow E_a are increases with concentration of juices. The flow activation energy E_a and parameter $\ln\eta_0$ can be directly calculated from the slope and intersect of the straight line by the Arrhenius relationship function ($\ln\eta \approx 1/T$) (Arrhenius plot $\ln\eta$ vs. $1/T$, see Figure 21). The intercepts and slopes of the linear plots ($\ln\eta \approx 1/T$) are flow activation energy E_a and parameter $\ln\eta_0$, respectively. As one can see from Figure 21, $\ln\eta$ *vs.* $1/T$ curves are straight line only for the low concentrations (see also Erickson et al. [219]). Therefore, the curvature of the $\ln\eta$ *vs.* $1/T$ curves at high concentration can be taking into account by relation (32). Figure 13 compare the present results for viscosity with values calculated from Eqs. (31) and (32). As one can see, at low concentrations (below 26 °Brix) both models good represent the experimental data. However, at high concentrations extended Arrhenius model (32) considerable accurate reproduced measured values of the viscosity of tangerine and lemon juices than original Arrhenius model (31). Therefore, Eq. (32) can be recommended for future used to represent experimental viscosity data for fruit juices at high temperatures and high concentrations.

4.2. Concentration Dependence of the Viscosity of Fruit Juices

Figures 8 and 9 show the concentration dependence of the viscosity of fruit juices along various selected isotherms at atmospheric pressure. Figure 8 demonstrate the effect of concentration on the viscosity of pomegranate and pear juices at various fixed temperatures. As one can see from Figure 8, the viscosity of pomegranate and pear fruit juices observed considerably increases (up to 2.2 % to 3.5 %) at concentration above 25 °Brix, especially at low temperatures. The viscosity of tangerine and lemon juices (see Figure 9) in the concentration range from (15 to 45) °Brix changes by factor 3.2 to 4.2. These figures also demonstrate how the behavior of the concentration dependence of the viscosity of fruit juices depends on temperature. As Figures 8 and 9 shows, the viscosity of fruit juices monotonically increases with the concentration. However, the effect of concentration on the viscosity of juices strongly depends on temperature and concentration. For example, at concentrations x<20 °Brix the viscosity is little affected (by factor 1.2) by concentration, while at high concentrations the effect of concentration stronger (by factor 3.5). The rate of the viscosity changes with concentration is depends on temperature also. At low temperatures (below 343 K) the slopes of the $\eta - x$ curves are small (changes by factor 3), while at high temperatures (above 343 K) the rapid changes (by factor 4) of the viscosity with concentration are observed. The concentration coefficient of viscosity, $(\partial \ln \eta / \partial x)_T$, for the juices was calculated using the measured values of the viscosity of fruit juices. The values of concentration coefficient of viscosity for tangerine juice is changes within (0.3 to 4.5) °Brix^{-1} depending on concentration and temperature. The highest rate, $(\partial \ln \eta / \partial x)_T$, up to 4.5 °Brix^{-1} was found in the low temperature range and high concentrations.

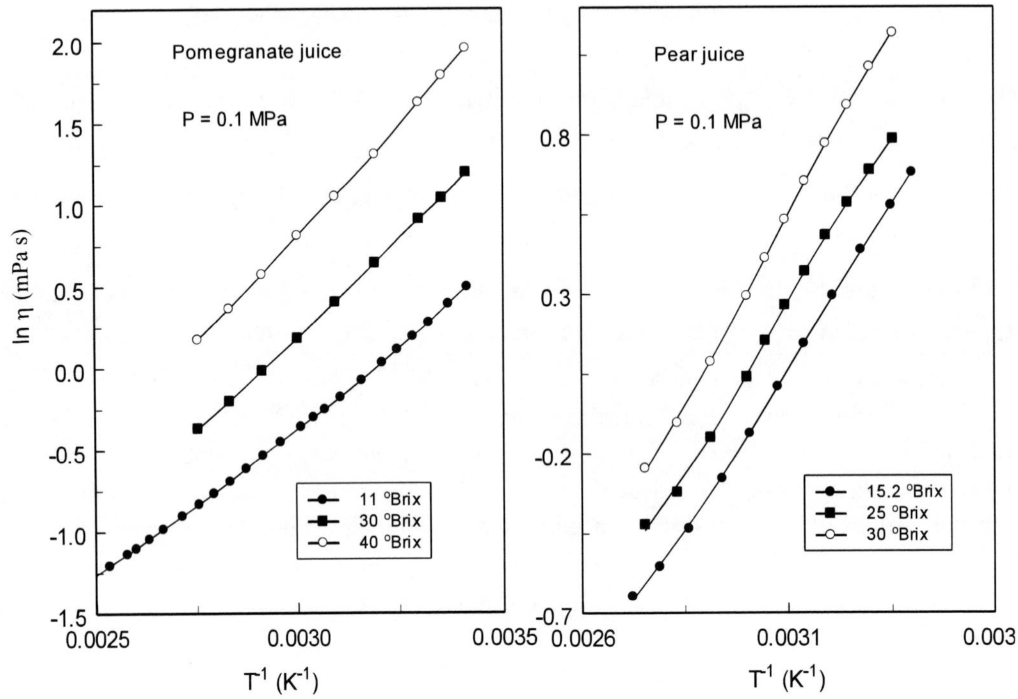

Figure 21. Experimental $ln\,\eta$ as a function of T^{-1} (Arrhenius plot) for pomegranate and pear juices (Magerramov et al. [14]).

There are different theoretical models to represent the concentration dependence of liquid foods and aqueous solutions (see Table 4). Below we briefly discussed the most often used models to describe the effect of concentration on the viscosity of fluids and fluid mixtures and their applicability for fruit juices.

Leyendekkers and Hunter [129,130] and Leyendekkers [131] have applied the TTM (Tammann-Tait-Gibson) model to the calculation of viscosity of the aqueous electrolyte solutions. According TTG model the viscosity equation can be present as

$$\eta_S = \eta_{wis} \exp[f(x)],\ f(x) = a_1 x + a_2 x^2, \tag{34}$$

where η_S and η_{wis} represent the viscosities of the solution (or juice) and the water in solution (or in juice), respectively, and x is the concentration. This relation can be used also to represent the concentration dependence of the viscosity of juices. Figures 11 and 14 depicts the values of the viscosity of pear, tangerine, and lemon juices calculated with Eq. (34) together with other models. The values of parameters of Eq. (34) for some fruit juices derived from the present measurements are given in Table 6. Ibarz et al. [108] also used this relation to accurate represent measured values of the viscosity for pear juice. The agreement between measured and calculated values of viscosity is excellent (AAD is within 0.5 to 1.0 %).

Table 6. The values of parameters $\ln\eta_{wis}$ and a_i (Eqs. 34) for fruit juices as a function of temperature

T (K)	Tangerine juice $\ln\eta_{wis}$ (mPa s)	$a_1\times10^3$ (°Brix^{-1})	$a_2\times10^3$ (°Brix^{-2})	Lemon juice $\ln\eta_{wis}$ (mPa s)	$a_1\times10^3$ (°Brix^{-1})	$a_2\times10^3$ (°Brix^{-2})
303.15	0.38913	-14.9364	1.32523	0.24826	-3.5141	0.88719
313.15	0.09069	-8.2186	1.12571	-0.20719	14.8562	0.53334
323.15	-0.20402	-0.4041	0.91634	-0.31373	7.8867	0.58774
333.15	-0.46844	5.5330	0.75972	-0.61370	18.2529	0.34286
343.15	-0.67651	8.0157	0.68460	-0.66400	8.7517	0.48471
353.15	-0.86352	9.0915	0.64927	-0.74775	2.2142	0.59102
363.15	-1.06047	11.1707	0.61624	-0.93747	4.8031	0.55168
373.15	-1.21220	11.4476	0.62303	-1.12172	8.1858	0.50707
383.15	-1.40096	15.1601	0.57764	-1.28241	10.9391	0.46989
393.15	-1.54684	16.7374	0.56530	-1.43307	13.6984	0.43332
***T* (K)**	**Pomegranate juice $\ln\eta_{wis}$ (mPa s)**	**a_1 (°Brix^{-1})**	**a_2 (°Brix^{-2})**	**Pear juice $\ln\eta_{wis}$ (mPa s)**	**a_1 (°Brix^{-1})**	**a_2 (°Brix^{-2})**
293.15	0.8609	-5.8990	2.303	-	-	-
298.15	0.7103	-5.6930	2.237	1.2596	-8.5280	2.6796
313.15	0.2447	-4.2933	1.838	0.7090	-6.1100	2.1005
333.15	-0.1575	-3.7152	1.587	0.3459	-6.2035	2.0054
353.15	-0.5411	-2.8335	1.302	-0.0667	-5.3504	1.7390
363.15	-0.7754	-1.6360	0.993	-0.5167	-2.0361	0.9744

Goldsack and Franchetto [132,133] proposed the simplified form of the Eq. (33) to describe the concentration dependence of the aqueous solutions

$$\eta = \frac{\eta_0 \exp(xE)}{1 + xV}, \tag{35}$$

where η is the viscosity of the solution or juice at a concentration x and temperature T, η_0 is the viscosity of the solvent (pure water) at temperature T, x is the concentration, and E and V are the adjustable parameters. The temperature dependence of the viscosity of fruit juices can be explained in terms of the temperature dependence of the E and V parameters of an Eq. (35). Unfortunately, the theory cannot to predict the temperature dependence of the E and V. Therefore, the values of the parameters E and V can be extracted from the experimental data as a function of temperature by fitting each isotherm to the Eq. (35). The results of the application of Eq. (35) to the measured viscosities of pomegranate, pear, tangerine, and lemon juices are presented in Table 7. This model has been used by Chirife [128] and Chirife and Buera [134] to fit viscosity data of various sugar and sugar mixtures up to very high concentrations.

Table 7. The values of parameters V and E (Eq. 35) for fruit juices as a function of temperature

Tangerine juice				Lemon juice			
T (K)	η_0 (mPa s)	E (°Brix^{-1})	V (°Brix^{-1})	T (K)	η_0 (mPa s)	E (°Brix^{-1})	V (°Brix^{-1})
303.15	24.5624	0.09662	4.50	303.15	18.6009	0.08545	3.00
333.15	18.8733	0.08579	5.50	333.15	0.93089	0.09209	0.15
363.15	1.17754	0.08080	0.49	363.15	0.95924	0.07136	0.32

Pomegranate juice				Pear juice			
T (K)	η_0 (mPa s)	E (°Brix^{-1})	V (°Brix^{-1})	T (K)	η_0 (mPa s)	E (°Brix^{-1})	V (°Brix^{-1})
293.15	324.27	0.1022	67.988	298.15	180.890	0.0843	25.322
303.15	128.25	0.0970	30.662	313.15	161.211	0.0813	28.984
313.15	85.799	0.0930	23.984	323.15	78.5376	0.0800	17.134
323.15	32.125	0.0910	10.723	333.15	42.5676	0.0760	10.492
363.15	16.011	0.0795	8.1656	343.15	36.0353	0.0750	10.532
-	-	-	-	363.15	9.4179	0.0690	3.1565

The existing theoretical result which describes the concentration dependence of the viscosity of aqueous solutions is valid only at very dilution. Falkenhagen – Onsager – Fuoss [135,136] and Debye-Hückel-Onsager [137,138] theory predicts a square root concentration, $\frac{\eta}{\eta_0} \propto \sqrt{x}$ (limiting law), dependence of the viscosity of solutions at infinite dilution ($x \to 0$). This theory correctly explains the rise of viscosity with concentration in the limit of very low (dilute solutions) concentrations. The dilute solution theories [135-138] of viscosity are not practicable because of their very limited concentration range. Jones and Dole [139] proposed an empirical extension of the previous model [135] to high concentrations as

$$\frac{\eta}{\eta_0} = 1 + A\sqrt{x} + Bx. \tag{36}$$

In Eq. (36) η and η_0 are the viscosities of an electrolyte solution and pure solvent (water), respectively, A is an always positive constant, and x is the concentration. Several authors [140-143,133,144-151], included a quadratic term Dc^2 (extended Jones-Dole equation)

$$\frac{\eta}{\eta_0} = 1 + A\sqrt{x} + Bx + Dx^2, \tag{37}$$

to extend the Jones-Dole equation for more concentrated solutions. Abdulagatov et al. [127, 141-143,152] added one more term $Fc^{2.5}$ for application Eq. (37) to higher concentration (up to saturation)

$$\frac{\eta}{\eta_0} = 1 + A\sqrt{x} + Bx + Dx^2 + Fx^{2.5}. \tag{38}$$

The measured relative viscosities for pomegranate, pear, tangerine and lemon juices were fitted with the Eqs. (37) (Magerramov et al. [14,15]). The derived values of the parameters are given in Table 8 as a function of temperature. Good agreement (within 0.5 to 1.2 %) was found between measured and calculated with Eq. (37) values of viscosity.

Kestin and Shankland [75] and Grimes et al. [74] omitted the square-root term owing to its small magnitude to describe the concentration dependence of the experimental viscosity data for aqueous solutions. The experimental viscosity data for aqueous solutions were fitted to

Table 8. The values of parameters *A*, *B*, and *D* (Eq. 37) for fruit juices as a function of temperature

Tangerine juice				Lemon juice			
T (K)	*A* (°Brix$^{-1/2}$)	*B* (°Brix^{-1})	*D* (°Brix^{-2})	*T* (K)	*A* (°Brix$^{-1/2}$)	*B* (°Brix^{-1})	*D* (°Brix^{-2})
303.15	2.2595	-0.7144	0.013450	303.15	2.1389	-0.6362	0.010566
313.15	1.7283	-0.5398	0.010497	313.15	1.3524	-0.3983	0.007366
323.15	1.2532	-0.3866	0.007977	323.15	1.1645	-0.3372	0.006196
333.15	0.9540	-0.2918	0.006367	333.15	0.5575	-0.1524	0.003620
343.15	0.7997	-0.2442	0.005512	343.15	0.7314	-0.2042	0.004083

Table 8 – (Continued)

353.15	0.6815	-0.2105	0.004915	353.15	0.8112	-0.2308	0.004329
363.15	0.5931	-0.1877	0.004566	363.15	0.7101	-0.2045	0.004001
373.15	0.5859	-0.1889	0.004589	373.15	0.6514	-0.1900	0.003863
	Pomegranate juice					**Pear juice**	
T **(K)**	***A*** **(°Brix$^{-1/2}$)**	***B*** **(°Brix^{-1})**	***D*** **(°Brix^{-2})**	***T*** **(K)**	***A*** **(°Brix$^{-1/2}$)**	***B*** **(°Brix^{-1})**	***D*** **(°Brix^{-2})**
298.15	1.4779	-0.5033	0.01029	298.15	1.9165	-0.5829	0.01043
303.15	1.3383	-0.4545	0.00940	303.15	1.9028	-0.5755	0.01028
313.15	1.1312	-0.3799	0.00792	313.15	1.5249	-0.4516	0.00830
323.15	1.0153	-0.3383	0.00705	323.15	1.4000	-0.4132	0.00759
333.15	0.9378	-0.3086	0.00634	333.15	1.2335	-0.3594	0.00654
343.15	0.8223	0.2672	0.00551	343.15	1.1462	-0.3333	0.00601
353.15	0.7149	-0.2310	0.00482	353.15	1.0755	-0.3099	0.00549
363.15	0.5871	-0.1859	0.00400	363.15	0.6807	-0.1774	0.00342

$$\frac{\eta}{\eta_0} = 1 + d_1 x + d_2 x^2 + d_3 x^3, \tag{39}$$

where $d_i = \sum_{j=0}^{3} d_{ij} t^j$ are the function of temperature.

Thomas [153] has extended the Einstein relation (Einstein [154]) for the hydrodynamic effect to high concentrations by showing that for suspensions the relative viscosity is given by the relation

$$\frac{\eta}{\eta_0} = 1 + 2.5\phi + 10.05\phi^2 = 1 + 2.5V_k x + 10.05V_k^2 x^2 . \tag{40}$$

Table 9. The values of V_k (Eq. 40) for fruit juices as a function of temperature

T, K	$V_k \times 10^3$	*T*, K	$V_k \times 10^3$
Tangerine juice		**Pomegranata juice**	
303.15	0.3639	293.15	0.2805
313.15	0.3257	298.15	0.2691
323.15	0.2909	303.15	0.5670
333.15	0.2601	313.15	0.2309
343.15	0.2370	323.15	0.2123
353.15	0.2166	333.15	0.1924
363.15	0.2010	343.15	0.1752
373.15	0.1916	353.15	0.1600
393.15	0.1786	363.15	0.1484

Lemon juice		Pear juice	
303.15	0.2903	298.15	0.2687
313.15	0.2663	303.15	0.2725
323.15	0.2330	308.15	0.2696
333.15	0.2039	313.15	0.2643
343.15	0.1883	318.15	0.2538
353.15	0.1762	323.15	0.2435
363.15	0.1680	328.15	0.2308
373.15	0.1636	333.15	0.2179
383.15	0.1581	353.15	0.1828
393.15	0.1575	363.15	0.1840

As was shown by Breslau and Miller [155], this relation can be used to represent concentration dependence of the relative viscosity for concentrated aqueous electrolyte solutions if V_k is taken as an adjustable parameter. Abdulagatov et al. [122-127,140-143,152] used Eq. (40) to determine the values of V_k as a function of temperatures for some aqueous solutions from measured values of viscosity. Therefore, the relation (40) can be used to estimate the values of the hydrodynamic volume V_k (rigid molar volume) using the experimental relative viscosity data. Moulik and Rakshit [156] also used Eq. (40) to correlate the concentration dependence of the viscosity of 72 different aqueous solutions at high concentrations. Sahu and Behera [157] also represented experimental relative viscosity of aqueous solutions by extending the limiting Einstein equation as

$$\frac{\eta}{\eta_0} = 1 + 2.5\overline{V}x + k_1\overline{V}^2x^2 + k_2\overline{V}^3x^3 + k_3\overline{V}^4x^4, \qquad (41)$$

where $\overline{V}$ is the volume of solution, x is the concentration. The measured viscosity values for pomegranate, pear, tangerine and lemon juices were fitted to the Eq. (40) (Magerramov et al. [14,15]). Note that this model is containing just one adjusting parameter V_k. The derived values of the parameter V_k for these juices are presented in Table 9 as a function of temperature.

4.3. Pressure Dependence of the Viscosity of Fruit Juices

Experimental viscosities of pomegranate and pear juices as a function of pressure are shown in Figure 10. The viscosity is little affected, (up to 1.5-1.7 %) at high temperatures (406 K) and up to 0.4-0.6 % at low temperatures (298 K), by pressure (at pressure changing between 0.1 and 10 MPa) along the constant temperature and constant concentration. The pressure dependence of the experimental viscosity of both juices in the range from 0.1 to 10 MPa is almost linear (see Figure 10). The values of experimental viscosity along an isotherm and constant concentration can be correlated within the experimental precision as a function of pressure by means of a linear expression (Kestin et al. [60], Kestin and Shankland [75])

$$\eta(T,x,P)=\eta_0(T,x)[1+\beta(T,x)(P-P_0)], \tag{42}$$

where $\eta_0(T,x)$ is the viscosity at P_0=0.101325 MPa (atmospheric pressure), can be correlated in terms of temperature and concentration, and $\beta(T,x)=\frac{1}{\eta_0}\left(\frac{\partial\eta}{\partial P}\right)_{T,x}$ is the pressure coefficient of viscosity. This equation was successfully used by Kestin et al. [60] and Kestin and Shankland [75] to represent pressure dependence of viscosity of the aqueous electrolyte solutions.

4.4. Combined Effect of the Temperature and Concentration on the Viscosity of Fruit Juices

Both the temperature and concentration variations of the viscosity of fruit juices were combined by Rao [18] and Cepeda and Villarán [97] in a single exponential model (modification of the relation 31) for depectinised juice

$$\eta=exp\left(a+\frac{b}{T}+cx\right)\text{ or }\eta=exp(a+cx)exp\left(\frac{b}{T}\right) \tag{43}$$

This relation was used by Jusczak and Fortuna [100] to represent measured values of viscosity of cherry juice. They also proposed other model (combination of the power and exponential functions) to combine the temperature and concentration dependence of viscosity

$$\eta=\eta_0x^{\alpha}\exp\left(\frac{E_a}{RT}\right). \tag{44}$$

Rao et al. [112] and Ibarz et al. [107] used an exponential-type and a power-type relation to describe the effect of concentration on viscosity of fruit juices at constant temperature. Bayindirli [93,95] reported the model to describe the temperature and concentration effects on viscosity of grape juices as

$$\eta=\eta_0\exp\left(\frac{(a+b/T)x}{100-(c+dT)x}\right). \tag{45}$$

The experimental values of flow activation parameter E_a in Arrhenius equation for crab apple juice were fitted by Cepeda and Villarán [97] to a third degree polynomial equation. Alvarado and Romero [92] used exponential dependence on concentration of the parameter,

$\eta_0 = \eta_1 \exp(ax)$ in Arrhenius equation in order to study of the combined effect of the temperature and concentration to the viscosity of juices. Ibraz et al. [108] proposed following form of the equation to describe the combined effect of temperature and concentration on the pear juice

$$\eta = K_2 \exp\left(\frac{E_a}{RT} + K_3 x + K_4 x^2\right) \text{ or } \eta = K_2\, exp\left(K_3 x + K_4 x^2\right) exp\left(\frac{E_a}{RT}\right) \tag{46}$$

Kaya and Sözer [114] and Altan and Maskan [184] proposed a simple equation for describing the combined effect of temperature and soluble solids content on the pomegranate juice

$$\eta = \eta_2\, exp\left(\frac{E_a}{RT} + Cx\right). \tag{47}$$

In order to describe the combined effect of temperature and concentration on the viscosity of fruit juices we used theoretically based Eqs. (32), (34) to (41) for the aqueous solutions. Because the theory cannot predict the concentration dependence of the parameters $\ln \eta_0$, b and c in Eqs. (31), (32) and temperature dependence of the parameters (V, E, A, B, C, D, V_k, and k_i) in Eqs. (34) to (41), we empirically extended these models to study of the combined effect of temperature and concentration on the viscosity of fruit juices by taken into account the concentration and temperature dependences of these parameters. These parameters (in Eqs. 32, 34 to 41) were considered as a simple polynomial function of concentration and temperature

$$ln\eta_0 = \sum_{i=0}^{n} a_i x^i \text{ and } b = \sum_{i=0}^{n} b_i x^i, \tag{48}$$

$$Y(A,B,C,D,V_k,k_i) = \sum_{i=0}^{n} a_i T^i. \tag{49}$$

We experimentally studied the concentration and temperature dependences of the adjustable parameters in theoretically based Eqs. (31), (32), (34) to (41). As Tables 7 to 9 shows, the temperature dependences of theoretically and physically meaning parameters V_k, V, and E is very simple function of temperature and can be very readily described by the polynomial functions. The parameters V_k, V, and E are monotonically decreases with temperature and can be presented as simple polynomial function. In the first approaches these parameters can be presented as linear function of temperature (or first order polynomial function), although to more accurately representation of the experimental data in some cases high order polynomial functions (second, for example) are needed. Equations (31), (32), (34)-

(41) together with (48) and (49) are providing the best description (within 0.8 to 2.0 %) of the experimental viscosity data for fruit juices.

The Arrhenius Eq. (31) with concentration dependences coefficients (Eq. 48) was applied to the measured values of the viscosity of pomegranate and pear juices. The derived values of the coefficients a_i and b_i in Eq. (48) are summarized in Table 10. Equation (31) together with (48) describes the experimental viscosity data for pomegranate and pear juices with accuracy of 2.0 %. Figure 14 compare the concentration dependence of the measured and calculated with various models the values of viscosity for tangerine and lemon juices at two selected temperatures of (303.15 and 363.15) K. As one can see from this figure, Eq. (34) and (37) excellent represents the present measurements for tangerine and lemon juices. These models can be recommended to future used for the describing of experimental viscosity data for liquid foods.

Table 10. Parameters a_i and b_i for Eq. (48)

	Pomegranate juice (R^2=0.998)				
	0	1	2	3	4
a_i	1.0662×10^{0}	-1.0327×10^{0}	7.5160×10^{-2}	-2.3096×10^{-3}	2.4463×10^{-5}
b_i	6.7579×10^{2}	2.6653×10^{2}	-2.0716×10^{1}	0.6811×10^{0}	-7.4490×10^{-3}
	Pear juice (R^2=0.998)				
	0	1	2	3	4
a_i	-3.4380×10^{0}	-0.4434×10^{0}	2.3646×10^{-2}	-4.175×10^{-4}	0.0×10^{0}
b_i	9.8756×10^{2}	1.6503×10^{2}	-8.894×10^{0}	0.1633×10^{0}	0.0×10^{0}

Table 11. Comparison accuracy and predictive capability of various combined models for the viscosity of lemon juice (K_i, a_i) parameters of the models)

	1	2	3	4	5	S^*
$\eta=\eta_0\ exp\left(\dfrac{(a_1+a_2/T)x}{100-(a_3+dT)x}\right)$						
a_i	$\ln\eta_0$=6.2208	225.596	-33317.26	30.54578	-0.015775	0.459×10^{-1}
$\eta=K_2\exp\left(\dfrac{E_a}{RT}+K_3x+K_4x^2\right)$						
K_i	$\ln K_2$=-6.9749	E_a/R=2167.48	K_3=0.008528	K_4=0.0005404	-	0.534×10^{-2}
$\eta=\eta_0\exp\left(\dfrac{b}{T}\right)$, $b=\sum_{i=0}^{4}a_ix^i$						
a_i	-6.2173	0.002522	1745.58	13.6980	-	0.583×10^{-2}
$\eta=exp\left(a_1+\dfrac{a_2}{T}+a_3x\right)$, $\eta=\eta_2\ exp\left(\dfrac{E_a}{RT}+Cx\right)$						
a_i	$\ln a_1$ =-7.4375	2167.48	0.04214	-	-	0.699×10^{-2}

$\eta = \eta_0 x^{\alpha} \exp\left(\frac{E_a}{RT}\right)$						
a_i	$\ln\eta_0$=-10.171	E_a / R=2167.48	1.1982	-	-	0.152×10^{-1}
$\eta = \eta_0 \exp[f(x)],\ f(x) = a_1x + a_2x^2$						
a_i	0.02352	0.0003062	-	-	-	0.216×10^{-1}
$\frac{\eta}{\eta_0} = 1 + a_1x + a_2x^2 + a_3x^3$						
a_i	0.08634	-0.004037	0.0001075	-	-	0.515×10^{-2}
$\frac{\eta}{\eta_0} = 1 + 2.5\phi + 10.05\phi^2 = 1 + 2.5V_kx + 10.05V_k^2x^2$						
V_k	0.01043	-	-	-	-	0.759×10^{-2}
$\frac{\eta}{\eta_0} = 1 + 2.5\overline{V}x + a_1\overline{V}^2x^2 + a_2\overline{V}^3x^3 + a_3\overline{V}^4x^4$						
a_i	0.03693	-0.00625	0.0002126	-0.00000165	-	0.524×10^{-2}
$\frac{\eta}{\eta_0} = 1 + a_1\sqrt{x} + a_2x + a_3x^2$						
a_i	0.717976	-0.206593	0.004243	-	-	0.510×10^{-2}
$\eta = \frac{\eta_0 \exp(xE)}{1 + xV}$						
E, V	0.09178	-0.10738	-	-	-	0.130×10^{-1}
$\eta = \eta_0 \exp\left(\frac{b}{T} + \frac{c}{T^2}\right),\ \ln\eta_0 = a_1x,\ b = a_2 + a_3x,\ c = a_4 + a_5x$						
a_i	0.09358	-2528.299	-49.8041	729457.81	10993.444	0.319×10^{-2}

[*] Error function $S = \frac{1}{N}\sum_i \left(Y_i^{cal} - Y_i^{exp}\right)$

Table 11 is providing the comparison accuracy of the models for lemon juice. As one can see from the table, Eqs. (37) and (39) are provide the best representation of the measured values of the viscosity of lemon juice. These models based on the pure water viscosity and contain only 3 adjustable parameters. Reasonable representation of the temperature and concentration effect on the viscosity of lemon juice was observed also for the one-parametric model (40) which based on the extended Einstein relation. The predictive (extrapolating properties) capability of the model (Eq. 40) is much better than other models.

Bálint [208] developed combined model by using the combination polynomial and power functions for the viscosity of whey

$$\eta = 0.0638(9/5t + 32)^{0.9982}\left(1.0042 + 3.11x + 14.7x^2\right). \tag{50}$$

Recently, an artificial network (ANN) model was developed for the prediction of viscosity of fruit juices as function of concentration and temperature by Rai et al. [220]. The accuracy of the model is within 3.78 to 4.20 mPa·s. Peacock [211] proposed the another model for the viscosity of sucrose solutions in the form

$$log_{10}\,\eta = a_0 N - a_1(30 - T)(a_2 + a_3 N^{1.25})/(91 + T), \tag{51}$$

where $N = x(1900 - 18x)$. The range applicability of the model is from 10 to 80 °C and between 0 and 85 °Brix.

5. Conclusion

In this chapter the different techniques employed for the measurement of viscosity of liquids and liquid foods were discussed. These were the capillary-flow technique, the oscillating-disc technique and the falling-body method. From the discussion of the techniques it is apparent that measurements performed with the capillary-flow viscometer and the oscillating-disc viscometer enjoy a low degree of uncertainty. Hence, measurements would be expected to attain an uncertainty of better than 2 %. Measurements performed with the falling-body viscometer would be expected to attain a higher uncertainty.

The temperature, pressure, and concentration dependences of the viscosity of fruit juices were studied. The values of the flow activation energy E_a of the temperature dependence Arrenius equation were calculated for the viscosity of pomegranate, pear, tangerine, and lemon juices as a function of concentration and pressure. In order to represent combined effect of concentration and temperature on the viscosity of fruit juices the various models were examined.

A new correlation and prediction models for the viscosity was developed. The applicability of the various theoretical based models used previously for aqueous solutions to describe the effect of temperature and concentration on viscosity of fruit juices was studied. The measured values of viscosity of fruit juices were used to test and confirm the accuracy and predictive capability of various theoretical and semi-empirical viscosity models.

An accuracy and predictive capability of the semitheoretical models for the viscosity of fruit juices proposed in this work are much better than various multiparametric correlations. It was found that the prediction models (Eq. 31 to 41) developed in this work for the viscosity of fruit juices can be adopted with satisfaction. The models (Eq. 32,34,35,37, and 40) with temperature and concentration depending parameters are accurately represent the combined effect of concentration and temperature on the viscosity of fruit juices in wide temperature and concentration ranges and can be recommended for the future scientific and engineering used.

Appendix: Experimental Viscosity Data for Fruit Juices

Table 1A. Experimental viscosity (mPa·s) of natural pomegranate juice as a function of temperature and pressure for 11.0 °Brix

T (K)	0.1 MPa	5 MPa	10 MPa
292.95	1.642	-	1.646
296.85	1.480	-	-
301.05	1.318	-	-
304.55	1.213	-	1.216
308.05	1.119	-	-
311.55	1.032	1.034	-
316.55	0.928	-	0.932
321.85	0.837	-	-
325.95	0.777		0.782
328.95	0.740	-	-
332.35	0.699	-	0.704
337.95	0.637	-	-
343.05	0.587	-	0.593
348.15	0.541	-	-
353.05	0.500	0.502	-
358.15	0.465	-	-
362.95	0.435	-	0.440
368.45	0.405	-	-
374.85	0.374 [a]	-	0.379
379.95	0.352 [a]	0.354	-
384.85	0.332 [a]	-	0.337
388.15	0.321 [a]	-	-
394.75	0.299 [a]	-	0.304
402.95	0.275 [a]	0.277	0.279

[a]At pressure of 0.3 MPa.

Table 2A. Experimental viscosity (mPa·s) of pomegranate juice as a function of temperaturte and concentration

T (K)	23 °Brix	30 °Brix	35 °Brix	40 °Brix
293.15	2.017	3.307	4.968	7.082
298.15	1.765	2.828	4.248	5.994
303.15	1.555	2.488	3.593	5.081
313.15	1.231	1.902	2.659	3.702
323.15	1.001	1.498	2.051	2.863
333.15	0.827	1.200	1.606	2.252
343.15	0.697	0.985	1.288	1.778
353.15	0.597	0.817	1.055	1.443
363.15	0.533	0.692	0.875	1.192

Table 3A. Experimental viscosity (mPa·s) of pear juice as a function of temperature and pressure for 15.2 °Brix

T (K)	0.1 MPa	5 MPa	10 MPa
294.10	1.975	1.977	1.979
298.60	1.781	-	1.784
305.12	1.550	-	1.554
311.60	1.342	-	1.346
318.44	1.154	1.157	-
325.04	1.009	1.011	-
332.40	0.872	0.875	-
340.00	0.757	-	0.762
349.71	0.647	-	0.651
358.63	0.574	-	0.579
367.23	0.523	0.526	0.528
374.80	0.488[a]	-	0.493
382.50	0.460[a]	-	0.465
391.30	0.427[a]	-	0.432
402.71	0.381[a]	-	0.386

[a] At pressure of 0.3 MPa.

Table 4A. Experimental viscosity (mPa·s) of pear juice as a function of temperature and concentration

T (K)	20 °Brix	25 °Brix	30 °Brix
298.15	1.902	2.194	3.061
303.15	1.721	1.990	2.749
308.15	1.551	1.795	2.438
313.15	1.403	1.621	2.162
318.15	1.252	1.448	1.921
323.15	1.122	1.303	1.703
328.15	1.012	1.164	1.510
333.15	0.920	1.040	1.341
343.15	0.761	0.861	1.091
353.15	0.646	0.725	0.902
363.15	0.590	0.655	0.782

Table 5A. Experimental viscosity (mPa·s) of tangerine juice as a function of temperature and concentration

T (K)	15 °Brix	21 °Brix	26°Brix	35°Brix	40°Brix
303.15	1.608	1.904	2.420	4.608	6.627
313.15	1.262	1.482	1.887	3.356	4.695
323.15	1.010	1.179	1.502	2.540	3.419
333.15	0.818	0.954	1.219	1.966	2.600
343.15	0.677	0.791	1.006	1.580	2.074
353.15	0.567	0.658	0.840	1.304	1.696
363.15	0.477	0.556	0.712	1.107	1.435
373.15	0.412 [a]	0.482	0.620	0.966	1.262
383.15	0.357 [a]	0.423	0.548	0.862	1.127
393.15	0.315 [a]	0.375	0.492	0.771	1.020

[a] At pressure of 0.3 MPa.

Table 6A. Experimental viscosity (mPa·s) of lemon juice as a function of temperature and concentration

T, K	17°Brix	22°Brix	30°Brix	40°Brix	45°Brix
303.15	1.563	1.816	2.571	4.599	6.600
313.15	1.233	1.423	2.106	3.390	4.710
323.15	0.999	1.133	1.596	2.547	3.433
333.15	0.832	0.922	1.286	1.983	2.430
343.15	0.699	0.763	1.056	1.587	2.030
353.15	0.595	0.635	0.885	1.325	1.729
363.15	0.510	0.543	0.764	1.146	1.480
373.15	0.444 [a]	0.475	0.677	1.015	1.310
383.15	0.393 [a]	0.420	0.607	0.910	1.176
393.15	0.350 [a]	0.378	0.549	0.822	1.060

[a] At pressure of 0.3 MPa.

References

[1] Moressi, M.; Spinosi, M. Engineering factors in the production of concentrated fruit juices.1. Fluid physical properties of orange juices. *J. Food. Technol.* 1980, *15*, 265-276.

[2] Crandall, P.G.; Chen, C.S.; Carter, R.D. Models for predicting viscosity of orange juice concentrate. *Food Technology* 1982, *36*, 245-252.

[3] Famelart, M.-H.; Chapron, L.; Piot, M.; Brule, G.; Durier, C. High pressure –induced gel formation of milk and whey concentrates. *J. Food Eng.* 1998, *36*, 149-164.

[4] Farkas, D.F.; Hoover, D.G. High pressure processing. *J. Food Sci. Supplem.* 2000, *65*, 47-64.

[5] Farr, D. High pressure technology in the food industry. Trends in Food Science & Technology 1990, 14-16.

[6] Felipe, X.; Capellas, M.; Law, A.J.R. Comparison of the effects of high-pressure treatments and heat pasteurization on the whey proteins in goat's milk. *J. Agr. Food Chem.* 1997, *45*, 627-631.

[7] Delza, R.; Rosenthal, A.; Abadio, F.B.D.; Silva, C.H.O.; Castillo, C. Application of high pressure technology in the fruit juice processing: benefits perceived by consumers. *J. Food Eng.* 2005, *67*, 241-246.

[8] Desrumaux, A.; Marcand, J. Formation of sunflower oil emulsions stabilized by whey proteins with high pressure homogenization (up to 350 MPa): effect of pressure on emulsion characteristics. *Int. J. Food Sci. & Techn.* 2002, *37*, 263-269.

[9] Garcia, F.; Butz, P.; Bognar, A.; Tauscher, B. Antioxidative capacity, nutrient content and sensory quality of orange juice and an orange-lemon-carrot juice product after high pressure treatment and storage in different packaging. *European Food Res. Tech.* 2001, *213*, 290-296.

[10] Magerramov, M.A. Density of the concentrates of peach and pomegranate juices at elevated state parameters. *J. Eng. Phys. Thermophys.* 2007, *79*, 811-816.

[11] Magerramov, M.A.; Abdulagatov, A.I.; Azizov, N.D.; Abdulagatov, I.M. *J. Food and Bioprocess Technology: An International Journal* 2007, in press.

[12] Magerramov, M.A.; Abdulagatov, A.I.; Azizov, N.D.; Abdulagatov, I.M. Thermal conductivity of peach, raspberry, cherry, and plum juices as a function of temperature and concentration. *J. Food Proc. Eng.* 2006, *29*, 304-326.

[13] Magerramov, M.A.; Abdulagatov, A.I.; Azizov, N.D.; Abdulagatov, I.M. Thermal conductivity of pear, sweet-cherry, apricot, and cherry-plum juices as a function of temperature and concentration. *J. Food Sci. E.-Food Eng. and Phys. Properties* 2006, *71* 238-244.

[14] Magerramov, M.A.; Abdulagatov, A.I.; Azizov, N.D.; Abdulagatov, I.M. Effect of temperature, concentration, and pressure on the viscosity of pomegranate and pear juice concentrates. *J. Food Engineering* 2007, *80*, 476-489.

[15] Magerramov, M.A.; Abdulagatov, A.I.; Azizov, N.D.; Abdulagatov, I.M. Viscosity of tangerine and lemon juices as a function of temperature and concentration. *Int. J. Food Sci. and Technology* 2007, *42*, 804-819.

[16] Quashou, M.S.; Vachon, R.I.; Touloukian, Y.S. *Thermal conductivity of foods*. Part 1; ASHRAE Transactions: New York, NY, 1972; Vol. 78, pp 165-182.

[17] 17. Rha, C. *Theory, Determination and Control of Physical Properties of Food Materials*; D. Riedel Pub. Co.: Dordrecht, Holland, 1975.

[18] Rao, M.A. Viscoelastic properties of fluid and semi solid foods. In: *Physical and Chemical Properties of Food*; Editor M.R. Okos; ASAE: New York, NY, 1986; 14-34.

[19] Rao, M.A. *Rheology of Fluid and Semisolid Foods. Principles and Applications*; Aspen Publishers, Inc.: Gaithersburg, Maryland, 1999.

[20] Rahman, *Food Properties Hand Book*; CRC Press: Boca Raton, FL, 1995.

[21] Cuevas, R.; Cheryan, M. Thermal conductivity of liquid foods-review. *J. Food Proc. Eng.* 1979, *2*, 283-306.

[22] Chen, C.S. Physical and rheological properties of juices. In: *Fruit Juice Processing Technology*; Editor S. Nagy; C.S. Chen; Ph.E. Shaw; Agscience, Inc.: Auburndale Florida, Chapter 3, 1993; pp 56-82.

[23] Choi, I.; Okos, M.R. The thermal properties of liquid foods. Paper no 83-6516. *Winter Meeting*; ASAE: Chicago, IL, 1983.

[24] Choi, Y.; Okos, M. Effect of temperature and composition on the thermal properties of foods. In: *Food Engineering and Process Applications, Transport Phenomena*; Editors M.L. Maguer, P. Jelen; EASP: New York, NY, 1986; Vol.1, pp 93-101.

[25] Choi, Y.; Okos, M. Thermal properties of liquid foods-Review. In: *Physical and Chemical Properties of Food*; Editor M.R. Okos; ASAE: New York, NY, 1986; pp 35-77.

[26] Bourne, M.C. *Food Texture and Viscosity: Concept and Measurement*; Academy Press: New York, NY, 1982.

[27] Sweat, V.E. Thermal properties of foods. In: *Engineering Properties of Foods*; Editors M.A. Rao; S.S.H. Rizvi; Marcel Dekker, Inc.: New York, NY, Chapter 1,1986; pp 49-87.

[28] Steffe, J.F.; Mohamed, I.O.; Ford, E.W. Rheological properties of fluid foods: Data compilation. In: *Physical and Chemical Properties of Food*; Editor M.R. Okos; ASAE: New York, NY, 1986; pp 1-13.

[29] Saravacos, G.D.; Maroulis, Z.B. *Transport Properties of Foods*; Marcel Dekker, Inc.: New York, NY, 2002.

[30] Polley, S.L.; Snyder, O.P.; Kotur, P. A compilation of thermal properties of foods. *Food Technology* 1980, *34*, 76-108.

[31] Padmanabhan, M. Measurement of extensional viscosity of viscoelastic liquid foods. *J. Food Eng.* 1995, *25*, 311-327.

[32] Krokida, M.K.; Maroulis, Z.B.; Saravacos, G.D. Rheological properties of fluid fruit and vegetable puree products: Compilation of literature data. *Int. J. Food Properties* 2001, *4*, 179-200.

[33] Golubev, I.F. *Viscosity of Gases and Gaseous Mixtures*; Phys. Math. Press: Moscow, Russia, 1959.

[34] Golubev, I.F.; Agaev, N.A. *Viscosity of Hydrocarbons*; Azernashr: Baku, Azerbaijan, 1964.

[35] Golubev, I.F.; Gnesdilov, N.E. *Viscosity of Gaseous Mixtures*; GSSSD: Moscow, Russia, 1971.

[36] Guseinov, K.D. Study of the thermodynamic and transport properties of some organic liquids in the wide range of parameters of state. *Ph. D. Thesis*, API: Baku, Azerbaijan, 1979.

[37] Abdulagatov, I.M.; Rasulov, S.M. Viscosity of n-pentane and n-heptane and their mixtures within the temperature range from 298 K up to critical points at the saturation vapor pressure. *Ber. Bunsenges. Phys. Chem.* 1996, *100*, 148-154.

[38] Saravacos, G.D. Effect of temperature on viscosity of fruit juices and purees. *J. Food Science* 1970, *35*, 122-125.

[39] Rouse, A.H.; Albrigo, L.G.; Huggart, R.L.; Moore, E.L. Viscometric measurements and pectic content of frozen concentrated orange juices for citrus futures. *Ann. Meeting of the Florida State Horticultyral Society* 1974, *87*, 293-296.

[40] Rao, M.A.; Anantheswaran, R.C. Rheology of fluids in food processing's. *Food Tech.* 1982, *36*, 116-126.

[41] Wakeham, W.A.; Nagashima, A.; Sengers, J.V. (Editors) *Measurements of the Transport Properties of Fluids*; Blackwell Scientific Publications: Oxford, Vo. III, 1991.

[42] Hagenbach, S. *Ann. Phys., Lpz.* 1860, *109*, 385-426.

[43] Barr, G. *A Monograph of Viscosity*; Oxford University Press: London, 1931.

[44] Kestin, J.; Sokolov, M.; Wakeham, W.A. Theory of capillary viscometers. *Appl. Sci. Res.* 1973, *27*, 241-264.

[45] Van Wazer, J.R.; Lyons, J.W.; Kim, K.Y.; Colwell, R.E. *Viscosity and Flow Measurements*; Intersciences: New York, NY, 1963.

[46] Abdulagatov, I.M.; Azizov, N.D. Viscosity for Aqueous Li_2SO_4 Solutions at Temperatures from 298 to 575 K and at Pressures up to 30 MPa. *J. Chem. Eng. Data* 2003, *48*, 1549-1556.

[47] Rivkin, S.L.; Kremenevskaya, E.A.; Romashin, S.N.; Tractuev, O.M. Experimental investigation of density and viscosity of aqueous boron solutions. In: *Proc. 10th Int. Conf. Prop. Steam*; Editors, V.V. Sytchev; A.A. Aleksandrov; Mir Publ.: Moscow, 1984; Vol.2, pp 289-298.

[48] Puchkov, L.V.; Sargaev, P.M. Viscosity of lithium, sodium, potassium and ammonium nitrates solutions at temperature up to 275 °C. *Russ. J. Appl. Chem.* 1973, *46*, 2637-2640.

[49] Semenyuk, E.N.; Zarembo, V.I.; Feodorov, M.K. Experimental apparatus for the measurements of viscosity of aqueous solutions at temperatures 273-673 K and at pressures up to 200 MPa. *Russ. J. Appl. Chem.* 1977, *50*, 315-319.

[50] Mashovets, V.P.; Puchkov, L.V.; Sargaev, P.M.; Feodorov, M.K. Experimental apparatus for the viscosity measurements of aqueous solutions at temperatures up to 275 °C. *Russ. J. Appl. Chem.* 1971, *44*, 90-94.

[51] Pepinov, R.I.; Yusufova, V.J.; Lobkova, N.V.; Panakhov, I.A. Viscosity of aqueous potassium chloride solutions over a wide range of state parameters. In: *Proc. 10th Int. Conf. Prop. Steam*; Editors; V.V. Sytchev; A.A. Aleksandrov, Mir Publ.: Moscow, 1984; Vol. 2, pp 196-202.

[52] Kestin, J.; Sengers, J.V.; Kamgar-Parsi, B.; Levelt Sengers, J.M.H. Thermophysical properties of fluid H_2O. *J. Phys. Chem. Ref. Data* 1984, *13*, 175-189.

[53] *International Organization of Standardization (IOS) 4787* Laboratory glassware-Volumetric glassware-Methods for use and testing capacity, IOS: Geneve, 1994.

[54] Coleman, HW; Steele, WG *Experimentation and Uncertainty Analysis for Engineers*; John Wiley & Sons: New York, NY, 1989.

[55] DiPippo, R.; Kestin, J.; Whitelaw, J.H. A high-temperature oscillating-disk viscometer. *Physica* 1966, *32*, 2064-2080.

[56] Kestin, J.; Paul, R.; Shankland, I.R.; Khalifa, H.E. A high-temperature, high-pressure oscillating –disk viscometer for concentrated ionic solutions. *Ber. Bunsenges. Phys. Chem.* 1980, *84*, 1255-1260.

[57] Kestin, J.; Khalifa, H.E.; Ro, S.T.; Wakeham, W.A. Preliminary data on the pressure effect on the viscosity of sodium chloride-water solutions in the range 10-40 °C. *J. Chem. Eng. Data* 1977, *22*, 207-214.

[58] Kestin, J.; Khalifa, H.E.; Sookiazian, H.; Wakeham, W.A. Experimental investigation of the effect of pressure on the viscosity of water in the temperature range 10-150 °C. *Ber. Bunsenges. Phys. Chem.* 1978, *82*, 180-188.

[59] Kestin, J.; Khalifa, H.E.; Abe, Y.; Grimes, C.E.; Sookiazian, H.; Wakeham, W.A. Effect of pressure on the viscosity of aqueous sodium chloride solutions in the temperature range 20-150 °C. *J. Chem. Eng. Data* 1978, *23*, 328-336.

[60] Kestin, J.; Shankland, I.R.; Paul, R. The viscosity of aqueous KCl solutions in the temperature range 25–200°C and the pressure range 0.1–30 MPa. *Int. J. Thermophys.* 1981, *2*, 301-314.

[61] Kestin, J.; Shankland, I.R. A re-evaluation of the relative measurements of viscosity with oscillating –disk viscometers. *J. Appl. Math. Phys.* 1981, *32*, 533-545.

[62] Correia, R.J.; Kestin, J.; Khalifa, H.E. Measurements and calculation of the viscosity of mixed aqueous solutions of NaCl and KCl in the temperature range 25-150 C and the pressure range 0-30 MPa. *Ber. Bunsenges. Phys. Chem.* 1979, *83*, 20-24.

[63] Kestin, J.; Khalifa, H.E. Measurement of logarithmic decrements through the measurement of time. *Appl. Sci. Res.* 1976, *32*, 483-493.

[64] Newell, G.F. Theory of oscillation type viscometers V: Disk oscillating between fixed plates. *Z. Angew. Math. Phys.* 1959, *10*, 160-174.

[65] Kestin, J.; Wang, H.E.; Providence, R.I. Corrections for the oscillating-disk viscometer. *J. Appl. Mech.* 1957, *79*, 197-206.

[66] Kestin, J.; Newell, G.F. Theory of oscillation type viscometers: The oscillating cup Part I. *Z. Angew. Math. Phys.* 1957, *8*, 433-442.

[67] Kestin, J.; Moszynski, J.R.; Providence, R.I. An Instrument for the measurement of the viscosity of steam and compressed water. *Trans. ASME* 1958, *80*, 1009-1014.

[68] Kestin, J.; Leidenfrost, W.; Liu, C.Y. *Z.* On relative measurements of the viscosity of gases by the oscillating-disk method. *Angew. Math. Phys.* 1959, *10*, 558-564.

[69] Nieuwoudt, J.C.; Kestin, J.; Sengers, J.V. On the theory of oscillating-body viscometers. *Physica A* 1987, *142*, 53-74.

[70] Nieuwoudt, J.C. An extension of the theory of oscillating cup viscometers. *Int. J. Thermophys.* 1990, *11*, 525-535.

[71] Tørklep, K.; Øye, H.A. Viscostiy of molten alkaline-earth chlorides. *J. Chem. Eng. Data* 1982, *27*, 387-391.

[72] Iwasaki, H.; Kestin, J. The viscosity of argon-helium mixtures at 20 °C and 1, 25, and 50 atm.. *Physica* 1963, *29*, 1345-1372.

[73] Kestin, J.; Sokolov, M.; Wakeham, W.A.Viscosity of liquid water in the range -8 °C to 150 °C. *J. Phys. Chem. Ref. Data* 1978, *7*, 941-948.

[74] Grimes, C.G.; Kestin, J.; Khalifa, H.E. Viscosity of aqueous potassium chloride solutions in the temperature range 25-150°C and the pressure range 0-30 MPa. *J. Chem. Eng. Data* 1979, *24*, 121-126.

[75] Kestin, J.; Shankland, I.R. Viscosity of aqueous NaCl solutions in the temperature range 25–200 °C and in the pressure range 0.1–30 MPa. *Int. J. Thermophys.* 1984, *5*, 241-263.

[76] Kawata, M.; Kurase, K.; Nagashima, A.; Yoshida, K. In: *Experimental Thermodynamics. III. The Measurement of Transport Properties of Fluids*; Editors, W.A. Wakeham; A. Nagashima; J.V. Sengers; Blackwell Scientific: Oxford, 1991; pp 49-75.

[77] Faxen, H. Die bewegung einer starren Kugel längs der Achse eines mit zäher Flüssigkeit gefüllten Rohres. *Arkiv f. Mat. Astron. Och Fysik* 1923, *17*, 1-28.

[78] Fidleris, V.; Whitemore, R.L. experimental determination of the wall effect for spheres falling axially in cylindrical vessels. *Brit. J. Appl. Phys.* 1961, *12*, 490-494.

[79] Sutterby, J.L. Falling sphere viscometer. *Trans. Soc. Rheol.* 1973, *17*, 559-573.

[80] Oseen, C.W. Uber. Die electromagnetischen schwingungen an dunnen ringen. *Arkiv f. Mat. Astron. Och Fysik* 1913, *9*, 1-15.

[81] Huner, B.; Hussey, R.G. Cylinder drag at low Reynolds number. *Phys. Fluids* 1977, *20*, 1211-1218.

[82] Maxworthy, T. Accurate measurements of sphere drag at low Reynolds numbers. *J. Fluid Mech.* 1965, *23*, 369-372.

[83] Proudman, I.; Pearson, J.R.A. Expansions at small Reynolds numbers for the flow past a sphere and a circular cylinder. *J. Fluid Mech.* 1957, *2*, 237-262.

[84] Maude, A.D. End effects in a falling-sphere viscometer. *Brit. J. Appl. Phys.* 1961, *12*, 293-295.

[85] Flude, M.J.C.; Daborn, J.E. Viscosity measurement by means of falling spheres compared with capillary viscometry. *J. Phys. E.* 1982, *15*, 1313-1321.

[86] Tanner, R.I. End effects in falling-ball viscometry. *J. Fluid Mech.* 1963, *17*, 161-170.

[87] Isdale, J.D.; Easteal, A.J.; Wolf, L.A. Shear viscosity of methanol and methanol + water mixtures under pressure. *Int. J. Thermpohys.* 1985, *6*, 439-450.

[88] Tanaka, Y.; Matsuda, Y.; Fujuwara, H. Viscosity of (water + alcohol) mixtures under high pressure. *Int. J. Thermpohys.* 1987, *8*, 147-163.

[89] Melikov, R.A. *Ph.D. Thesis*, Azerbaijan Power Engineering Research Institute, Baku, 1996.

[90] Melikov, R.A. In: *Scientific Transactions of Azerbaijan State Oil Academy. Power Engineering of Oil and Gas Industry* 1999, *4*, 144-147.

[91] Melikov, R.A. In: *Proc. Conference, "Ratsional'noe Ispol'zovanie Energo-Resursov I Nadezhnost Electrooborudovanii"*, Azerbaijan State Oil Academy: Baku, Azerbaijan, 2000; pp 360-363.

[92] Alvarado, J.D.; Romero, C.H. Physical properties of fruits I-II. Density and viscosity of juices as functions of soluble solids content and temperature. *Latin Amer. Applied Research* 1989, *19*, 15-21.

[93] Bayindirli, L. Mathematical analysis of variation of density and viscosity of apple juice with temperature and concentration. *J. Food Processing & Preservation* 1992, *16*, 23-28.

[94] Bayindirli, L.; Özsan, O. Modeling of thermophysical properties of sourchery juice. *Gida* 1992, *17*, 405-407.

[95] Bayindirli, L. Density and viscosity of grape juice as a function of concentration and temperature. *J. Food Processing & Preservation* 1993, *17*, 147-151.

[96] Bayindirli, L.; Sahin, S.; Artik, N. The effect of clarification methods on pomegranate juice quality. *Fruit Processing* 1994, *4*, 267-270.

[97] Cepeda, E.; Villarán, M.C. Density and viscosity of Malus floribunda juice as a function of concentration and temperature. *J. Food Eng.* 1999, *41*, 103-107.

[98] Constenla, D.T., Lozano J.E.; Crapiste, G.H. Thermophysical properties clarified apple juice as a function of concentration and temperature. *J. Food Science* 1989, *54*, 663-668.

[99] Juszczak, L.; Fortuna, T. Viscosity of concentrated strawberry juice. Effect of temperature and soluble solids content. *J. Polish Agr. University* 2003, *6*, 1-7.

[100] Juszczak, L.; Fortuna, T. Effect of temperature and soluble solids content on the viscosity of cherry juice concentrate. *Int. Agrophys.* 2004, *18*, 17-21.

[101] Ibarz, A.; Gonzalez, C.; Esplugas, S. Rheology of clarified fruit juices. III: Orange juices. *J. Food Eng.* 1994, *21*, 485-494.

[102] Ibarz, A.; Garvin, A.; Costa, J. Rheological behavior of sloe (*prunus spinosa*) fruit juices. *J. Food Eng.* 1996, *27*, 423-430.

[103] Ibarz, A.; Garvin, A.; Costa, J. Rheological behavior of loquat (*eriobotrya japonica*) juices. *J. Food Eng.* 1996, *27*, 175-184.

[104] Ibarz, A.; Pagán, J. Rheology of raspberry juices. I: *J. Food Eng.* 1987, *6*, 269-289.

[105] Ibarz, A.; Gonzalez, C.; Esplugas, S.; Vicente, M. Rheology of clarified fruit juices. I: Peach juices. *J. Food Eng.* 1992, *15*, 49-61.

[106] Ibarz, A.; Pagán, J.; Miguelsanz, R. Rheology of clarified fruit juices. II: Blackcurrant juices. *J. Food Eng.* 1992, *15*, 63-73.

[107] Ibarz, A.; Vicente, M.; Graell, J. Rheological behavior of apple juice and pear juice and their concentrates. *J. Food Eng.* 1987, *6*, 257-267.

[108] Ibarz, A.; Pagan, J.; Gutierrez, J.; Vicente, M. Rheological properties of clarified pear juices concentrates. *J. Food Eng.* 1989, *10*, 57-63.

[109] Barros, S.M. *Quality summary. Citrus juice products from FMC citrus juice extractors*; Citrus Machinery Div., FMC Corp.: Lakeland, Fla., 1977; 1978; 1979.

[110] Rao, M.A.; Cooley, H.J.; Ortloff, C.; Chung, K.; Wijts, S.C. Influence of rheological properties of fluid and semisolid foods on the performance of a filler. *J. Food Proc. Eng.* 1993, *16*, 289-304.

[111] Rao, K.L.; Eipeson, W.E.; Rao, P.N.S.; Patwardhan, M.V.; Ramanathan, P.K. Rheological properties of mango pulp and concentrate. *J. Food Sci. Tech.* 1985, *22*, 30-33.

[112] Rao, M.A.; Cooley, H.J.; Vitali, A.A. Flow properties of concentrated juices at low temperatures. *Food Technology* 1984, *38*, 113-119.

[113] Vitali, A.A.; Rao, M.A. Flow properties of low-pulp concentrated orange juice: Effect of temperature and concentration. *J. Food Sciences* 1984, *49*, 882-888.

[114] Kaya, A.; Sözer, N. Rheological behavior of sour pomegranate juice concentrates (*Punica granatum L.*). *Int. J. Food Science and Technology* 2005, *40*, 223-227.

[115] Kaya, A. Rheology of mulberry pekmez. *J. Texture Studies* 2001, *32*, 335-342

[116] Saravacos, G.D.; Kostaropoulos, A.E. Transport properties in processing of fruits and vegetables. *Food Technology*, September, 1995, 99-105.

[117] Saravacos, G.D. In: *Engineering Properties of Foods*. Editors; M.A. Rao; S.S.H. Rizvi; Marcel Dekker, Inc.: 1986, pp 89-132.

[118] Glasstone, S.; Laidler, K.; Eyring, E. *Theory of Rate Processes*; McGraw-Hill: New York, NY, 1941.

[119] Erday-Grúz, T. *Transport Phenomena in Aqueous Solutions*. John Wiley & Sons Inc.: New York, NY, 1974.

[120] Millat, J.; Dymond, J.H.; Nieto de Castro, C.A. Editors, *Transport Properties of Fluids. Their Correlation, Prediction and Estimation*; IUPAC, Cambridge University Press: New York, NY, 1996.

[121] Stokes, R.H.; Mills, R. *Viscosity of Electrolytes and Related Properties*; Pergamon Press, Inc.: New York, NY, 1965.

[122] Abdulagatov, I.M.; Azizov, N.D. Viscosity of aqueous LiI solutions at 293 - 525 K and 0.1-40 MPa. *Thermochimica Acta* 2005, *439*, 8-20.

[123] Abdulagatov, I.M.; Azizov, N.D. Viscosity of aqueous calcium chloride solutions at high temperatures and high pressures. *Fluid Phase Equilibria* 2006, *240*, 204-219.

[124] Abdulagatov, I.M.; Azizov, N.D. Experimental study of the effect of temperature, pressure, and concentration on the viscosity of aqueous NaBr solutions. *J. Sol. Chem.* 2006, *35*, 705-738.

[125] Abdulagatov, I.M.; Azizov, N.D. Experimental study of the effect of temperature, pressure, and concentration on the viscosity of aqueous $SrCl_2$ solutions. *J. Chem. Eng. Data* 2007, *52*, 841-850.

[126] Abdulagatov, I.M.; Azizov, N.D. Experimental study of the effect of temperature, pressure, and concentration on the viscosity of aqueous KBr. *J. Sol. Chemistry* 2007, in press.

[127] Abdulagatov, I.M.; Zeinalova, A.B.; Azizov, N.D. Viscosity of aqueous $Ni(NO_3)_2$ solutions at temperatures from (297 to 475) K and at pressures up to 30 MPa and concentration between (0.050 and 2.246) $mol{\cdot}kg^{-1}$. *J. Chem. Thermodyn.* 2006, *38*, 179-189.

[128] Chirife, J. Microbial growth at reduced water activities: some physico-chemical properties of compatible soluties. *J. Appl. Bacteriol.* 1984, *56*, 259-268.

[129] Leyenndekkers, J.V.; Hunter, R.J. Refractive index of aqueous electrolyte solutions. Extrapolation to other temperatures, pressures, and wavelengths and to multicomponent systems. *J. Chem. Eng. Data* 1977, *22*, 427-431.

[130] Leyenndekkers, J.V.; Hunter, R.J. The viscosity of aqueous electrolyte solutions and the TTG model. *J. Phys. Chem.* 1977, *81*, 1657-1663.

[131] Leyenndekkers, J.V. The viscosity of aqueous electrolyte solutions and the TTG model. *J. Sol. Chem.* 1979, *8*, 853-869.

[132] Goldsack, D.E.; Franchetto, R.C. The viscosity of concentrated electrolyte solutions. I. Concentrated dependence at fixed temperature. *Can. J. Chem.-Rev. Can. Chim.* 1977, *55*, 1062-1072.

[133] Goldsack, D.E.; Franchetto, R.C. The viscosity of concentrated electrolyte solutions. II. Temperature dependence. *Can. J. Chem.-Rev. Can. Chim.* 1978, *56*, 1442-1450.

[134] Chirife, J.; Buera, M.P. A simple model for predicting the viscosity of sugar and oligosaccharide solutions. *J. Food Eng.* 1997, *33*, 211-226.

[135] Falkenhagen, H.; Dole, M. Die innere reibung von elektrolytischen losungen und ihre deutung nach der Debyeschen theorie. *Phys. Z.* 1929, *30*, 611-622.

[136] Onsager, L.; Fuoss, R.M. Irreversible processes in electrolytes. Diffusion, conductance, and viscous flow in arbitrary mixtures of strong electrolytes. *J. Phys. Chem.* 1932, *36*, 2689-2778.

[137] Onsager, L. Z. The theory of electrolytes. *Z. Phys.* 1926, *27*, 388-392.

[138] Debye, P. and Hückel, H. Bemerkungen zu einem satze über die kataphoretische wanderungsgeschwindigkeit suspendierter teilchen. *Z. Phys.* 1924, *25*, 49-52.

[139] Jones, G.; Dole, M. The viscosity of aqueous solutions of strong electrolytes with special reference to barium chloride. *J. Am. Chem. Soc.* 1929, *51*, 2950-2964.

[140] Abdulagatov, I.M.; Azizov, N.D. Densities, Apparent Molar Volumes, and Viscosities of Concentrated Aqueous $NaNO_3$ Solutions at Temperatures from 298 to 607 K and at Pressures up to 30 MPa. *J. Sol. Chem.* 2005, *34*, 645-685.

[141] Abdulagatov, I.M.; Zeinalova, A.B.; Azizov, N.D., Viscosity of aqueous electrolyte solutions at high temperatures and high pressures. Viscosity B-coefficient. Sodium iodide. *J. Chem. Eng. Data* 2006, *51*,1645-1659.

[142] Abdulagatov, I.M.; Azizov, N.D.; Zeinalova, A.B. Density, apparent and partial molar volumes, and viscosity of aqueous Na_2CO_3 solutions at high temperatures and high pressures. *Z. Phys. Chem.* 2007, *221*, 1-38.

[143] Abdulagatov, I.M.; Azizov, N.D.; Zeinalova, A.B. Viscosities, densities, apparent and partial molar volumes of concentrated aqueous $MgSO_4$ solutions at high temperatures and high pressures. *J. Phys. Chem. Liquids* 2007, *45*, 127-148.

[144] Kaminsky, M. *Z.* Experimentelle untersuchungen über die konxentrations- und temperaturabhangigkeit der zähigkeit wäβriger lösungen starker electrolyte. I. Mitteilang: KJ-, NH4Cl- und Na_2SO_4-lösungen. *Phys. Chem.*1955, *5*, 154-191.

[145] Kaminsky, M. *Z.* Experimental study of the concentration and temperature dependence of the viscosity of aqueous solutions of strong electrolyte. I. *Phys. Chem.* 1956, *8*, 173-191.

[146] Kaminsky, M. *Z.* Concentration and temperature dependence of the viscosity of aqueous solutions of strong electrolytes. III. KCl, K_2SO_4, $MgCl_2$, $BeSO_4$, and $MgSO_4$ solutions. *Phys. Chem. N.F.* 1957, *12*, 206-231.

[147] Kaminsky, M. *Disc. Faraday Soc.* 1958, *24*, 171-179.

[148] Desnoyers, J.E.; Arel, M.; Leduc, P.A. Conductance and viscosity of n-alkylamine hydrobromides in water at 25 °C: influence of hydrophobic hydration. *Can. J. Chem.* 1969, *47*, 547-553.

[149] Desnoyers, J.E.; Perron, G. The viscosity of aqueous solutions of alkali and tetraalkylammonium halides at 25 °C. *J. Sol. Chem.* 1972, *1*, 199-212.

[150] Feakins, D.; Lawrence, D.G. The relative viscosities of solutions of sodium and potassium chlorides and bromides in N-methylformamide at 25, 35, and 45 °C. *J. Chem. Soc. A.* 1966, 212-219.

[151] Robertson, C.T.; Tyrrell, H.J.U. Viscosity B coefficients for some substituted anilinium cations in aqueous solutions at 25 and 35 °C. *J. Chem. Soc. A.* 1969, 1938-1942.

[152] Abdulagatov, I. M.; Zeinalova, A.B.; Azizov, N.D. Experimental viscosity B-coefficients for aqueous LiCl solutions. *J. Mol. Liquids* 2006, *126*, 75-88.

[153] Thomas, D.G. Transport characteristics of suspension: VIII. A note on the viscosity of Newtonian suspensions of uniform spherical particles. *J. Colloid Sci.* 1965, *20*, 267-277.

[154] Einstein, A. Berichtigung zu meiner Arbeit: "Eine neue Bestimmung der Molekül-dimensionen." *Ann. Phys.* 1911, *34*, 591-592.

[155] Breslau, B.R.; Millero, I.F. On the viscosity of concentrated aqueous electrolyte solutions. *J. Phys. Chem.* 1970, *74*, 1056-1061.

[156] Moulik, S.P.; Rakshit, A.K. A.K. Viscosity of aqueous electrolyte solutions as a function of *B*-coefficients. *J. Ind. Chem. Soc.* 1975, *52*, 450-453.

[157] Sahu, B.; Behera, B. Viscosity of concentrated aqueous solutions of I:I electrolytes. *Ind. J. Chem. A* 1980, *19*, 1153-1157.

[158] Altan, A.; Kus, S.; Kaya, A. Rheological behavior and time dependent characterization of gilaboru juice (*viburnum opulus L.*). *Food Sci. Tech. Int.* 2005, *11*, 129-137.

[159] Gochiyaev, B.R. Determination of the viscosity and density of apple juice. *Izv. Vyssh. Ucheb. Zaved., ser. Pish. Tekhnol.* 1964, *4*, 93-95.

[160] Saravacos, G.D. Tube viscometry of fruit purees and juices. *J. Food Science* 1968, *22*, 1585-1588.

[161] Schwartz, M.; Costell, E. Influencia de la temperature y la concentracion en la viscpsidad de los zumos de manzana y de uva. *Revista de Agroquimica y Technologia de Alimentos* 1989, *29*, 239-245.

[162] Moresi, M.; Spinosi, M. Engineering factors in the production of concentrated fruit juices. 1. Fluid physical properties of orange juices. *J. Food. Technol.* 1980, *15*, 265-276.

[163] Steverson, E.M. In: *Quality summary. Citrus juice products from FMC citrus juice extractors*. Citrus Machinery Div., FMC Corp.: Lakeland, Fla., 1977; 1978; 1979.

[164] Mizrahi, S.; Berk, Z. Flow behavior of concentrated orange juice: Mathematical treatment. *J. Texture Studies* 1972, *3*, 69-79.

[165] Mizrahi, S.; Berk, Z. Flow behavior of concentrated orange juice. *J. Texture Studies* 1970, *1*, 342-355.

[166] Mizrahi, S.; Firstenberg, R. Effect of orange juice composition on flow behavior of six-fold concentrate. *J. Texture Studies* 1975, *6*, 523-532.

[167] Ezell, G.H. Viscosity of concentrated orange and grapefruit juices. *Food Technology* 1959, *13*, 9-13.

[168] Varshney, N.N.; Kumbhar, B.K. Effect of concentration and temperature on rheological properties of pineapple and orange juices. *J. Food. Sci. Tech. India* 1978, *15*, 53-55.

[169] Hernandez, E.; Chen, C.S.; Johnson, J.; Carter, R.D. Viscosity changes in orange juices. *J. Food Eng.* 1995, *25*, 387-396.

[170] Dubois, C.W.; Murdock, D.I. The effect of concentration on quality of frozen orange juice with particular refernce to 58.5° and 42 °Brix products. Chemical and Physiological aspects. *Food Technol.* 1955, *9*, 60-63.

[171] Berk, Z. Viscosity of orange juice concentrates: Effect of ultrasonic treatment and concentration. *Food Technol.* 1964, *18*, 153-154.

[172] Rouse, A.H.; Albrigo, L.G.; Huggart, R.L.; Moore, E.L. Viscometry affected by pectic constituents in 45 °Brix frozen concentrated orange juice. *Ann. Meeting of the Florida State Horticultyral Society* 1973, *86*, 249-254.

[173] Ingram, M. *The viscosity of concentrated orange juice*; The Hebrew University: Jerusalem, 1948.

[174] Moresi, M.; Spinosi, M. Engineering factors in the production of concentrated fruit juices. II. Fluid physical properties of grape juices. *J. Food Tech.* 1984, *19*, 519-533.

[175] Khalil, K.E.; Ramakrishna, P.; Nanjundaswamy, A.M.; Patwardhan, M.V. Rheological behavior of clarified banana juice: Effect of temperature and concentration. *J. Food Eng.* 1989, *10*, 231-240.

[176] Fito, P.J.; Clemente, G.; Sanz, F.J. Rheological behavior of tomato concentrate (hot break and cold break). *J. Food Eng.* 1983, *2*, 51-62.

[177] Foda, Y.H.; McCollum, J.P. Viscosity as affected by various constituents of tomato juice. *J. Food Sci.* 1970, *35*, 333-338.

[178] Saravacos, G.D.; Oda, Y.; Moyer, J.C. *Tube viscometry of tomato concentrates*; NY State Agr. Exp. Station Bull., Cornell University: Geneva, NY, 1967.

[179] Harper, J.C.; El-Sahrigi, A.F. Viscometric behavior of tomato concentrates. *J. Food Sci.* 1965, *30*, 470-476.

[180] Molwane, S.D.; Gunjal, B.B. Viscometric characteristics of cold-break and hot-break extracted tomato juice concentrates. *J. Food Sci. Tech.* 1985, *22*, 353-357.

[181] Krapivin, N.I.; Fedotkin, I.M. *Konserv. Ovoshch. Prom.* 1977, *39*, 40-46.

[182] Luh, B.S.; Villarreal, F.; Leonard, S.J.; Yamaguchi, M. Effect of ripeness level on consistency of canned tomato juice. *Food Technology* 1960, *12*, 635-639.

[183] Giner, J.; Ibarz, A.; Garza, S.; Xhian-Quan, S. Rheology of clarified cherry juices. *J. Food Eng.* 1996, *30*, 147-154.

[184] Altan, A.; Maskan, M. Rheological behavior of pomegranate (*Punica granatum L.*) juice and concentrate. J. Texture Studies 2005, *36*, 68-77.

[185] Peleg, H.; Noble, A.C. Effect of viscosity, temperature and pH on astringency in cranberry juice. *Food Quality and Preference* 1999, *10*, 343-347.

[186] Vitali, A.A.; Roig, S.M.; Rao, M.A. Viscosity behavior of concentrated passion fruit juice. *Confructa* 1974, *19*, 201-106.

[187] Garciá, R.; Rivera, J.; Rolz, C. Rheological properties of some tropical fruit products and their enzymic clarification. *Proc. IV Int. Cong. Food Sci. Tech.* 1974, *2*, 18-26.

[188] Lopez, A.; Ibarz, A.; Pagan, J.; Vilavella, M. Rheology of wine musts during fermentation. *J. Food Eng.* 1989, *10*, 155-161.

[189] Oomah, B.D.; Sery, G.; Godfrey, D.V.; Beveridge, T.H.J. Rheology of sea buckthorn (*hippophae rhamnoides* L.) juice. *J. Agric. Chem.* 1999, *47*, 3546-3550.

[190] Lau, A.K.; March, A.C.; Lo, K.V.; Cumming, D.B. Physical properties of celery juice. *Can Agric Eng.* 1992, *34*,105-110.

[191] Manohar, B.; Ramakrishna, P.; Udayasankar, K. Some physical properties of tamarind (*Tamarindus indica L.*) juice concentrates. *J. Food Eng.* 1991, *13*, 241-258.

[192] Maskan, M. Rheological behavior of liquorice (*Glycyrrhiza glabra*) extract. *J. Food Eng.* 1999, *39*, 389-393.

[193] Gunjal, B.B.; Waghmare, N.J. Flow characteristics of pulp, juice and nectar of 'baneshan' and 'neelum' mangoes. *J. Food. Sci. Tech. India* 1987, *24*, 20-23.

[194] Sogi, D.S. Effect of concentration and temperature on the viscosity of watermelon juice. *J. Food Science and Technology* 2003, *40*, 509-511.

[195] Simpson, M. Viscosity as related to pectin content in strawberry juices. *Horticultural Experimental Station and Products Laboratory*; 1958, pp 126-129.

[196] Vitali, A.A.; Rao, M.A. Flow behavior of guava puree as a function of temperature and concentration. *J. Texture Srudies* 1982, *13*, 275-289.

[197] Brekke, J.E.; Myers, A.L. Viscometric behavior of guava purees and concentrates. *J. Food Science* 1978, *43*, 272-273.

[198] Manohar, B.; Ramakrishna, P.; Ramteke, R.S. Effect of pectin content on flow properties of mango pulp concentrates. *J. Texture Studies* 1990, *21*, 179-190.

[199] Singh, N.I.; Eipeson, W.E. Rheological behavior of clarified mango juice concentrates. *J. Texture Studies* 2000, *31*, 287-295.

[200] Watson, E.L. Rheological behavior of apricot purees and concentrates. *Can. Agr. Eng.* 1968, *10*, 8-11.

[201] Harper, J.C.; Lebermann, K.W. Rheological behavior of pear purees. *Proc. 1st Int. Cong. Food Sci. Tech.* 1962, *1*, 719-728.

[202] Elfak, A.M.; Pass, G.; Phillips, G.O.; Morley, R.G. The viscosity of dilute solutions of guar gum and locust bean gum with and without added sugars. *J. Sci. Food Agric.* 1978, *28*, 895-899.

[203] Soesanto, T.; Williams, M. Volumetric interpretation of viscosity for concentrated and dilute sugar solutions. *J. Phys. Chem.* 1981, *85*, 3338-3341.

[204] Rao, M.A. Rheology of liquid foods-A review. *J. Texture Studies* 1977, *8*, 135-168.

[205] Mizrahi, S. A review of the physicochemical approach to the analysis of the structural viscosity of fluid fruit product. *J. Texture Studies* 1979, *10*, 67-82.

[206] Jones, G.; Talley, S.K. The viscosity of aqueous solutions as a function of the concentration. II. Potassium bromide and potassium chloride. *J. Am. Chem. Soc.* 1933, *55*, 4124-4125.

[207] Charm, S.E. In: *The Fundamentals of Food Engineering*; Conn., Avi Pub., Co.: Westport, 1963; Chapter 3, pp 47-106.

[208] Bálint, A. Prediction of physical properties of foods for unit operations. *Periodica Polytechnica Ser. Chem. Eng.* 2001, *45*, 35-40.

[209] Bayindirli, L.; ve Ersan, C. Mathematical modeling of variation of density and viscosity of clear fruit juices with temperature and concentration. *Gida Teknolojisi* 1998, *3*, 66-69.

[210] Fernéndez-Martin, F. Influence of temperature and concentration on some physical properties of milk and milk concentrates. II. Viscosity. *J. Dairy Res.* 1972, *39*, 75-82.

[211] Peacock, S. Prediction physical properties of factory juices and syrups. *Int. Sugar Jnl.* 1995, *97*, 571-577.

[212] Elfak, A.M.; Pass, G.; Phillips, G.O. The viscosity of dilute solutions of ϑ-carrageenan and sodium carboxymethylcellulose. *J. Sci. Food Agric.* 1978, *29*, 557-562.

[213] Odigboh, E.U.; Mohsenin, N.N. Effect of concentration on the viscosity profile of cassava starch pastes during the cooking-cooling process. *J. Texture Studies* 1975, *5*, 441-457.

[214] Geller, V.Z.; Pugach, A.K.; Mkhitaryan, G.G. Density and effective viscosity of apple juice at various concentrations. *Pishevaya Promyshlennost* 1992, *1*, 45-56.

[215] Holdsworth, S.D. Applicability of rheological models to the interpretation of flow and processing behavior of fluid food products. *J. Texture Studies* 1971, *2*, 393-418.

[216] Autio, K.; Houska, M. Measurement of flow curves for model liquids and real food systems with two commercial viscometers. *J. Food Eng.* 1991, *13*, 57-66.

[217] Alviar, M.S.B.; Reid, D.S. Determination of reological behavior of tomato concentrates using back extrusion. *J. Food Science* 1990, *55*, 554-555.

[218] McCarthy, K.L.; Seymour, J.D. A fundamental approach for the relationship between the bostwick measurements and Newtonian fluid viscosity. *J. Texture Sciences* 1994, *24*, 1-10.

[219] Erickson, E.R.; Berntsen, R.A.; Eliason, M.A. Viscosity of corn syrup. *J. Chem. Eng. Data* 1966, *11*, 485-488.

[220] Rai, P.; Majumdar, G.C.; DasGupta, S., De, S. Prediction of the viscosity of clarified fruit juices using artificial neural network: a combined effect of concentration and temperature. J. Food Engineering 2005, 68, 527-533.

In: Fruit Juices: Properties, Consumption and Nutrition
Editor: Pauline G. Scardina
ISBN: 978-1-60741-505-3

Chapter 8

Effects of Permeation on Mass Transfer Coefficient for Laminar Non-Newtonian Fluid Flow in Membrane Modules during Clarification/Concentration of Fruit Juice*

Sirshendu De**, *Sunando DasGupta and S. Ranjith Kumar
Department of Chemical Engineering; Indian Institute of Technology, Kharagpur; Kharagpur - 721 302; India

Abstract

Membrane based clarification and concentration of fruit juice has become a popular unit operation in modern fruit juice processing industries. The well known membrane modules used for this purpose are tubular and spiral wound modules. Therefore, design of these modules is of utmost industrial importance. The key parameter for design of membrane modules is mass transfer coefficient. Most of the fruit juices have non-Newtonian rheology, e.g., power law, ellis fluid, etc. Till today, the mass transfer coefficient for such systems used is approximated from the corresponding relations developed for Newtonian fluids. Hence, a detailed fluid flow modeling with non-Newtonian rheology is urgently warranted. In the present work, this aspect is attempted. The expressions of the mass transfer coefficients are derived from the first principles for laminar, non-Newtonian fluid flow in a porous conduit. The effects of the permeation are incorporated quantitatively in the mass transfer coefficient from a theoretical basis. The

* A version of this chapter was also published in *Progress in Food Engineering Research and Developments*, edited by Vivian N. Pletney published by Nova Science Publishers, Inc. It was submitted for appropriate modifications in an effort to encourage wider dissemination of research.

* Corresponding author: Sirshendu De; Tel: + 91 – 3222 – 283926; Fax: +91 – 3222 – 2755303; E Mail: sde@che.iitkgp.ernet.in

analysis is carried out for various non-Newtonian rheologies. Effects of the operating conditions, i.e., Reynolds number, permeate flux, etc. on mass transfer coefficient are also investigated. Two flow geometries are considered. Flow through a tube and that through a rectangular thin channel, which are useful for the design of the tubular and spiral wound cross flow membrane modules. The developed relations of mass transfer coefficients would be of tremendous help to the design engineers.

1. Introduction

The mass transfer coefficient is an important parameter for designing membrane separation modules, where the flow occurs through a porous conduit. Therefore, accurate estimation of the mass transfer coefficient is necessary. These coefficients are generally calculated from the Sherwood number correlations, obtained from the heat and mass transfer analogies. The major limitations of these correlations are, (i) they are applicable for non-porous conduits, (ii) the effects of pressure on the mass transfer coefficient are not incorporated, (iii) it is assumed that the mass transfer boundary layer is fully developed and (iv) the property variations with concentration remain unaccounted. Therefore, the standard correlations lead to inaccurate estimation of the mass transfer coefficient. One way to avoid this is to carry out a detailed numerical simulation of the fluid and the mass transfer in the membrane modules [1,2] and the subsequent estimation of the mass transfer coefficient. But, this method is not attractive to the engineers due to the extensive computation effort and complications. The available mass transfer coefficient correlations had been reviewed in detail [3,4]. The shortcomings of these correlations as stated earlier have been extensively discussed in detail in both the reviews. The alternative approaches, like velocity variation technique [3] or osmotic pressure model [4,5], are also examined. But, both of these methods have their own limitations.

The effect of the permeation is extremely important in the mass transfer. The effect is two fold; first, it enhances the mass transfer and second, it stabilizes the laminar flow by delaying the onset of laminar to turbulent transition [3].

Membrane based separation processes are used extensively in various process industries, e.g., food processing [6], dairy products [7], clarification and concentration of fruit juice [8,9], polymer concentration, separation and fractionation [10], biomedical applications [10], protein concentration and separation [11], etc. Most of the fruit juices, polymeric solutions, blood, etc. follow non-Newtonian rheology. Power law is the commonest rheology of these non-Newtonian process streams [12]. The Sherwood number relations for the non-Newtonian fluids are scarce in literature. Most of the available relations are empirical or semi-empirical in nature and these are for power law fluids only [13-15]. The generalized expressions of Sherwood number including the effects of membrane permeation for Newtonian laminar flow as well as the turbulent flow regimes are already developed [16,17]. The Sherwood number relations for the entire range of the power law fluids, from pseudoplastic to dilatant, have been developed both for the laminar and turbulent flow regimes [18,19]. The present work is aimed at the developing expressions of the Sherwood numbers for three non-Newtonian fluids, namely, Ellis, Reiner-Philippoff and Eyring fluids in a tube. The analysis is applicable for laminar cross flow in reverse osmosis (RO) as well as in ultrafiltration (UF).

2. Theory

2.1. Flow Through a Tube

The theoretical developments of the tubular flow for Ellis, Eyring and Reiner-Philippoff fluids are presented herein. The flow geometry is shown in figure 1.

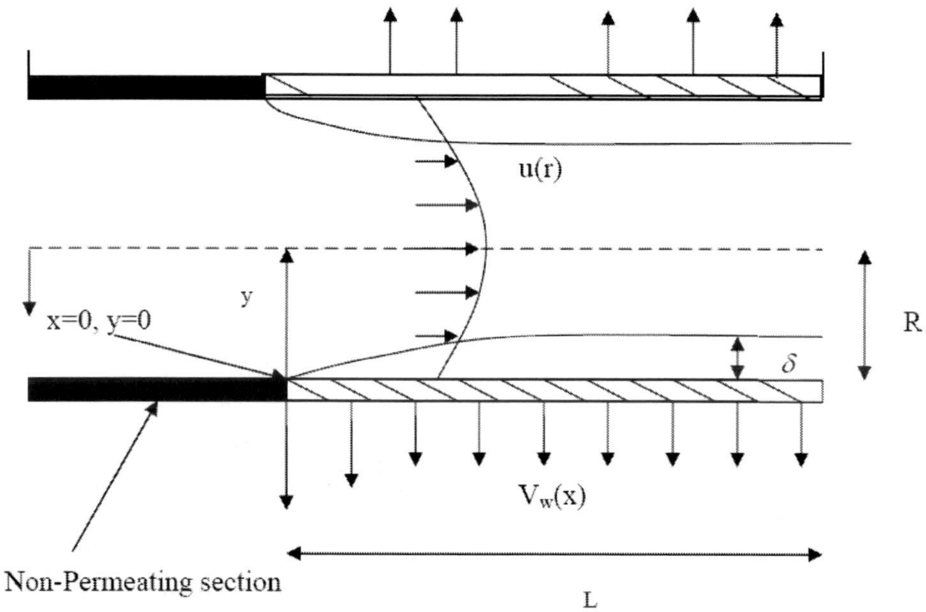

Figure 1. Schematic of the flow geometry in the tube.

2.1.1. Ellis Fluid

The rheology of the Ellis fluid is [20],

$$-\frac{dv_x}{dr} = \left(\varphi_0 + \varphi_1 \left|\tau_{rx}\right|^{\alpha-1}\right)\tau_{rx} \tag{1}$$

The laminar velocity profile of the Ellis fluid can be obtained by solving the x-component equation of motion and using Eq.(1),

for $0 \le r \le R,$

$$v_x = \left\{\frac{F\varphi_0 R^2}{2}\left(1-\left(\frac{r}{R}\right)^2\right) + \frac{F^\alpha}{\alpha+1}\varphi_1 R^{\alpha+1}\left(1-\left(\frac{r}{R}\right)^{\alpha+1}\right)\right\} \tag{2}$$

where, $F = (-\frac{dP}{dx})$. F, can be expressed as a function of average velocity (u_0) over the cross-section of the channel as,

$$u_0 = \frac{\int_0^R v_x r dr}{\int_0^R r dr} \qquad or,$$

$$u_0 = \left\{ F\varphi_0 \left(\frac{R^2}{4} \right) + \frac{F^\alpha}{\alpha+3} \varphi_1 \left(R^{\alpha+1} \right) \right\} \tag{3}$$

The steady state solute mass balance in the concentration boundary layer is obtained as,

$$v_x \frac{\partial c}{\partial x} + v_r \frac{\partial c}{\partial r} = \frac{D}{r} \frac{\partial}{\partial r} (r \frac{\partial c}{\partial r}) \tag{4}$$

by neglecting the diffusive flux compared to the convective flux in the axial direction.

Considering a thin concentration boundary layer adjacent to the wall, the curvature effects may be neglected and the problem may be treated as though the wall were flat [20]. If the distance from the wall is denoted as y=R-r, the fluid may be regarded as being confined between a flat mass-transfer surface extending from y=0 to y=∞. Therefore, the solute mass balance equation (Eq. (4)) can be expressed as,

$$v_x \frac{\partial c}{\partial x} + v_y \frac{\partial c}{\partial y} = D \frac{\partial^2 c}{\partial y^2} \tag{5}$$

The x-component velocity profile is expressed by Eq. (2). By substituting r=R-y in Eq. (2) and neglecting $\frac{y^2}{R^2}$ and the higher order terms in the binomial expansion of the Eq. (2) (since the thickness of the concentration boundary layer is small), the simplified velocity profile becomes,

$$for\ 0 \le y \le R,\ v_x = \left\{ F\varphi_0 R^2 + F^\alpha \varphi_1 R^{\alpha+1} \right\} y/R \tag{6}$$

Since the x-component velocity v_x is large enough compared to the permeate flux, the y-component velocity can be approximated as [21], assuming no solute adsorption on the membrane surface,

$$v_y = -v_w \tag{7}$$

The initial and boundary conditions of Eq. (5) are,

at $x = 0$, $c = c_0$ (8)

at $y = \infty$, $c = c_0$ (9)

At the membrane surface, the net solute flux towards the membrane is zero at the steady state. Therefore, the boundary condition at the membrane surface is,

$$\text{at } y = 0, \quad v_w\left(c - c_p\right) + D\frac{\partial c}{\partial y} = 0 \tag{10}$$

Eq. (10) can be expressed in terms of real retention of the membrane ($R_r = 1 - \frac{c_m}{c_p}$), which is constant for a membrane solute system [22],

$$\text{at } y = 0, \quad v_w c R_r + D\frac{\partial c}{\partial y} = 0 \tag{11}$$

Inserting the velocity profiles, Eqs. (6) and (7) in Eq. (5) and after non-dimensionalization, the following equation is obtained,

$$A_1 y^* \frac{\partial c^*}{\partial x^*} - Pe_w\left(x^*\right)\frac{\partial c^*}{\partial y^*} = \frac{\partial^2 c^*}{\partial y^{*2}} \tag{12}$$

where,

$x^* = \frac{x}{L}$, $y^* = \frac{y}{d}$, $c^* = \frac{c}{c_0}$, $Pe_w = \frac{v_w d}{D}$, $A_1 = \left\{F\varphi_0 R + F^\alpha \varphi_1 R^\alpha\right\}\left(\frac{d^3}{LD}\right)$ and $d = 2R$.

The rheological parameter A1 can be expressed in terms of Reynolds and Schmidt numbers as,

$$A_1 = \left\{F\varphi_0 R + F^{\alpha}\varphi_1 R^{\alpha}\right\}\left(\frac{d}{u_0}\right)\left(\frac{u_0 d^2}{LD}\right) \quad or,$$

$$A_1 = \frac{1}{u_0}\left\{F\varphi_0\frac{d^2}{2} + F^{\alpha}\varphi_1\frac{d^{\alpha+1}}{2^{\alpha}}\right\}\left(\operatorname{Re} Sc\frac{d}{L}\right)$$

or $$A_1 = A_{11}\left(\operatorname{Re} Sc\frac{d}{L}\right) \tag{13}$$

where, the non-dimensional rheological parameter becomes,

$$A_{11} = \frac{F\varphi_0\frac{d^2}{2} + F^{\alpha}\varphi_1\frac{d^{\alpha+1}}{2^{\alpha}}}{u_0} \tag{14}$$

and $\operatorname{Re} = \dfrac{\rho u_0 d}{\mu_{eff}}$, $Sc = \dfrac{\mu_{eff}}{\rho D}$

The effective viscosity is generally expressed for the non-Newtonian fluid as [12],

$$\mu_{eff} = \frac{Fd^2}{32u_0} \tag{15}$$

The derivation of Eq. (15) is presented in the appendix. The non-dimensional boundary conditions for Eq. (5) become,

at $x^* = 0$, $c^* = 1$ (16)

at $y^* = \infty$, $c^* = 1$ (17)

and at $y^* = 0$, $Pe_w c^* R_r + \dfrac{\partial c^*}{\partial y^*} = 0$ (18)

Eq. (12) is a parabolic partial differential equation with one of the boundary at infinity. Hence, it admits a similarity solution. The similarity parameter in this case is derived in the appendix and is expressed as,

$$\eta = A_1^{1/3} \frac{y^*}{x^{*1/3}} \tag{19}$$

In terms of the similarity parameter, Eq (12) becomes an ordinary differential equation,

$$\frac{d^2c^*}{d\eta^2} + \left(\frac{\eta^2}{3} + B_1\right)\frac{dc^*}{d\eta} = 0 \tag{20}$$

where, B1 is a constant and is given as,

$$B_1 = \frac{Pe_w}{A_1^{1/3}} x^{*1/3}$$

$$or$$

$$B_1 = \frac{Pe_w}{A_{11}^{1/3} (\mathrm{Re}\ Sc \frac{d}{L})^{1/3}} x^{*1/3} \tag{21}$$

The transformed boundary conditions become,

$$\text{at } \eta = \infty,\ c^* = 1 \tag{22}$$

$$\text{at } \eta = 0,\ \frac{dc^*}{d\eta} + B_1 R_r c^* = 0 \tag{23}$$

The solution of Eq. (20) with the boundary conditions, Eqs. (22) and (23) is,

$$c^*(\eta) = K_1 \int \exp\left(-\frac{\eta^3}{9} - B_1\eta\right) d\eta + K_2 \tag{24}$$

The integration constants, K_1 and K_2 are obtained using Eqs. (22) and (23) as,

$$K_1 = -\frac{B_1 R_r}{1 - B_1 R_r I_1} \tag{25}$$

and
$$K_2 = \frac{1}{1 - B_1 R_r I_1} \tag{26}$$

where,
$$I_1 = \int_0^\infty \exp\left(-\frac{\eta^3}{9} - B_1 \eta\right) d\eta \tag{27}$$

The constant B1, can be expressed in terms of length averaged dimensionless permeate flux $\left(\overline{Pe_w}\right)$ from Eq. (21),

$$\overline{Pe_w} = \int_0^1 Pe_w dx^* = 1.5 A_{11}^{1/3} \left(\mathrm{Re}\, Sc \frac{d}{L}\right)^{1/3} B_1$$

or,

$$B_1 = 0.67 \frac{\overline{Pe_w}}{(A_{11}^{1/3})(\mathrm{Re}\, Sc \frac{d}{L})^{1/3}} \tag{28}$$

Estimation of the Mass Transfer Coefficient

The definition of mass transfer coefficient is,

$$k(c_m - c_0) = -D\left(\frac{\partial c}{\partial y}\right)_{y=0} \tag{29}$$

In terms of the similarity parameter, Eq. (29) is expressed as

$$Sh\left(c_m^* - 1\right) = -\frac{A_{11}^{1/3}\left(\mathrm{Re}\, Sc \frac{d}{L}\right)^{1/3}}{x^{*1/3}} \left(\frac{dc^*}{d\eta}\right)_{\eta=0} \tag{30}$$

c_m^* and $\left(\frac{dc^*}{d\eta}\right)_{\eta=0}$ are expressed in terms of the integration constants K_1 and K_2 as,

$$Sh = -\frac{A_{11}^{1/3}\left(\mathrm{Re}\, Sc \frac{d}{L}\right)^{1/3}}{x^{*1/3}} \frac{K_1}{K_2 - 1} \tag{31}$$

Substituting K_1 and K_2 from Eqs. (25) and (26), the Sherwood number profile along the membrane length becomes,

$$Sh(x^*) = \frac{A_{11}^{1/3}}{x^{*1/3} I_1} (\mathrm{Re}\, Sc \frac{d}{L})^{1/3} \tag{32}$$

The definite integral I_1, can be expressed in terms of non-dimensional, length averaged flux ($\overline{Pe_w}$) using Eqs. (27) and (28),

$$I_1 = \int_0^\infty \exp\left(-\frac{\eta^3}{9} - 0.67 \frac{\overline{Pe_w}}{A_{11}^{1/3} (\mathrm{Re}\, Sc \frac{d}{L})^{1/3}} \eta \right) d\eta \text{ or,}$$

$$I_1 = \int_0^\infty \exp\left(-\frac{\eta^3}{9} - 0.67 \lambda_{eff1} \eta \right) d\eta \tag{33}$$

where, $$\lambda_{eff1} = \frac{\overline{Pe_w}}{A_{11}^{1/3} (\mathrm{Re}\, Sc \frac{d}{L})^{1/3}} \tag{34}$$

The length averaged Sherwood number becomes, (from Eq. (32)),

$$\overline{Sh_L} = \int_0^1 Sh(x^*) dx^* = \frac{1.5}{I_1} (A_{11})^{1/3} (\mathrm{Re}\, Sc \frac{d}{L})^{1/3} \tag{35}$$

Based on the extent of permeation, results of various cases are discussed below.

Case 1: No Permeation

In this case, $\overline{Pe_w} = 0$ and hence, $I_1 = \int_0^\infty \exp\left(-\frac{\eta^3}{9} \right) d\eta = 1.8575$

Therefore, the expression for average Sherwood number is,

$$\overline{Sh_L} = 0.81 (A_{11})^{1/3} (\mathrm{Re}\, Sc \frac{d}{L})^{1/3} \tag{36}$$

Case 2: With Permeation (RO/UF System)

To trap the effects of suction as well as the non- Newtonian behavior, I_1 is evaluated numerically for various values of λ_{eff1} (in the range of λ_{eff1}, between nearly 0 and 16, typically encountered in RO/UF), and the inverse of the integral is plotted against λ_{eff1}, in figure 2. The results are fitted in polynomial function of λ_{eff1} with a correlation coefficient more than 0.99, as

$$\frac{1}{I_1} = 0.54\left[1 + 0.74\lambda_{eff1} + 0.12\lambda_{eff1}^2 - 8.4 \times 10^{-3}\,\lambda_{eff1}^3\right] \tag{37}$$

The expression of the average Sherwood number from Eq. (35) is then,

$$\overline{Sh}_L = 0.81 \times (A_{11})^{1/3}\left(\mathrm{Re}\,Sc\,\frac{d}{L}\right)^{1/3}\left[1 + 0.74\lambda_{eff1} + 0.12\lambda_{eff1}^2 - 8.4 \times 10^{-3}\,\lambda_{eff1}^3\right] \tag{38}$$

Case 3: $\varphi_1 = 0$, Newtonian Fluid

In this case, φ_0 becomes inverse of the viscosity (μ) of the solution. Hence, the pressure gradient ($-\frac{dP}{dx} = F$) from Eq. (3) becomes,

$$F = \frac{4u_0\mu}{R^2}, \tag{39}$$

The rheological parameter A_{11} is simplified from Eq. (14),

$$A_{11} = \frac{Fd^2}{2\mu u_0} \tag{40}$$

Using Eq.(39), the value of A_{11} is obtained as 8. Therefore, from Eq.(38), the expression of the length averaged Sherwood number becomes,

$$\overline{Sh_L} = 1.62\left(\mathrm{Re}\,Sc\,\frac{d}{L}\right)^{1/3}\left[1 + 0.74\lambda_{eff1} + 0.12\lambda^2{}_{eff1} - 8.4 \times 10^{-3}\,\lambda^3{}_{eff1}\right] \tag{41}$$

where from Eq. (34), λ_{eff1} is, $\lambda_{eff1} = 0.5\dfrac{\overline{Pe_w}}{(\mathrm{Re}\,Sc\,\frac{d}{L})^{1/3}}$ (42)

Hence, Eq. (41) can be written as,

$$\overline{Sh_L} = 1.62\left(\mathrm{Re}\,Sc\frac{d}{L}\right)^{1/3}\left[1 + 0.37\frac{\overline{Pe_w}}{(\mathrm{Re}\,Sc\frac{d}{L})^{1/3}} + 0.03\frac{\overline{Pe_w}^2}{(\mathrm{Re}\,Sc\frac{d}{L})^{2/3}} - 1.05\times10^{-3}\frac{\overline{Pe_w}^3}{(\mathrm{Re}\,Sc\frac{d}{L})}\right] \quad (43)$$

It may be noticed that this result coincides with the reported one for the mass transfer coefficient with permeation for Newtonian fluid [16] in a porous tube.

For, no permeation i.e., $\overline{Pe_w}$ =0 and Eq. (43) becomes,

$$\overline{Sh_L} = 1.62\left(\mathrm{Re}\,Sc\frac{d}{L}\right)^{1/3} \quad (44)$$

which is identical with the Leveque solution [3].

Case 4: $\varphi_0 = 0$, Power Law Fluid

In this case, the pressure gradient is obtained from Eq. (3) as,

$$F = \left\{\frac{2^{\alpha+1}u_0(\alpha+3)}{\varphi_1 d^{\alpha+1}}\right\}^{\frac{1}{\alpha}} \quad (45)$$

From Eq. (14), rheological parameter A_{11} becomes,

$$A_{11} = \frac{F^{\alpha}\varphi_1 d^{\alpha+1}}{u_0 2^{\alpha}} \quad (46)$$

Using Eqs. (45) and (46), A_{11} becomes

$$A_{11} = 2(\alpha+3) \quad (47)$$

Therefore, the expression of average Sherwood number is (from Eq. 38),

$$\overline{Sh_L} = 1.02(\alpha+3)^{1/3}\left(\mathrm{Re}\,Sc\frac{d}{L}\right)^{1/3}\left[1+0.74\lambda_{eff1}+0.12\lambda^2{}_{eff1}-8.4\times10^{-3}\lambda^3{}_{eff1}\right] \quad (48)$$

where, λ_{eff1} is (from Eq. 34),

$$\lambda_{eff1} = \frac{0.794\overline{Pe}_w}{(\alpha+3)^{1/3}(\mathrm{Re}\,Sc\frac{d}{L})^{1/3}} \quad (49)$$

It may be noted here that in the definition of Re and Sc, the viscosity is μ_{eff}. The expression of μ_{eff} is shown in the appendix.

2.1.2. Reiner-Philippoff Fluid

The rheological equation for Reiner-Philippoff fluid is [20],

$$-\frac{dv_x}{dr} = \left(\frac{1}{\mu_\infty + \dfrac{\mu_0-\mu_\infty}{1+\left(\tau_{rx}/\tau_s\right)^2}}\right)\tau_{rx} \quad (50)$$

An analysis of the equation of motion in x-direction yields the following equation,

$$\frac{1}{r}\frac{d}{dr}\left(r\,\tau_{rx}\right) = -\frac{dP}{dx} = F \quad (51)$$

The solution of the above equation using Eq. (50) yields the laminar velocity profile as,

$$v_x = \frac{F}{\mu_0}\left\{\frac{R^2}{2}\left(1-\left(\frac{r}{R}\right)^2\right) - C\ln\left((2\mu_0-\mu_\infty)+\mu_0 a^2 r^2\right) + C\ln\left((2\mu_0-\mu_\infty)+\mu_0 a^2 R^2\right)\right\} \quad (52)$$

where, $a = -F/\tau_s$

and $C = \left(\dfrac{\mu_0-\mu_\infty}{2\mu_0 a^2}\right)$

The term F can be related with u_0 using the definition of average velocity (Eq. 3) in the tube as follows,

$$u_0 = \frac{2F}{\mu_0 R^2}\left\{\frac{R^4}{8} + \frac{CR^2}{2} - C\left(\frac{2\mu_0 - \mu_\infty}{2\mu_0 a^2}\right)\ln\left(1 + \frac{\mu_0 a^2}{(2\mu_0 - \mu_\infty)}R^2\right)\right\} \tag{53}$$

Inside the very thin concentration boundary layer, $r=R-y$ and $y << R$, hence, $\frac{y^2}{R^2}$ and higher order terms are neglected, to get the approximate velocity profile as,

$$v_x = \frac{F}{\mu_0}Ry \tag{54}$$

The solute mass balance equation and its boundary conditions within the concentration boundary layer remain in the same form as Eqs. (12), Eqs.(16-18). Only, A_1 is replaced by A_2.

$$A_2 = A_{22}\,\mathrm{Re}\,Sc\frac{d}{L} \tag{55}$$

where, $$A_{22} = \frac{Fd^2}{2\mu_0 u_0} \tag{56}$$

In the definition of Re and Sc in Eq. (55), μ_{eff} is expressed by Eq. (15), where F can be calculated from Eq. (53) for a known u_0, rheological parameters and tube radius.

The concentration profile is obtained by solving Eq. (12) and Eqs. (16-18) using the similarity method with the similarity parameter,

$$\xi = A_2^{1/3}\frac{y^*}{x^{*1/3}} \tag{57}$$

Using the similar calculation steps as discussed in detail for the Ellis fluid, profile of Sherwood number along the membrane length becomes,

$$Sh(x^*) = \frac{(A_{22})^{1/3}}{I_2 x^{*1/3}}(\mathrm{Re}\,Sc\frac{d}{L})^{1/3} \tag{58}$$

where, $$I_2 = \int_0^\infty \exp\left(-\frac{\xi^3}{9} - 0.67\lambda_{eff2}\xi\right)d\xi \tag{59}$$

and $$\lambda_{eff2} = \frac{\overline{Pe_W}}{(A_{22})^{1/3}(\mathrm{Re}\,Sc\frac{d}{L})^{1/3}} \tag{60}$$

The length averaged Sherwood number becomes,

$$\overline{Sh_L} = 1.5\frac{(A_{22})^{1/3}}{I_2}\left(\mathrm{Re}\,Sc\frac{d}{L}\right)^{1/3} \tag{61}$$

Based on the extent of permeation, following simplifications are discussed.

Case 1

No permeation: $\overline{Pe_W}$ =0 and I_2=1.8575. Hence, the average Sherwood number is,

$$\overline{Sh_L} = 0.81(A_{22})^{1/3}\left(\mathrm{Re}\,Sc\frac{d}{L}\right)^{1/3} \tag{62}$$

Case 2: With Permeation

In this case, I_2 is evaluated by numerical integration for various values of λ_{eff2} and $1/I_2$ is plotted with λ_{eff2} in figure 2. The expression of the length averaged Sherwood number is given by Eq. (38), replacing A_{11} by A_{22} and λ_{eff1} by λ_{eff2}.

Case 3: $\mu_0 = \mu_\infty = \mu$, Newtonian fluid

In this case, as for Ellis fluid, A_{22}= 8 and the length averaged Sherwood number becomes similar to Eq. (41), replacing λ_{eff1} by λ_{eff2}, while λ_{eff2} is expressed by Eq. (42). Therefore, the final expression for the length averaged Sherwood number is identical with Eq. (43).

2.1.3 Eyring Fluid

The rheological equation for the Eying fluid is [20],

$$\tau_{rx} = ASinh^{-1}\left(-\frac{1}{B}\frac{dv_x}{dr}\right) \tag{63}$$

An analysis of x-component equation of motion results in Eq. (51). Using Eqs. (51) and (63), the expression of the x-component velocity profile becomes,

$$v_x = \frac{B}{K}\{Cosh(KR) - Cosh(Kr)\} \tag{64}$$

where, $K = \frac{F}{A}$

The relation between the cross sectional average velocity u_0 and F can be obtained as before (from Eq. 3),

$$u_0 = \frac{2B}{KR^2}\left\{\frac{R}{K}Sinh(KR) + \frac{1}{K^2}(1 - Cosh(KR)) - \frac{R^2}{2}Cosh(KR)\right\} \tag{65}$$

Inside the concentration boundary layer, $r=R-y$ and $y << R$, hence $\frac{y^2}{R^2}$ and higher order terms are neglected, to get the velocity profile as,

$$v_x = [BSinh(KR)]y \tag{66}$$

The solute mass balance equation and its boundary conditions within the concentration boundary layer remain in the same form as Eq. (12) and Eqs. (16-18), with A_1 is replaced by A_3,

$$A_3 = A_{33}\,\mathrm{Re}\,Sc\frac{d}{L} \tag{67}$$

where,

$$A_{33} = \frac{Bd}{u_0}Sinh(\frac{Kd}{2}) \tag{68}$$

The definition of Re and Sc, in Eq. (68), μ_{eff} is expressed by the Eq. (15), where F can be calculated from Eq. (65) for a known value of u_0 , rheological parameters and channel height.

The concentration profile is obtained by solving Eq. (12) and Eqs. (16-18) using the similarity method with similarity parameter,

$$\phi = A_3^{1/3}\frac{y^*}{x^{*1/3}} \tag{69}$$

Using the similar calculation steps as discussed in detail for the Ellis fluid, the Sherwood number profile along the membrane length becomes,

$$Sh(x^*) = \frac{(A_{33})^{1/3}}{I_3 x^{*1/3}} \left(\mathrm{Re}\, Sc \frac{d}{L} \right)^{1/3} \tag{70}$$

where, $$I_3 = \int_0^\infty \exp\left(-\frac{\phi^3}{9} - 0.67\lambda_{eff3}\phi \right) d\phi \tag{71}$$

and $$\lambda_{eff3} = \frac{\overline{Pe_W}}{(A_{33})^{1/3} (\mathrm{Re}\, Sc \frac{d}{L})^{1/3}} \tag{72}$$

The length averaged Sherwood number becomes,

$$\overline{Sh_L} = 1.5 \frac{(A_{33})^{1/3}}{I_3} \left(\mathrm{Re}\, Sc \frac{d}{L} \right)^{1/3} \tag{73}$$

The simplifications with various extents of permeation are as follows,

Case 1: No Permeation, $\overline{Pe_W} = 0$

The length averaged Sherwood number becomes

$$\overline{Sh_L} = 0.81 (A_{33})^{1/3} \left(\mathrm{Re}\, Sc \frac{d}{L} \right)^{1/3} \tag{74}$$

Case 2: With Permeation

As earlier, I_3 is evaluated numerically for various values of λ_{eff3} and $1/I_3$ versus λ_{eff3} is plotted in figure 2. The Sherwood number relationship is given by Eq. (38), replacing A_{11} and A_{33} and λ_{eff1} by λ_{eff3}.

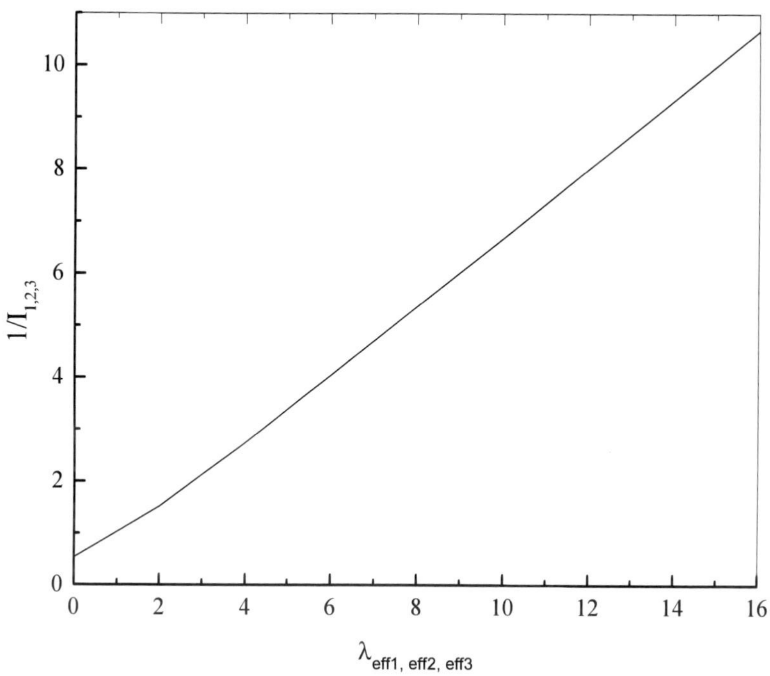

Figure 2. Variation of the definite integrals I1,2,3 with $\lambda_{eff1,\, eff2,\, eff3}$ for tubular geometry.

2.2. Flow through a Rectangular Channel

The theoretical developments of the rectangular thin channel for Ellis, Eyring and Reiner-Philippoff fluids are presented herein. The flow geometry is shown in figure 3.

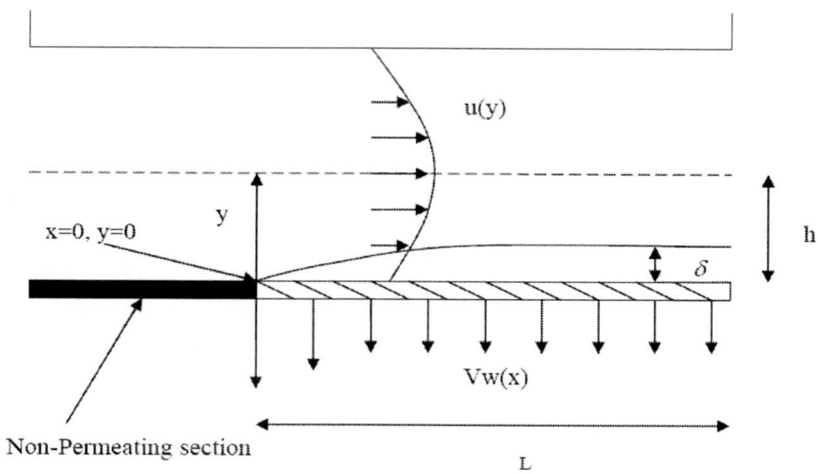

Figure 3. Schematic of the flow geometry in the rectangular channel.

2.2.1. Ellis Fluid

The rheology of the Ellis fluid is [20],

$$-\frac{dv_x}{dy} = \left(\varphi_0 + \varphi_1 \left|\tau_{yx}\right|^{\alpha-1}\right)\tau_{yx} \tag{75}$$

The laminar velocity profile of the Ellis fluid can be obtained by solving the x-component equation of motion using Eq.(75),

$$\text{for } 0 \le y \le h,\ v_x = \left[F\varphi_0 hy\left(1-\frac{y}{2h}\right) + \frac{F^\alpha}{\alpha+1}\varphi_1 h^{\alpha+1}\left\{1-\left(1-\frac{y}{h}\right)^{\alpha+1}\right\}\right] \tag{76}$$

$$\text{for } h \le y \le 2h,\ v_x = \left[F\varphi_0 hy\left(1-\frac{y}{2h}\right) + \frac{F^\alpha}{\alpha+1}\varphi_1 h^{\alpha+1}\left\{1-\left(\frac{y}{h}-1\right)^{\alpha+1}\right\}\right] \tag{77}$$

where, $F = (-\frac{dP}{dx})$. F, can be expressed as a function of average velocity (u_0) over the cross-section of the channel as,

$$u_0 = \frac{\int_0^{2h} v_x dy}{\int_0^{2h} dy}$$

or,

$$u_0 = \left\{F\varphi_0\left(\frac{h^2}{3}\right) + \frac{F^\alpha}{\alpha+2}\varphi_1\left(h^{\alpha+1}\right)\right\} \tag{78}$$

The solute mass balance in the concentration boundary layer is obtained as,

$$v_x\frac{\partial c}{\partial x} + v_y\frac{\partial c}{\partial y} = D\frac{\partial^2 c}{\partial y^2} \tag{79}$$

The x-component velocity profile is expressed by Eq. (76). Since the thickness of the concentration boundary layer is small, $\frac{y^2}{h^2}$ and the higher order terms in the binomial expansion of the Eq. (76) are neglected and the simplified velocity profile becomes,

$$\text{for } 0 \le y \le h,\ v_x = \left\{F\varphi_0 h^2 + F^{\alpha}\varphi_1 h^{\alpha+1}\right\}\frac{y}{h} \tag{80}$$

Since the x-component velocity v_x is large enough compared to the permeate flux, the y-component velocity can be approximated as expressed in Eq.(7). The boundary conditions of Eq.(79) are given in Eqs.(8-11). Inserting the velocity profiles and after non-dimensionalization, the following equation is obtained,

$$A_1^0 y^* \frac{\partial c^*}{\partial x^*} - Pe_w\left(x^*\right)\frac{\partial c^*}{\partial y^*} = \frac{\partial^2 c^*}{\partial y^{*2}} \tag{81}$$

where,

$$x^* = \frac{x}{L},\ y^* = \frac{y}{d_e},\ c^* = \frac{c}{c_0},\ Pe_w = \frac{v_w d_e}{D} \text{ and}$$

$$A_1^0 = \left\{F\varphi_0 h + F^{\alpha}\varphi_1 h^{\alpha}\right\}\left(\frac{d_e^{\ 3}}{LD}\right)$$

The equivalent diameter for a thin channel is defined as $d_e = 4h$ [23].The rheological parameter A_1^0 can be expressed in terms of Reynolds and Schmidt numbers as,

$$A_1^0 = \left\{F\varphi_0 h + F^{\alpha}\varphi_1 h^{\alpha}\right\}\left(\frac{d_e}{u_0}\right)\left(\frac{u_0 d_e^{\ 2}}{LD}\right)$$

or,

$$A_1^0 = \frac{1}{u_0}\left\{F\varphi_0\frac{d_e^{\ 2}}{4} + F^{\alpha}\varphi_1\frac{d_e^{\ \alpha+1}}{4^{\alpha}}\right\}\left(\operatorname{Re} Sc\frac{d_e}{L}\right)$$

$$\text{or } A_1^0 = A_{11}^0\left(\operatorname{Re} Sc\frac{d_e}{L}\right) \tag{82}$$

where, the non-dimensional rheological parameter becomes,

$$A_{11}^0 = \frac{F\varphi_0\dfrac{d_e^{\ 2}}{4} + F^{\alpha}\varphi_1\dfrac{d_e^{\ \alpha+1}}{4^{\alpha}}}{u_0} \tag{83}$$

and $\mathrm{Re} = \dfrac{\rho u_0 d_e}{\mu_{eff}}$, $Sc = \dfrac{\mu_{eff}}{\rho D}$

The effective viscosity is generally expressed for the non-Newtonian fluid as [12]

$$\mu_{eff} = \frac{F d_e^{\,2}}{32 u_0} \tag{84}$$

The derivation of Eq. (84) is presented in the appendix.

The non-dimensional boundary conditions for Eq. (81) are given by Eqs.(16-18). Eq. (81) is a parabolic partial differential equation with one of the boundary at infinity. Hence, it admits a similarity solution. The similarity parameter in this case is derived in the appendix and is expressed as,

$$\eta_0 = A_1^{0\,1/3} \frac{y^*}{x^{*1/3}} \tag{85}$$

In terms of the similarity parameter, Eq (81) becomes an ordinary differential equation,

$$\frac{d^2 c^*}{d\eta_0^{\,2}} + \left(\frac{\eta_0^{\,2}}{3} + B_1^0\right)\frac{dc^*}{d\eta_0} = 0 \tag{86}$$

where, B_1^0 is a constant and is given as,

$$B_1^0 = \frac{Pe_w}{A_1^{0\,1/3}} x^{*1/3}$$

or

$$B_1^0 = \frac{Pe_w}{A_{11}^{0\,1/3} (\mathrm{Re}\ Sc\ \frac{d_e}{L})^{1/3}} x^{*1/3} \tag{87}$$

The transformed boundary conditions become,

at $\eta_0 = \infty$, $c^* = 1$ (88)

$$\text{at } \eta_0 = 0, \quad \frac{dc^*}{d\eta_0} + B_1^0 R_r c^* = 0 \tag{89}$$

The solution of Eq. (86) with the boundary conditions, Eqs. (88) and (89) is,

$$c^*(\eta_0) = K_1^0 \int \exp\left(-\frac{\eta_0^3}{9} - B_1^0 \eta_0\right) d\eta_0 + K_2^0 \tag{90}$$

The integration constants, K_1^0 and K_2^0 are obtained using Eqs. (88) and (89) as,

$$K_1^0 = -\frac{B_1^0 R_r}{1 - B_1^0 R_r I_1^0} \tag{91}$$

$$\text{and } K_2^0 = \frac{1}{1 - B_1^0 R_r I_1^0} \tag{92}$$

$$\text{where, } I_1^0 = \int_0^\infty \exp\left(-\frac{\eta_0^3}{9} - B_1^0 \eta_0\right) d\eta_0 \tag{93}$$

The constant B_1^0, can be expressed in terms of length averaged dimensionless permeate flux $\left(\overline{Pe_w}\right)$ from Eq. (87),

$$\overline{Pe_w} = \int_0^1 Pe_w dx^* = 1.5 A_{11}^{0\,1/3} \left(\mathrm{Re}\, Sc \frac{d_e}{L}\right)^{1/3} B_1^0$$

or,

$$B_1^0 = 0.67 \frac{\overline{Pe_w}}{(A_{11}^{0\,1/3})(\mathrm{Re}\, Sc \frac{d_e}{L})^{1/3}} \tag{94}$$

Estimation of Mass Transfer Coefficient

From the definition of mass transfer coefficient, in terms of similarity parameter, Eq. (29) is expressed as

$$Sh\left(c_m^* - 1\right) = -\frac{A_{11}^{0\,1/3}\left(\mathrm{Re}\,Sc\dfrac{d_e}{L}\right)^{1/3}}{x^{*1/3}}\left(\frac{dc^*}{d\eta_0}\right)_{\eta_0=0} \tag{95}$$

c_m^* and $\left(\dfrac{dc^*}{d\eta_0}\right)_{\eta_0=0}$ are expressed in terms of the integration constants K_1^0 and K_2^0 as,

$$Sh = -\frac{A_{11}^{0\,1/3}\left(\mathrm{Re}\,Sc\dfrac{d_e}{L}\right)^{1/3}}{x^{*1/3}}\frac{K_1^0}{K_2^0 - 1} \tag{96}$$

Substituting K_1^0 and K_2^0 from Eqs. (91) and (92), the Sherwood number profile along the membrane length becomes,

$$Sh\left(x^*\right) = \frac{A_{11}^{0\,1/3}}{x^{*1/3} I_1^0}\left(\mathrm{Re}\,Sc\frac{d_e}{L}\right)^{1/3} \tag{97}$$

The definite integral I_1^0, can be expressed in terms of non-dimensional, length averaged flux ($\overline{Pe_w}$) using Eqs. (93) and (94),

$$I_1^0 = \int_0^\infty \exp\left(-\frac{\eta_0^{\,3}}{9} - 0.67\frac{\overline{Pe_w}}{A_{11}^{0\,1/3}\left(\mathrm{Re}\,Sc\dfrac{d_e}{L}\right)^{1/3}}\eta_0\right)d\eta_0 \quad \text{or,}$$

$$I_1^0 = \int_0^\infty \exp\left(-\frac{\eta_0^{\,3}}{9} - 0.67\lambda_{eff1}^0\eta_0\right)d\eta_0 \tag{98}$$

$$\text{where, } \lambda_{eff1}^0 = \frac{\overline{Pe_w}}{A_{11}^{0\,1/3}\left(\mathrm{Re}\,Sc\dfrac{d_e}{L}\right)^{1/3}} \tag{99}$$

The length averaged Sherwood number becomes, (from Eq. (97)),

$$\overline{Sh_L} = \int_0^1 Sh(x^*)dx^* = \frac{1.5}{I_1^0}\left(A_{11}^0\right)^{1/3}\left(\mathrm{Re}\,Sc\frac{d_e}{L}\right)^{1/3} \tag{100}$$

Based on the extent of permeation, results of various cases are discussed below.

Case 1: No Permeation

In this case, $\overline{Pe_w}$ =0 and hence, $I_1^0 = \int_0^{\infty} \exp\left(-\frac{\eta_0^{\ 3}}{9}\right) d\eta_0 = 1.8575$

Therefore, the expression for average Sherwood number is,

$$\overline{Sh_L} = 0.81(A_{11}^0)^{1/3}(\mathrm{Re}\,Sc\frac{d_e}{L})^{1/3} \tag{101}$$

Case 2: With Permeation (RO/UF System)

To trap the effects of suction as well as the non- Newtonian behavior, I_1^0 is evaluated numerically for various values of λ_{eff1}^0 (between nearly 0 and 16, typically encountered in RO/UF), and the inverse of the integral is plotted against λ_{eff1}^0, in figure 4. The results are fitted in polynomial function of λ_{eff1}^0 with a correlation coefficient more than 0.99, as

$$\frac{1}{I_1^0} = 0.54\left[1 + 0.743\lambda_{eff1}^0 + 0.105(\lambda_{eff1}^0)^2 - 9.66\times10^{-3}(\lambda_{eff1}^0)^3\right] \tag{102}$$

The expression of the average Sherwood number from Eq. (100) is then,

$$\overline{Sh}_L = 0.81\times(A_{11}^0)^{1/3}\left(\mathrm{Re}\,Sc\frac{d_e}{L}\right)^{1/3}\left[1 + 0.743\lambda_{eff1}^0 + 0.105(\lambda_{eff1}^0)^2 - 9.66\times10^{-3}(\lambda_{eff1}^0)^3\right] \tag{103}$$

Case 3: $\varphi_1 = 0$, Newtonian Fluid

In this case, φ_0 becomes inverse of the viscosity of the solution. Hence, the pressure gradient ($-\frac{dP}{dx} = F$) from Eq. (78) becomes,

$$F = \frac{3u_0\mu}{h^2}, \tag{104}$$

The rheological parameter A_{11}^0 is simplified from Eq. (83),

$$A_{11}^0 = \frac{Fd_e^{\ 2}}{4\mu u_0} \tag{105}$$

Using Eq.(104), the value of A_{11}^0 is obtained as 12. Therefore, from Eq.(103), the expression of the length averaged Sherwood number becomes,

$$\overline{Sh_L} = 1.85\left(\mathrm{Re}\,Sc\frac{d_e}{L}\right)^{1/3}\left[1+0.743\lambda_{eff1}^0+0.105(\lambda_{eff1}^0)^2-9.66\times10^{-3}(\lambda_{eff1}^0)^3\right] \tag{106}$$

where from Eq. (99), λ_{eff1}^0 is, $\lambda_{eff1}^0 = 0.44\dfrac{\overline{Pe_w}}{(\mathrm{Re}\,Sc\frac{d_e}{L})^{1/3}}$ (107)

Hence, Eq. (106) can be written as,

$$\overline{Sh_L} = 1.85\left(\mathrm{Re}\,Sc\frac{d_e}{L}\right)^{1/3}\left[1+0.32\frac{\overline{Pe_w}}{(\mathrm{Re}\,Sc\frac{d_e}{L})^{1/3}}+0.02\frac{\overline{Pe_w}^2}{(\mathrm{Re}\,Sc\frac{d_e}{L})^{2/3}}-8.05\times10^{-4}\frac{\overline{Pe_w}^3}{(\mathrm{Re}\,Sc\frac{d_e}{L})}\right] \tag{108}$$

It may be noticed that this result coincides with the reported one for the mass transfer coefficient with permeation for Newtonian fluid [16].

For, no permeation i.e., $\overline{Pe_w}=0$ and Eq. (108) becomes,

$$\overline{Sh_L} = 1.85\left(\mathrm{Re}\,Sc\frac{d_e}{L}\right)^{1/3} \tag{109}$$

which is identical with the Leveque solution [3].

Case 4: $\varphi_0 = 0$, Power Law Fluid

In this case, the pressure gradient is obtained from Eq. (78) as,

$$F = \left\{ \frac{4^{\alpha+1} u_0 (\alpha + 2)}{\varphi_1 d_e^{\ \alpha+1}} \right\}^{\frac{1}{\alpha}} \tag{110}$$

From Eq. (83), rheological parameter A_{11}^0 becomes,

$$A_{11}^0 = \frac{F^{\alpha} \varphi_1 d_e^{\ \alpha+1}}{u_0 4^{\alpha}} \tag{111}$$

Using Eqs. (110) and (111), A_{11}^0 becomes

$$A_{11}^0 = 4(\alpha + 2) \tag{112}$$

Therefore, the expression of average Sherwood number is (from Eq. 103),

$$\overline{Sh_L} = 1.28(\alpha + 2)^{1/3} \left(\mathrm{Re}\, Sc \frac{d_e}{L} \right)^{1/3} \left[1 + 0.73\lambda_{eff1}^0 + 0.105(\lambda_{eff1}^0)^2 - 9.66 \times 10^{-3} (\lambda_{eff1}^0)^3 \right] \tag{113}$$

where, λ_{eff1}^0 is (from Eq. 99),

$$\lambda_{eff1}^0 = \frac{0.63\overline{Pe}_w}{(\alpha + 2)^{1/3} (\mathrm{Re}\, Sc \frac{d_e}{L})^{1/3}} \tag{114}$$

It may be noted here that in the definition of Re and Sc, the viscosity is μ_{eff}. The expression of μ_{eff} is shown in the appendix.

2.2.2. Reiner-Philippoff Fluid

The rheological equation for Reiner-Philippoff fluid is [20],

$$-\frac{dv_x}{dy} = \left(\frac{1}{\mu_0 + \dfrac{\mu_0 - \mu_\infty}{1 + \left(\tau_{yx} / \tau_s \right)^2}} \right) \tau_{yx} \tag{115}$$

An analysis of the equation of motion in x-direction yields the following equation,

$$\frac{d\tau_{yx}}{dy} = -\frac{dp}{dx} = F \tag{116}$$

The solution of the above equation using Eq. (115) yields the laminar velocity profile as,

$$v_x = \frac{F}{\mu_0}\left\{hy\left(1-\frac{y}{2h}\right) - C\ln\left(\left(2\mu_0 - \mu_\infty\right) + \mu_0 a^2 (h-y)^2\right) + C\ln\left(\left(2\mu_0 - \mu_\infty\right) + \mu_0 a^2 h^2\right)\right\} \quad (117)$$

where, $a = -F/\tau_s$

and $C = \left(\dfrac{\mu_0 - \mu_\infty}{2\mu_0 a^2}\right)$

The term F can be related with u_0 using the definition of average velocity (Eq. 78) in the channel as follows,

$$u_0 = \frac{F}{\mu_0 h}\left\{\frac{h^3}{3} - Ch\ln\left(\left(2\mu_0 - \mu_\infty\right) + \mu_0 a^2 h^2\right) + 2Ch - 2C^{3/2}\tan^{-1}\left(\frac{h}{\sqrt{C}}\right)\right\} \quad (118)$$

Inside the Concentration Boundary layer, where $\dfrac{y^2}{h^2}$ and higher order terms are neglected, the velocity profile becomes,

$$v_x = \frac{F}{\mu_0} hy \quad (119)$$

The solute mass balance equation and its boundary conditions within the concentration boundary layer remain in the same form as Eqs. (81), (16-18). Only, A_1^0 is replaced by A_2^0.

$$A_2^0 = A_{22}^0 \operatorname{Re} Sc \frac{d_e}{L} \quad (120)$$

where, $$A_{22}^0 = \frac{F d_e^{\,2}}{4\mu_0 u_0} \quad (121)$$

In the definition of Re and Sc in Eq. (120), μ_{eff} is expressed by Eq. (84), where F can be calculated from Eq. (118) for a known u_0, rheological parameters and channel half height. The concentration profile is obtained by solving Eq. (81) and Eqs. (16-18) using the similarity method with the similarity parameter,

$$\xi_0 = A_2^{0\,1/3} \frac{y^*}{x^{*1/3}} \tag{122}$$

Using the similar calculation steps as discussed in detail for the Ellis fluid, profile of Sherwood number along the membrane length becomes,

$$Sh(x^*) = \frac{(A_{22}^0)^{1/3}}{I_2^0 x^{*1/3}} (\mathrm{Re}\, Sc \frac{d_e}{L})^{1/3} \tag{123}$$

where, $$I_2^0 = \int_0^\infty \exp\left(-\frac{\xi_0^{\ 3}}{9} - 0.67 \lambda_{eff\,2}^0 \xi_0 \right) d\xi_0 \tag{124}$$

and $$\lambda_{eff\,2}^0 = \frac{\overline{Pe_W}}{(A_{22}^0)^{1/3} (\mathrm{Re}\, Sc \frac{d_e}{L})^{1/3}} \tag{125}$$

The length averaged Sherwood number becomes,

$$\overline{Sh_L} = 1.5 \frac{\left(A_{22}^0\right)^{1/3}}{I_2^0} \left(\mathrm{Re}\, Sc \frac{d_e}{L} \right)^{1/3} \tag{126}$$

Based on the extent of permeation, following simplifications are discussed.

Case 1: No permeation

$\overline{Pe_W}$ =0 and I_2^0=1.8575. Hence, the average Sherwood number is,

$$\overline{Sh_L} = 0.81 \left(A_{22}^0\right)^{1/3} \left(\mathrm{Re}\, Sc \frac{d_e}{L} \right)^{1/3} \tag{127}$$

Case 2: With Permeation

In this case, I_2^0 is evaluated by numerical integration for various values of $\lambda_{eff\,2}$ and $1/I_2^0$ is plotted with $\lambda_{eff\,2}^0$ in figure 4. The expression of the length averaged Sherwood number is given by Eq. (103), replacing A_{11}^0 by A_{22}^0 and $\lambda_{eff\,1}^0$ by $\lambda_{eff\,2}^0$.

Case 3: $\mu_0 = \mu_\infty = \mu$, Newtonian Fluid

In this case, as for Ellis fluid, A_{22}^0 = 12 and the length averaged Sherwood number becomes similar to Eq. (106), while λ_{eff2}^0 is expressed by Eq. (107). Therefore, the final expression for the length averaged Sherwood number is identical with Eq. (108).

2.2.3. Eyring Fluid

The rheological equation for the Eying fluid is [20],

$$\tau_{yx} = ASinh^{-1}\left(-\frac{1}{B}\frac{dv_x}{dy} \right) \tag{128}$$

An analysis of x-component equation of motion results in Eq. (116). Using Eqs. (116) and (128), the expression of the x-component velocity profile becomes,

$$v_x = \frac{B}{K}\{Cosh(K(h-y)) - Cosh(Kh)\} \tag{129}$$

where, $K = \dfrac{F}{A} = \dfrac{\left(-\dfrac{dP}{dx}\right)}{A}$

The relation between the cross sectional average velocity u_0 and F can be obtained as before (from Eq.78),

$$u_0 = \frac{B}{2Kh}\left\{\frac{2}{K}Sinh(Kh) - 2hCosh(Kh)\right\} \tag{130}$$

Inside the Concentration Boundary layer, where $\dfrac{y^2}{h^2}$ and higher order terms are neglected, the velocity profile becomes,

$$v_x = B\,Sinh(Kh)\,y \tag{131}$$

The solute mass balance equation and its boundary conditions within the concentration boundary layer remain in the same form as Eq. (81) and Eqs. (16-18), with A_1^0 is replaced by A_3^0,

$$A_3^0 = A_{33}^0 \operatorname{Re} Sc \frac{d_e}{L} \tag{132}$$

where,

$$A_{33}^0 = \frac{Bd_e}{u_0} Sinh(\frac{Kd_e}{4}) \tag{133}$$

The definition of Re and Sc, in Eq. (133), μ_{eff} is expressed by the Eq. (84), where F can be calculated from Eq. (130) for a known value of u_0 , rheological parameters and channel height.

The concentration profile is obtained by solving Eq. (81) and Eqs. (16-18) using the similarity method with similarity parameter,

$$\phi_0 = A_3^{0\,1/3} \frac{y^*}{x^{*\,1/3}} \tag{134}$$

Using the similar calculation steps as discussed in detail for the Ellis fluid, the Sherwood number profile along the membrane length becomes,

$$Sh(x^*) = \frac{\left(A_{33}^0\right)^{1/3}}{I_3^0 x^{*\,1/3}} \left(\operatorname{Re} Sc \frac{d_e}{L}\right)^{1/3} \tag{135}$$

$$\text{where, } I_3^0 = \int_0^\infty \exp\left(-\frac{\phi_0{}^3}{9} - 0.67\lambda_{eff\,3}^0 \phi_0\right) d\phi_0 \tag{136}$$

$$\text{and } \lambda_{eff\,3}^0 = \frac{\overline{Pe_W}}{(A_{33}^0)^{1/3} (\operatorname{Re} Sc \frac{d_e}{L})^{1/3}} \tag{137}$$

The length averaged Sherwood number becomes,

$$\overline{Sh_L} = 1.5 \frac{\left(A_{33}^0\right)^{1/3}}{I_3^0} \left(\operatorname{Re} Sc \frac{d_e}{L}\right)^{1/3} \tag{138}$$

The simplifications with various extents of permeation are as follows,

Case 1: No Permeation, $\overline{Pe_W} = 0$

The length averaged Sherwood number becomes

$$\overline{Sh_L} = 0.81\left(A_{33}^0\right)^{1/3}\left(\mathrm{Re}\,Sc\,\frac{d_e}{L}\right)^{1/3} \tag{139}$$

Case 2: With Permeation

As earlier, I_3^0 is evaluated numerically for various values of λ_{eff3}^0 and $1/I_3^0$ versus λ_{eff3}^0 is plotted in figure 4. The Sherwood number relationship is given by Eq. (103), replacing A_{11}^0 by A_{33}^0 and λ_{eff1}^0 by λ_{eff3}^0.

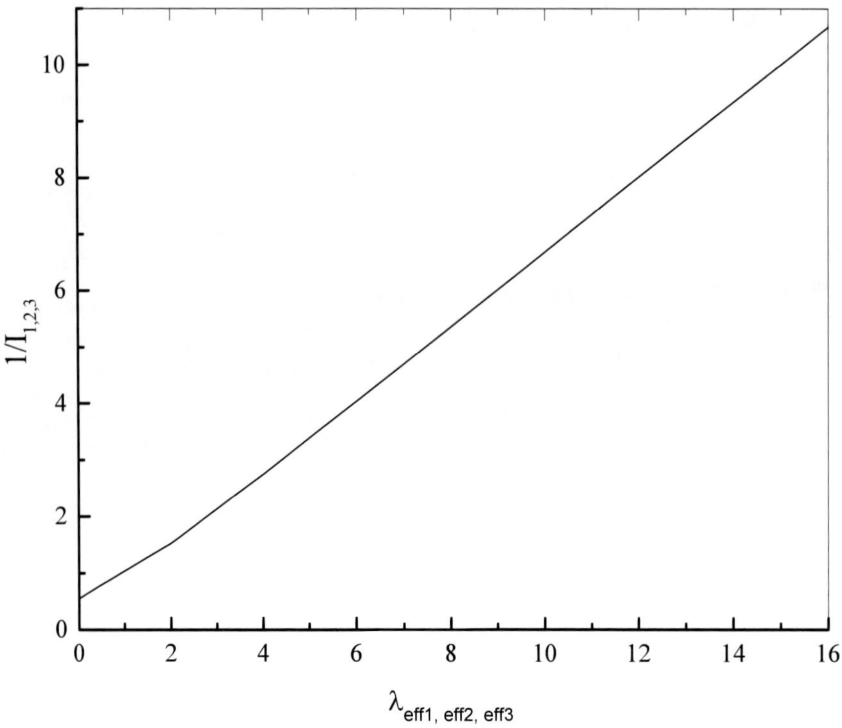

Figure 4. Variation of the definite integrals $I_{1,2,3}^0$ with $\lambda^0{}_{eff1,\,eff2,\,eff3}$ for rectangular channel.

3. Results and Discussion

3.1. Tubular Geometry

3.1.1. Ellis Fluid

Aqueous solution of carboxymethyl cellulose (CMC) follows Ellis fluid behavior. Various rheological parameters of the CMC solutions are given below [20],

$\varphi_0 = 0.2891$ cm^2 s^{-1} dyne^{-1}, $\varphi_1 = 0.028$ cm$^{2\alpha}$ s^{-1} dyne$^{-\alpha}$, α =1.707 for 0.6% CMC and $\varphi_0 = 0.421$ cm^2 s^{-1} dyne^{-1}, $\varphi_1 = 0.2724$ cm$^{2\alpha}$ s^{-1} dyne$^{-\alpha}$, α =1.185 for 1.5% CMC solution. In order to calculate the Sherwood number, first F (i.e., $-\frac{dP}{dx}$) is fitted with the average velocity (u_0), using the following steps,

i) a value of u_0 is assumed.

ii) using the rheological parameters and assumed values of u_0 and channel geometry R (0.001 m), F is obtained from Eq. (3) using Newton-Raphson iteration method.

iii) μ_{eff} is calculated using the F value from step (ii) by Eq. (15).

iv) Reynolds number is calculated from its definition $\frac{\rho u_0 d}{\mu_{eff}}$ and is checked whether it is lying within the laminar flow regime ($\mathrm{Re} \le 2200$).

Using the above method, F is evaluated for various value of u_0 and is fitted as a function of u_0. The tubular channel radius (R) is considered to be 0.001 m in this study. The relationship of F with u_0 is presented below,

$$F = -1.1\times 10^5 u_0^2 + 1.8\times 10^5 u_0 + 9.8\times 10^3, \text{ for 0.6\% CMC solution} \quad (140)$$

$$F = 2.8\times 10^5 u_0 + 5.5\times 10^3, \text{ for 1.5\% CMC solution} \quad (141)$$

where, F is in Pa/m and u_0 is in m/s.

Using Eq. (14), A_{11} is evaluated at u_0 =0.3 m/s and its values are,

$$A_{11} = 9.66, \text{ for 0.6\% CMC solution}$$
$$= 8.23, \text{ for 1.5\% CMC solution} \quad (142)$$

The profiles of Sherwood numbers along the channel length are obtained from Eq. (32),

$$Sh(x^*) = \frac{2.13}{I_1 x^{*1/3}} \left(\mathrm{Re} Sc \frac{d}{L} \right)^{1/3}, \text{ for 0.6\% CMC solution}$$

$$= \frac{2.02}{I_1 x^{*1/3}} \left(\mathrm{Re} Sc \frac{d}{L} \right)^{1/3}, \text{ for 1.5\% CMC solution} \tag{143}$$

The values of the permeation parameter, λ_{eff1} is obtained from Eq. (34),

$$\lambda_{eff1} = \frac{0.469 \overline{Pe_w}}{\left(\mathrm{Re}\, Sc \frac{d}{L} \right)^{1/3}} \text{ for 0.6\% CMC solution}$$

$$= \frac{0.495 \overline{Pe_W}}{\left(\mathrm{Re}\, Sc \frac{d}{L} \right)^{1/3}} \text{ for 1.5\% CMC solution} \tag{144}$$

The length averaged Sherwood numbers are obtained from Eq. (38) as,

$$\overline{Sh_L} = 1.73 \left(\mathrm{Re}\, Sc \frac{d}{L} \right)^{1/3} \left[1 + 0.35 \frac{\overline{Pe_W}}{\left(\mathrm{Re}\, Sc \frac{d}{L} \right)^{1/3}} + 0.026 \frac{\overline{Pe_W}^2}{\left(\mathrm{Re}\, Sc \frac{d}{L} \right)^{2/3}} - 8.67 \times 10^{-4} \frac{\overline{Pe_W}^3}{\left(\mathrm{Re}\, Sc \frac{d}{L} \right)} \right]$$

for 0.6% CMC solution

$$= 1.64 \left(\mathrm{Re}\, Sc \frac{d}{L} \right)^{1/3} \left[1 + 0.366 \frac{\overline{Pe_W}}{\left(\mathrm{Re}\, Sc \frac{d}{L} \right)^{1/3}} + 0.029 \frac{\overline{Pe_W}^2}{\left(\mathrm{Re}\, Sc \frac{d}{L} \right)^{2/3}} - 1.02 \times 10^{-3} \frac{\overline{Pe_W}^3}{\left(\mathrm{Re}\, Sc \frac{d}{L} \right)} \right]$$

for 1.5% CMC solution (145)

The variation of the Sherwood number along the channel length for values of $\mathrm{Re}\, Sc \frac{d}{L} = 10^3$ and 10^5 for $\overline{Pe_W} = 200$ is shown in figure 5. It is observed from the figure that, the Sherwood number decreases along the tube length. The decline is sharp in the upstream of the channel and gradual thereafter. This is due to the fact that the build up of the concentration boundary layer over the membrane surface becomes sluggish at the downstream of the channel because of the forced convection imposed by the cross flow. This reduces the concentration difference between the membrane surface and the bulk of the solution. Therefore, the Sherwood number and consequently, the mass transfer coefficient decreases along the channel length. It may be observed from figure 5 that the Sherwood number is more at higher $\mathrm{Re}\,Sc\frac{d}{L}$ at the same level of the permeate flux ($\overline{Pe_w}$). This indicates that at higher Reynolds number, forced convection is more due to higher cross flow velocity, which enhances the mass transfer coefficient. It may also be observed that the Sherwood number profiles for both concentrations of CMC solution almost coincide at $\mathrm{Re}\,Sc\frac{d}{L}=10^3$ and they differ marginally at $\mathrm{Re}\,Sc\frac{d}{L}=10^5$.

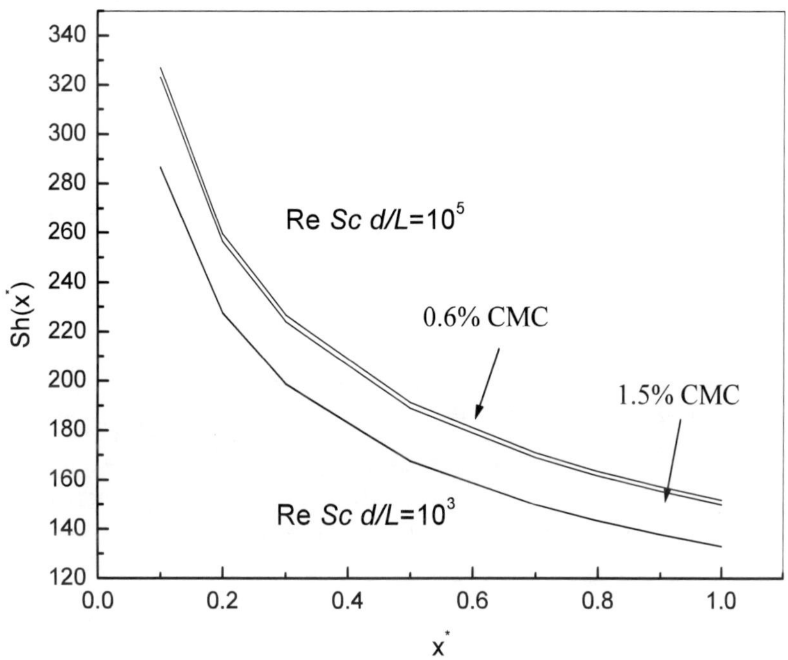

Figure 5. Variation of Sherwood number along the tube length for the Ellis fluid at $\overline{Pe_w}=200$.

The variation of the length averaged Sherwood number with the average wall Peclet number is presented in figure 6, for $\mathrm{Re}\,Sc\frac{d}{L}=10^3$ and 10^5. It is evident from the figure that the Sherwood number increases with the wall Peclet number. This implies the mass transfer coefficient increases with the extent of permeation. As permeation increases, the convective solute flux through the membrane increases and at the steady state, to maintain the solute balance, the backward diffusion from the surface to the bulk also increases. This leads to an enhancement of the mass transfer coefficient. It may also be observed that at lower $\mathrm{Re}\,Sc\dfrac{d}{L}$, Sherwood number for both concentrations of CMC becomes identical.

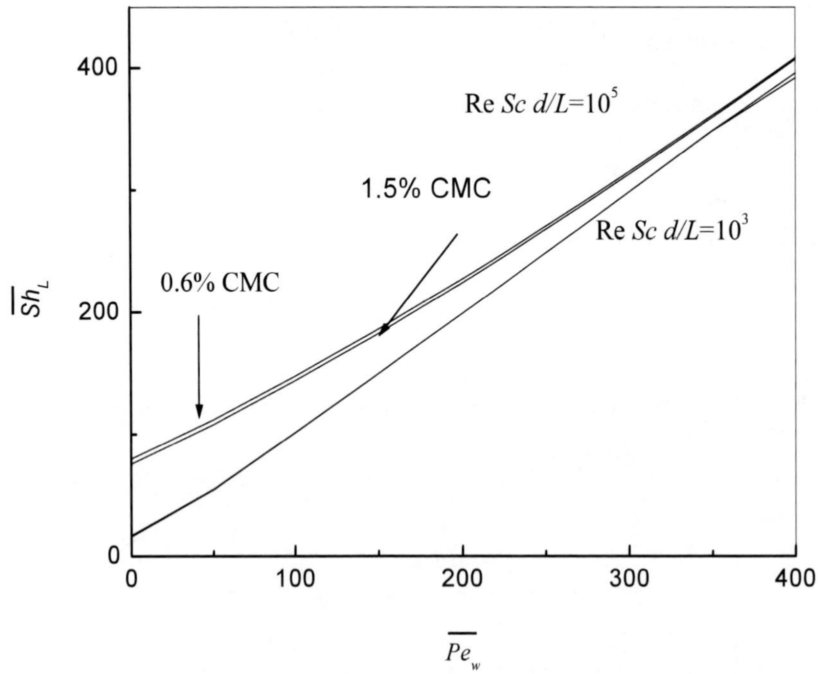

Figure 6. Variation of length averaged Sherwood number with the average dimensionless permeate flux for the Ellis fluid for flow through a tube.

The effects of permeation on Sherwood number can be quantified from Eq. (145). The ratio of Sherwood number with permeation to that without permeation ($\overline{Pe_W}$ =0) is presented below,

$$Q=\left[1+0.35\frac{\overline{Pe_W}}{\left(\mathrm{Re}\,Sc\dfrac{d}{L}\right)^{1/3}}+0.026\frac{\overline{Pe_W}^2}{\left(\mathrm{Re}\,Sc\dfrac{d}{L}\right)^{2/3}}-8.67\times10^{-4}\frac{\overline{Pe_W}^3}{\left(\mathrm{Re}\,Sc\dfrac{d}{L}\right)}\right],\quad \text{for 0.6\% CMC}$$

solution,

$$=\left[1+0.366\frac{\overline{Pe_W}}{\left(\mathrm{Re}\,Sc\dfrac{d}{L}\right)^{1/3}}+0.029\frac{\overline{Pe_W}^2}{\left(\mathrm{Re}\,Sc\dfrac{d}{L}\right)^{2/3}}-1.02\times10^{-3}\frac{\overline{Pe_W}^3}{\left(\mathrm{Re}\,Sc\dfrac{d}{L}\right)}\right],\quad \text{for 1.5\% CMC}$$

solution (146)

The variation of Q with the average wall Peclet number is shown in figure 7. It is observed from the figure that the permeation results in about 2 times increase in the Sherwood number for $\mathrm{Re}\,Sc\frac{d}{L}$=10^5 and $\overline{Pe_W}$ =400, whereas for $\mathrm{Re}\,Sc\frac{d}{L}$=10^3, at $\overline{Pe_W}$ =400, permeation causes about six fold increase in the Sherwood number.

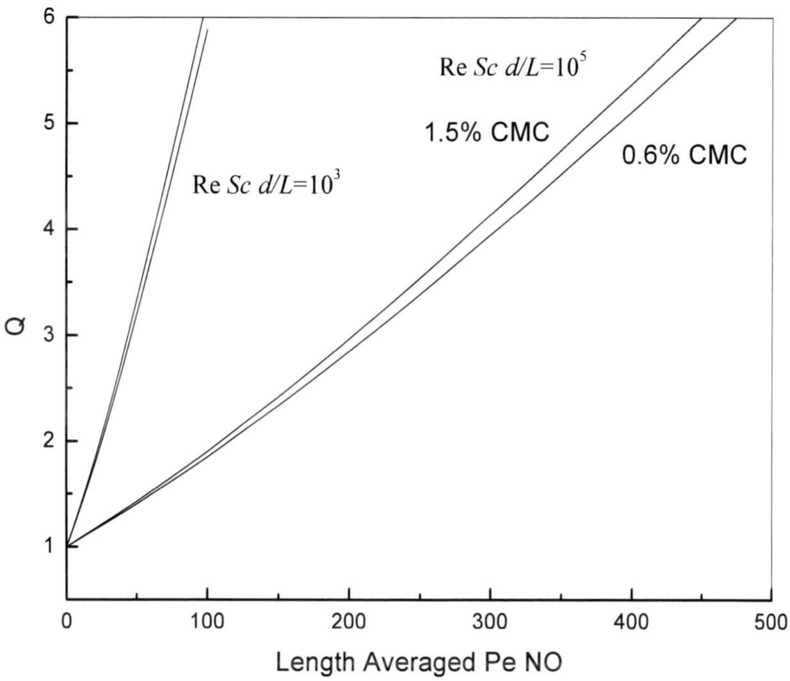

Figure 7. Variation of Q with the average dimensionless permeate flux for Ellis fluid for flow through a tube.

3.1.2. Reiner-Philippoff Fluid

A typical set of rheological parameters for Reiner-Philippoff fluid is given below [20],

$\mu_0 = 0.0215$ Kg/m.s, $\mu_\infty = 0.00105$ Kg/m.s and $\tau_s = 0.0073$ N/m^2.

As discussed in section 3.1 F versus u_0 relationship becomes,

$$F = 8.6\times10^4 u_0 + 0.014 \tag{147}$$

where, F is in Pa/m and u_0 is in m/s.

For a typical velocity, u_0 =1.18 m/s, rheological parameters and tube geometry, A_{22} is evaluated from Eq. (56) as 8. From Eq. (55) A_2 becomes,

$$A_2 = 8\left(\mathrm{Re}\,Sc\frac{d}{L}\right) \tag{148}$$

The Sherwood number profile along the tube length is obtained from Eq. (58) as,

$$Sh\left(x^*\right) = \frac{2\left(\mathrm{Re}\,Sc\frac{d}{L}\right)^{1/3}}{x^{*1/3} I_2} \tag{149}$$

The value of suction parameter $\lambda_{eff\,2}$ in this case is obtained from Eq. (60),

$$\lambda_{eff\,2} = 0.5\frac{\overline{Pe_W}}{\left(\mathrm{Re}\,Sc\frac{d}{L}\right)^{1/3}} \tag{150}$$

The length averaged Sherwood number is obtained from Eq. (38) as,

$$\overline{Sh_L} = 1.62\left(\frac{\mathrm{Re}\,Scd}{L}\right)^{1/3}\left[1 + 0.37\frac{\overline{Pe_W}}{\left(\mathrm{Re}\,Sc\frac{d}{L}\right)^{1/3}} + 0.03\frac{\overline{Pe_W}^2}{\left(\mathrm{Re}\,Sc\frac{d}{L}\right)^{2/3}} - 1.05\times10^{-3}\frac{\overline{Pe_W}^3}{\left(\mathrm{Re}\,Sc\frac{d}{L}\right)}\right] \tag{151}$$

The ratio (Q) of the average Sherwood number with permeation to that without permeation ($\overline{Pe_W}$ =0) is expressed as,

$$Q = \left[1 + 0.37\frac{\overline{Pe_W}}{\left(\mathrm{Re}\,Sc\frac{d}{L}\right)^{1/3}} + 0.03\frac{\overline{Pe_W}^2}{\left(\mathrm{Re}\,Sc\frac{d}{L}\right)^{2/3}} - 1.05\times10^{-3}\frac{\overline{Pe_W}^3}{\left(\mathrm{Re}\,Sc\frac{d}{L}\right)}\right] \tag{152}$$

The variation of the Sherwood number along the channel length for $\mathrm{Re}\,Sc\frac{d}{L}$ = 10^3 and 10^5 at the wall Peclet number, $\overline{Pe_W}$ =200, is shown in figure 8. The results show the usual trend. The variation of the length averaged Sherwood number with the average wall Peclet number is shown in figure 9. The ratio Q with the extent of suction ($\overline{Pe_W}$) is presented in figure 10. The figures show the expected trend.

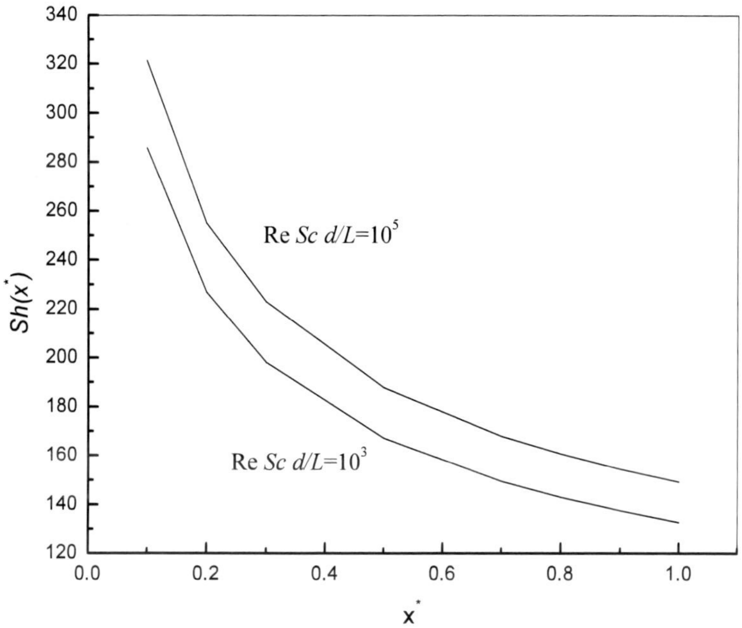

Figure 8. Variation of Sherwood number along the tube length for the Reiner-Philippoff fluid at $\overline{Pe_w} = 200$.

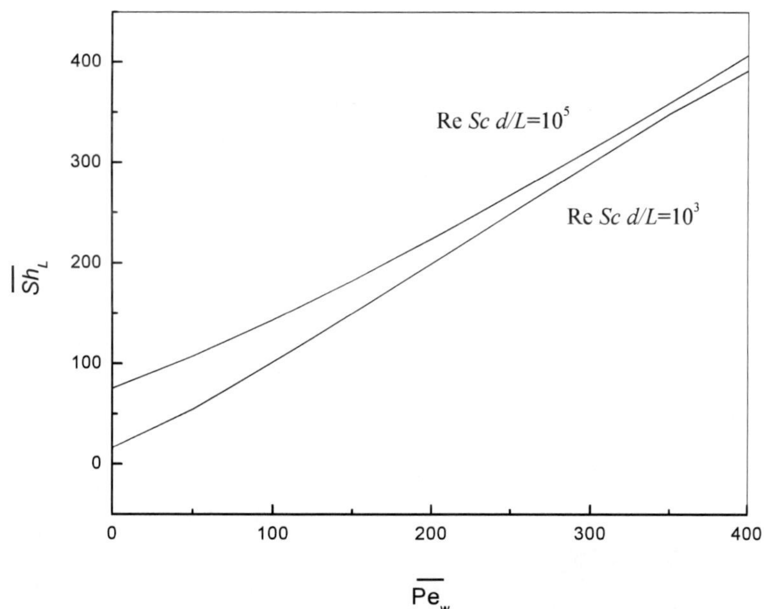

Figure 9. Variation of length averaged Sherwood number with the average dimensionless permeate flux for the Reiner-Philippoff fluid for flow through a tube.

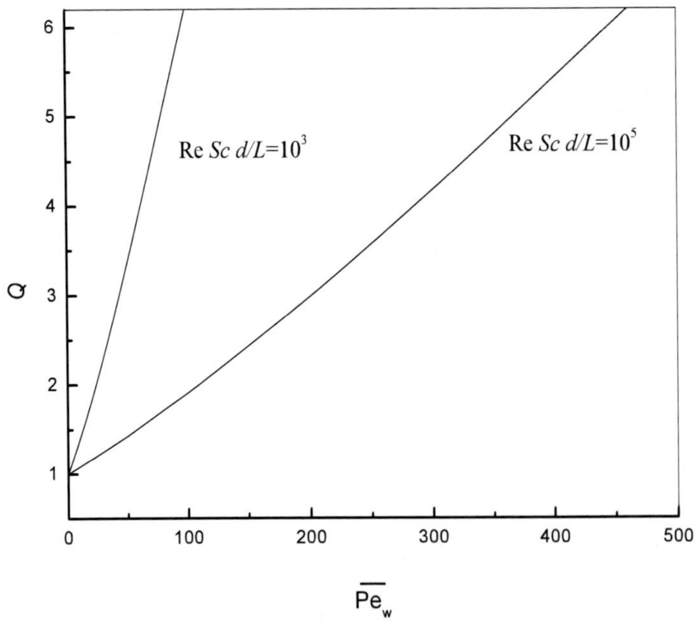

Figure 10. Variation of Q with the average dimensionless permeate flux for Reiner-Philippoff fluid for flow through a tube.

3.1.3. Eyring Fluid

The typical values of the rheological parameters for Eyring fluid are [23],

A= 600 N/m^2, B= 200 S^{-1}

The expression of F with u_0 is obtained as before,

$$F = 2.0\times10^7 u_0^{\ 3} - 2.2\times10^7 u_0^{\ 2} + 9.7\times10^6 u_0 + 1.5\times10^5 \tag{153}$$

For an average velocity of u_0 =0.3 ms^{-1} and R=0.001 m, the value of A_{33} is found out from the Eq. (68) as $A_{33} = 9.875$. From Eq. (67),

$$A_3 = 9.875\left(\mathrm{Re}\, Sc\frac{d}{L}\right) \tag{154}$$

The Sherwood number profile along the channel length is obtained from Eq. (70) as,

$$Sh\left(x^*\right) = \frac{2.15}{x^{*1/3} I_3}\left(\mathrm{Re}Sc\frac{d}{L}\right)^{1/3} \tag{155}$$

The value of the permeation parameter, λ_{eff3} is obtained from Eq. (72) as,

$$\lambda_{eff3} = 0.466 \frac{\overline{Pe_W}}{\left(\mathrm{Re}\, Sc \frac{d}{L}\right)^{1/3}} \tag{156}$$

The length averaged Sherwood number is obtained from Eq. (38) as,

$$\overline{Sh_L} = 1.74\left(\frac{\mathrm{Re}\, Scd}{L}\right)^{1/3}\left[1 + 0.345\frac{\overline{Pe_W}}{\left(\mathrm{Re}\, Sc\frac{d}{L}\right)^{1/3}} + 0.026\frac{\overline{Pe_W}^2}{\left(\mathrm{Re}\, Sc\frac{d}{L}\right)^{2/3}} - 1.06\times 10^{-3}\frac{\overline{Pe_W}^3}{\left(\mathrm{Re}\, Sc\frac{d}{L}\right)}\right] \tag{157}$$

Q, the ratio of average Sherwood number with suction to that without suction is given as

$$Q = \left[1 + 0.346\frac{\overline{Pe_W}}{\left(\mathrm{Re}\, Sc\frac{d}{L}\right)^{1/3}} + 0.023\frac{\overline{Pe_W}^2}{\left(\mathrm{Re}\, Sc\frac{d}{L}\right)^{2/3}} - 9.78\times 10^{-4}\frac{\overline{Pe_W}^3}{\left(\mathrm{Re}\, Sc\frac{d}{L}\right)}\right] \tag{158}$$

The variation of the Sherwood number along the channel length for $\mathrm{Re}\, Sc\frac{d}{L} = 10^3$ and 10^5 at the wall Peclet number, $\overline{Pe_W}$ =200, is shown in figure 11. The results show the usual trend. The variation of the length averaged Sherwood number with the average wall Peclet number is shown in figure 12. The ratio Q with the extent of suction ($\overline{Pe_W}$) is presented in figure 13. The figures show the expected result.

3.2. Rectangular Geometry

3.2.1. Ellis Fluid

Using the method described in section 3.1.1 for CMC solution F is evaluated for various value of u_0 and is fitted as a function of u_0. The rectangular channel half height (h) is considered to be 0.001 m in this study. The relationship of F with u_0 is presented below,

$$F = 9.58\times 10^4 u_0 + 1.5\times 10^4 \text{, for 0.6\% CMC solution} \tag{159}$$

$$F = 2.09\times 10^5 u_0 + 6.7\times 10^3 \text{, for 1.5\% CMC solution} \tag{160}$$

where, F is in Pa/m and u_0 is in m/s.

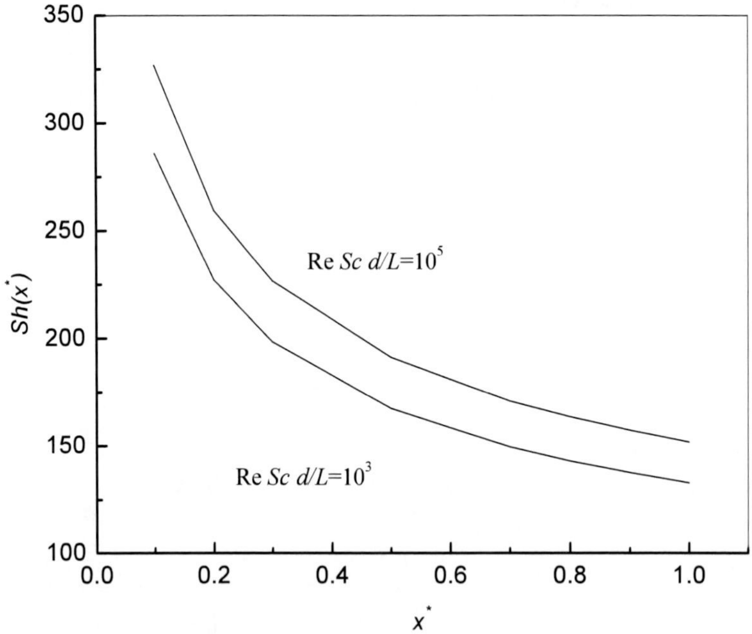

Figure 11. Variation of Sherwood number along the tube length for the Eyring fluid at $\overline{Pe_w} = 200$.

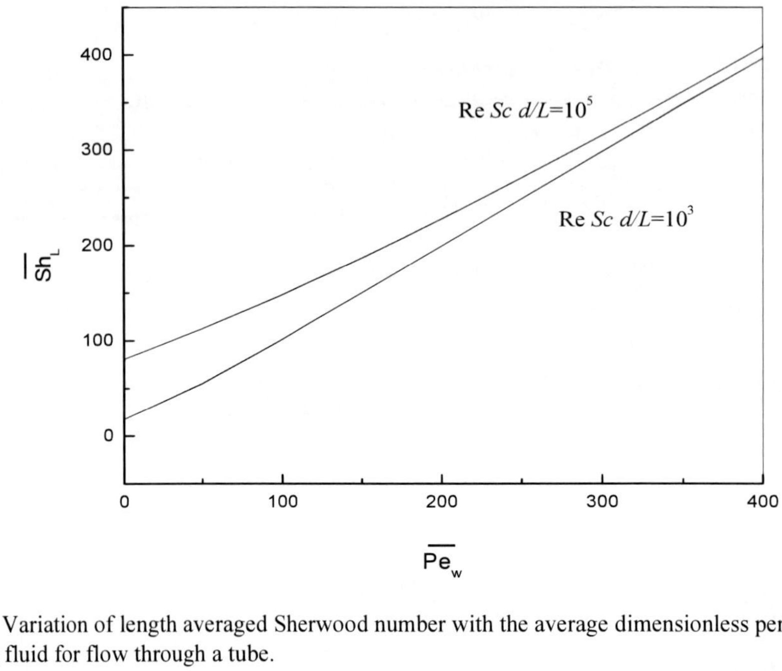

Figure 12. Variation of length averaged Sherwood number with the average dimensionless permeate flux for the Eyring fluid for flow through a tube.

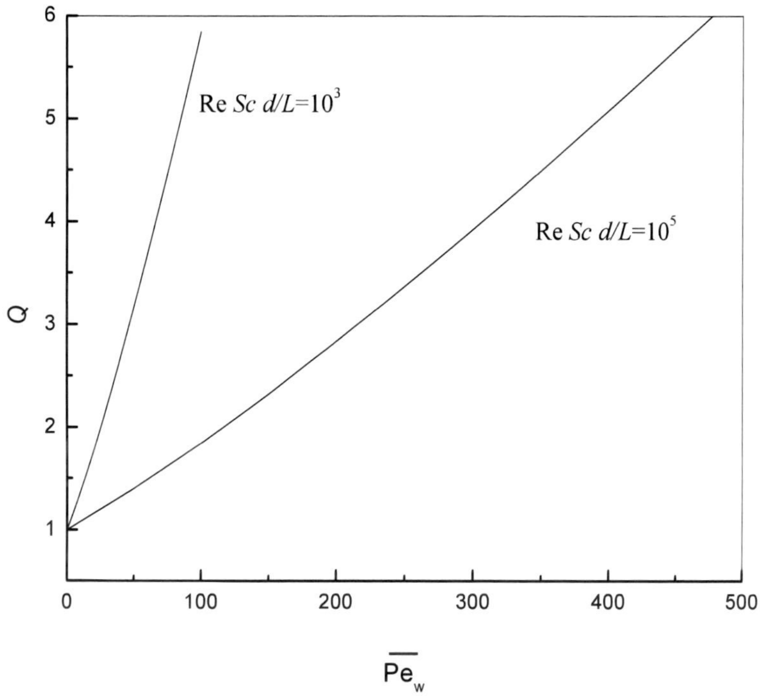

Figure 13. Variation of Q with the average dimensionless permeate flux for Eyring fluid for flow through a tube.

Using Eq. (83), A_{11}^{0} is evaluated at u_0 =0.3 m/s and its values are,

$$A_{11}^{0} = 12.33\text{, for 1.5\% CMC solution}$$

$$= 13.7\text{, for 0.6\% CMC solution} \tag{161}$$

The profiles of Sherwood numbers along the channel length are obtained from Eq. (97),

$$Sh(x^*) = \frac{2.39}{I_1^0 x^{*1/3}}\left(\mathrm{Re}Sc\frac{d_e}{L}\right)^{1/3}\text{, for 0.6\% CMC solution}$$

$$= \frac{2.31}{I_1^0 x^{*1/3}}\left(\mathrm{Re}Sc\frac{d_e}{L}\right)^{1/3}\text{, for 1.5\% CMC solution} \tag{162}$$

The values of the permeation parameter, λ_{eff1}^{0} is obtained from Eq. (99),

$$\lambda_{eff1}^{0} = \frac{0.418\overline{Pe}_w}{\left(\mathrm{Re}\,Sc\frac{d_e}{L}\right)^{1/3}}\text{ for 0.6\% CMC solution}$$

$$= \frac{0.433\overline{Pe_W}}{\left(\mathrm{Re}\, Sc \frac{d_e}{L}\right)^{1/3}} \text{ for 1.5\% CMC solution} \quad (163)$$

The length averaged Sherwood numbers are obtained from Eq. (103) as,

$$\overline{Sh_L} = 1.93\left(\frac{\mathrm{Re}\, Scd_e}{L}\right)^{1/3}\left[1 + 0.31\frac{\overline{Pe_W}}{\left(\mathrm{Re}\, Sc\frac{d_e}{L}\right)^{1/3}} + 0.018\frac{\overline{Pe_W}^2}{\left(\mathrm{Re}\, Sc\frac{d_e}{L}\right)^{2/3}} - 7.06\times 10^{-4}\frac{\overline{Pe_W}^3}{\left(\mathrm{Re}\, Sc\frac{d_e}{L}\right)}\right]$$

for 0.6% CMC solution

$$= 1.87\left(\frac{\mathrm{Re}\, Scd_e}{L}\right)^{1/3}\left[1 + 0.316\frac{\overline{Pe_W}}{\left(\mathrm{Re}\, Sc\frac{d_e}{L}\right)^{1/3}} + 0.02\frac{\overline{Pe_W}^2}{\left(\mathrm{Re}\, Sc\frac{d_e}{L}\right)^{2/3}} - 7.84\times 10^{-4}\frac{\overline{Pe_W}^3}{\left(\mathrm{Re}\, Sc\frac{d_e}{L}\right)}\right]$$

for 1.5% CMC solution (164)

The variation of the Sherwood number along the channel length for values of $\mathrm{Re}\, Sc\frac{d_e}{L}$ = 10^3 and 10^5 for $\overline{Pe_W}$ =200 is shown in figure 14. It is observed from the figure that, the Sherwood number decreases along the channel length. The decline is sharp in the upstream of the channel and gradual thereafter. This is due to the fact that the build up of the concentration boundary layer over the membrane surface becomes sluggish at the downstream of the channel because of the forced convection imposed by the cross flow. This reduces the concentration difference between the membrane surface and the bulk of the solution. Therefore, the Sherwood number and consequently, the mass transfer coefficient decreases along the channel length. It may be observed from figure 14 that the Sherwood number is more at higher $\mathrm{Re}\, Sc\frac{d_e}{L}$ at the same level of the permeate flux ($\overline{Pe_w}$). This indicates that at higher Reynolds number, forced convection is more due to higher cross flow velocity, which enhances the mass transfer coefficient. It may also be observed that the Sherwood number profiles for both concentrations of CMC solution almost coincide at $\mathrm{Re}\, Sc\frac{d_e}{L}$ =10^3 and they differ marginally at $\mathrm{Re}\, Sc\frac{d_e}{L}$ =10^5.

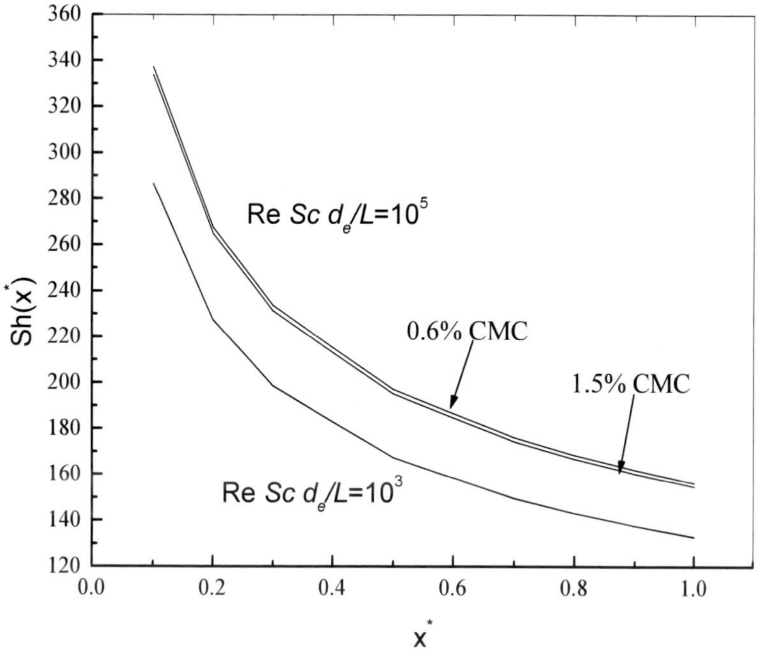

Figure 14. Variation of Sherwood number along the channel length for the Ellis fluid at $\overline{Pe_w} = 200$.

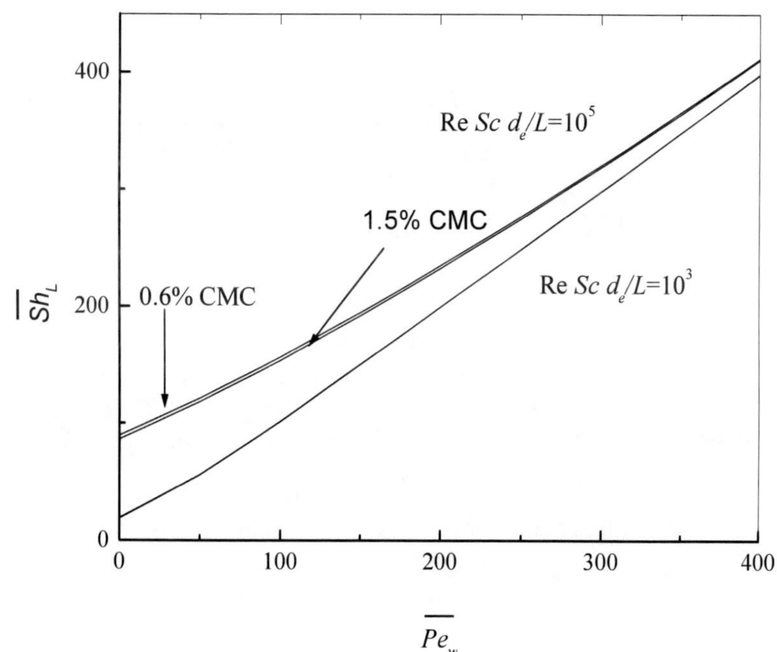

Figure 15. Variation of length averaged Sherwood number with the average dimensionless permeate flux for the Ellis fluid for flow through the rectangular channel.

The variation of the length averaged Sherwood number with the average wall Peclet number is presented in figure 15, for $\mathrm{Re}\, Sc \frac{d_e}{L}$ =10^3 and 10^5. It is evident from the figure that the Sherwood number increases with wall Peclet number. This implies the mass transfer coefficient increases with the extent of permeation. As permeation increases, the convective solute flux through the membrane increases and at the steady state, to maintain the solute balance, the backward diffusion from the surface to the bulk also increases. This leads to an enhancement of the mass transfer coefficient. It may also be observed that at lower $\mathrm{Re}\, Sc \frac{d_e}{L}$, Sherwood number for both concentrations of CMC becomes identical.

The effects of permeation on Sherwood number can be quantified from Eq. (164). The ratio of Sherwood number with permeation and without permeation ($\overline{Pe_W}$ =0) is presented below,

$$Q = \left[1 + 0.31 \frac{\overline{Pe_W}}{\left(\mathrm{Re}\, Sc \frac{d_e}{L} \right)^{1/3}} + 0.018 \frac{\overline{Pe_W}^2}{\left(\mathrm{Re}\, Sc \frac{d_e}{L} \right)^{2/3}} - 7.06 \times 10^{-4} \frac{\overline{Pe_W}^3}{\left(\mathrm{Re}\, Sc \frac{d_e}{L} \right)} \right], \text{ for 0.6\% CMC}$$

solution,

$$= \left[1 + 0.316 \frac{\overline{Pe_W}}{\left(\mathrm{Re}\, Sc \frac{d_e}{L} \right)^{1/3}} + 0.02 \frac{\overline{Pe_W}^2}{\left(\mathrm{Re}\, Sc \frac{d_e}{L} \right)^{2/3}} - 7.84 \times 10^{-4} \frac{\overline{Pe_W}^3}{\left(\mathrm{Re}\, Sc \frac{d_e}{L} \right)} \right], \text{ for 1.5\% CMC}$$

solution.

(165)

The variation of Q with the average wall Peclet number is shown in figure 16. It is observed from the figure that the permeation results in about 5 times increase in the Sherwood number for $\mathrm{Re}\, Sc \frac{d_e}{L}$ =10^5 and $\overline{Pe_W}$ =400, whereas for $\mathrm{Re}\, Sc \frac{d_e}{L}$ =10^3, at $\overline{Pe_W}$ =400, permeation causes about three fold increase in the Sherwood number.

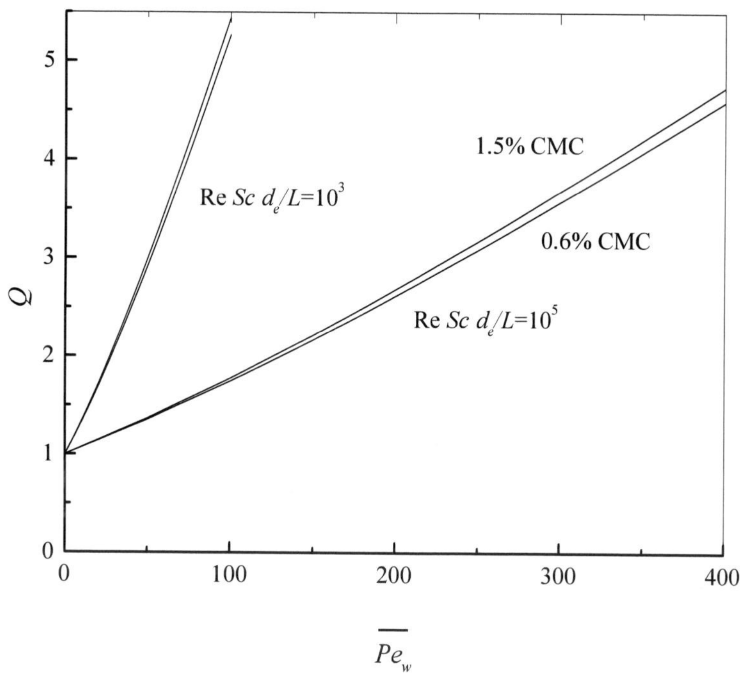

Figure 16. Variation of Q with the average dimensionless permeate flux for Ellis fluid for flow through the rectangular channel.

3.2.2. Reiner-Philippoff Fluid

For a typical set of rheological parameters for Reiner-Philippoff fluid, as discussed in section 3.1.2, F versus u_0 relationship becomes,

$$F = 6.45 \times 10^4 u_0 + 0.03 \tag{166}$$

where, F is in Pa/m and u_0 is in m/s.

For a typical velocity, u_0 =1.18 m/s, rheological parameters and channel height, A_{22}^0 is evaluated from Eq. (121) as 12.52. From Eq. (120), A_2^0 becomes,

$$A_2^0 = 12.52\left(\text{Re}\, Sc \frac{d_e}{L}\right) \tag{167}$$

The Sherwood number profile along the channel length is obtained from Eq. (123) as,

$$Sh\left(x^*\right)=\frac{2.32\left(\operatorname{Re}Sc\frac{d_e}{L}\right)^{1/3}}{x^{*1/3}I_2^0} \tag{168}$$

The value of suction parameter $\lambda^0_{eff\,2}$ in this case is obtained from Eq. (125),

$$\lambda^0_{eff\,2}=0.43\frac{\overline{Pe_W}}{\left(\operatorname{Re}Sc\frac{d_e}{L}\right)^{1/3}} \tag{169}$$

The length averaged Sherwood number is obtained from Eq. (103) as,

$$\overline{Sh_L}=1.88\left(\frac{\operatorname{Re}Scd_e}{L}\right)^{1/3}\left[1+0.32\frac{\overline{Pe_W}}{\left(\operatorname{Re}Sc\frac{d_e}{L}\right)^{1/3}}+0.02\frac{\overline{Pe_W}^2}{\left(\operatorname{Re}Sc\frac{d_e}{L}\right)^{2/3}}-7.68\times10^{-4}\frac{\overline{Pe_W}^3}{\left(\operatorname{Re}Sc\frac{d_e}{L}\right)}\right] \tag{170}$$

The ratio (Q) of the average Sherwood number with suction and without suction ($\overline{Pe_W}$ =0) is expressed as,

$$Q=\left[1+0.32\frac{\overline{Pe_W}}{\left(\operatorname{Re}Sc\frac{d_e}{L}\right)^{1/3}}+0.02\frac{\overline{Pe_W}^2}{\left(\operatorname{Re}Sc\frac{d_e}{L}\right)^{2/3}}-7.68\times10^{-4}\frac{\overline{Pe_W}^3}{\left(\operatorname{Re}Sc\frac{d_e}{L}\right)}\right] \tag{171}$$

The variation of the Sherwood number along the channel length for $\operatorname{Re}Sc\frac{d_e}{L}$ = 10^3 and 10^5 at the wall Peclet number, $\overline{Pe_W}$ =200, is shown in figure 17. The results show the usual trend. The variation of the length averaged Sherwood number with the average wall Peclet number is shown in figure 18. The ratio Q with the extent of suction ($\overline{Pe_W}$) is presented in figure 19. The figures show the expected trend.

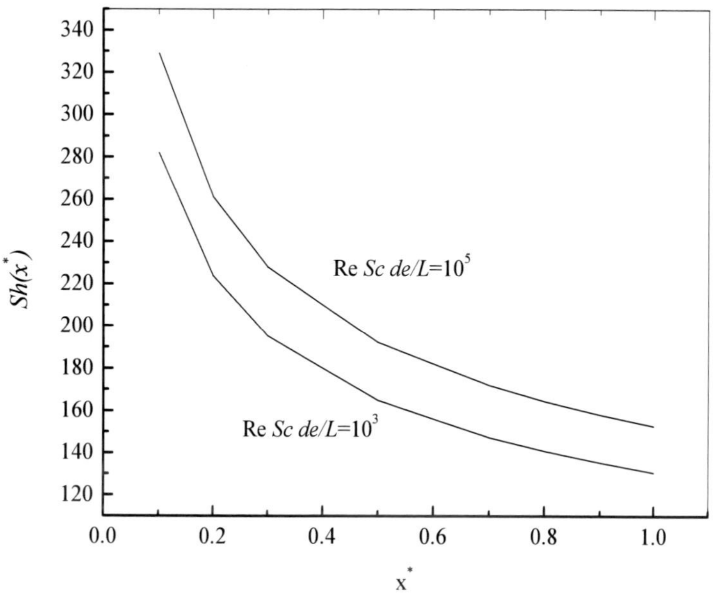

Figure 17. Variation of Sherwood number along the channel length for the Reiner-Philippoff fluid at $\overline{Pe_w} = 200$.

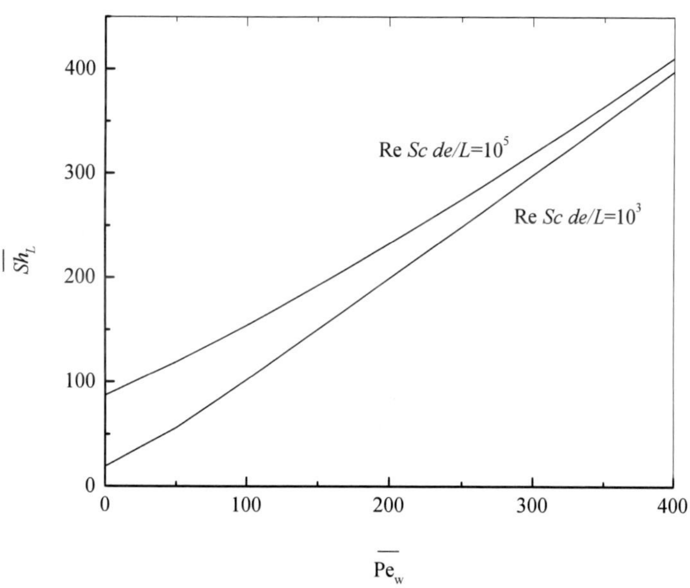

Figure 18. Variation of length averaged Sherwood number with the average dimensionless permeate flux for the Reiner-Philippoff fluid for flow through the rectangular channel.

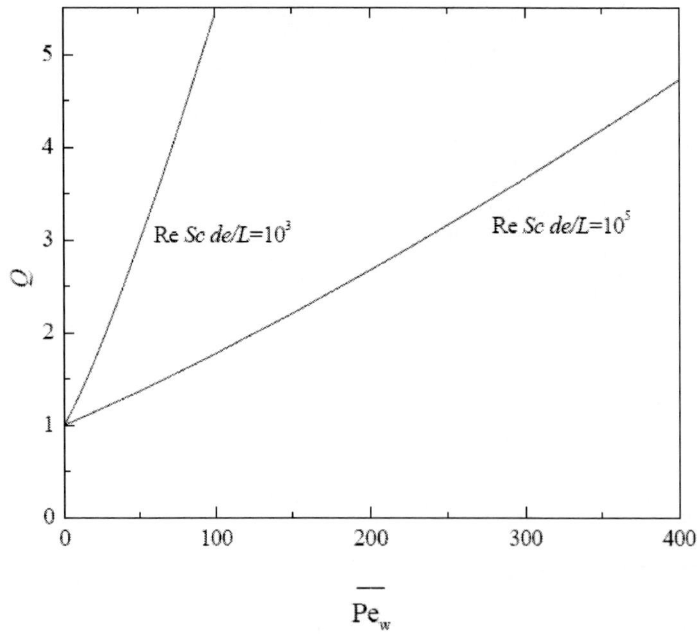

Figure 19. Variation of Q with the average dimensionless permeate flux for Reiner-Philippoff fluid for flow through the rectangular channel.

3.2.3. Eyring Fluid

For typical values of the rheological parameters for Eyring fluid as discussed in section 3.1.3, the expression of F with u_0 is obtained as before,

$$F = 3\times10^5 + 5.44\times10^6 u_0 - 4.65\times10^6 u_0^{\ 2} \tag{172}$$

For an average velocity of u_0 =0.3 ms^{-1} and h=1 mm, the value of A_{33}^0 is found out from the Eq. (133) as $A_{33}^0 = 16.54$. From Eq. (132),

$$A_3^0 = 16.5353\left(\mathrm{Re}\, Sc\frac{d_e}{L}\right) \tag{173}$$

The Sherwood number profile along the channel length is obtained from Eq. (135) as,

$$Sh\left(x^*\right) = \frac{2.55}{x^{*1/3} I_3^0}\left(\mathrm{Re}\, Sc\frac{d_e}{L}\right)^{1/3} \tag{174}$$

The value of the permeation parameter, λ_{eff3}^0 is obtained from Eq. (137) as,

$$\lambda^0_{eff3} = 0.39 \frac{\overline{Pe_W}}{\left(\operatorname{Re} Sc \frac{d_e}{L}\right)^{1/3}} \tag{175}$$

The length averaged Sherwood number is obtained from Eq. (103) as,

$$\overline{Sh_L} = 2.06\left(\frac{\operatorname{Re} Scd_e}{L}\right)^{1/3}\left[1 + 0.28\frac{\overline{Pe_W}}{\left(\operatorname{Re} Sc \frac{d_e}{L}\right)^{1/3}} + 0.016\frac{\overline{Pe_W}^2}{\left(\operatorname{Re} Sc \frac{d_e}{L}\right)^{2/3}} - 5.73\times10^{-4}\frac{\overline{Pe_W}^3}{\left(\operatorname{Re} Sc \frac{d_e}{L}\right)}\right] \tag{176}$$

Q, the ratio of average Sherwood number with suction to that without suction is given as

$$Q = \left[1 + 0.28\frac{\overline{Pe_W}}{\left(\operatorname{Re} Sc \frac{d_e}{L}\right)^{1/3}} + 0.016\frac{\overline{Pe_W}^2}{\left(\operatorname{Re} Sc \frac{d_e}{L}\right)^{2/3}} - 5.73\times10^{-4}\frac{\overline{Pe_W}^3}{\left(\operatorname{Re} Sc \frac{d_e}{L}\right)}\right] \tag{177}$$

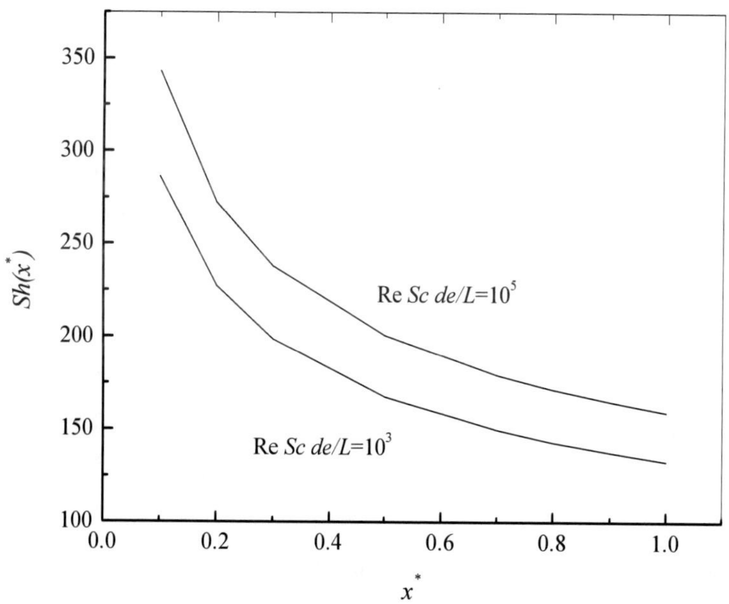

Figure 20. Variation of Sherwood number along the channel length for the Eyring fluid at $\overline{Pe_w} = 200$.

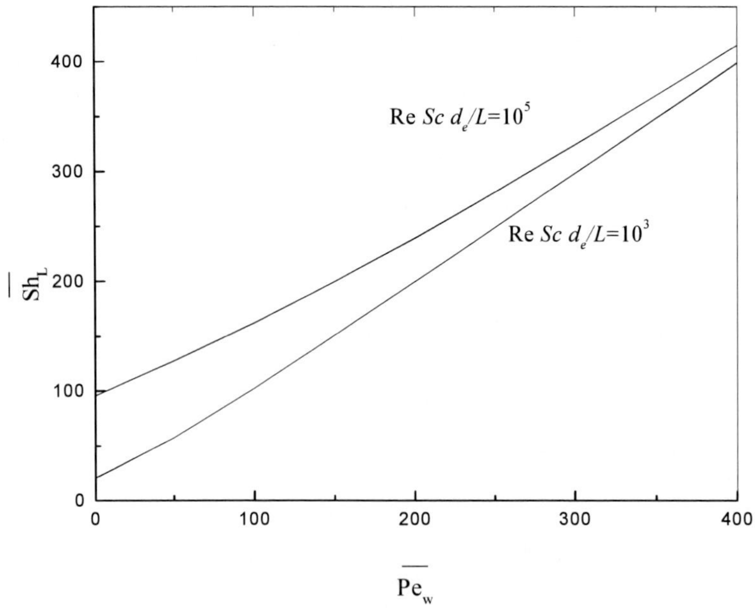

Figure 21. Variation of length averaged Sherwood number with the average dimensionless permeate flux for the Eyring fluid for flow through the rectangular channel.

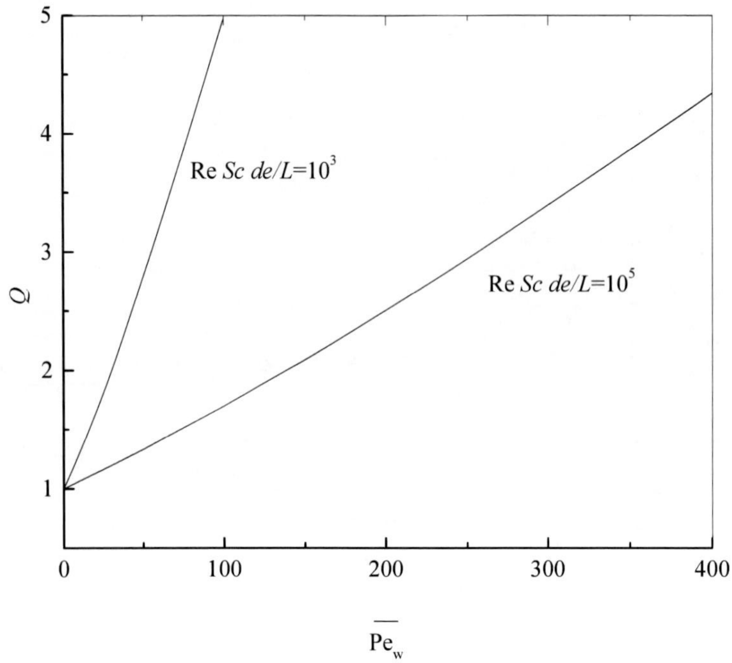

Figure 22. Variation of Q with the average dimensionless permeate flux for Eyring fluid for flow through the rectangular channel.

The variation of the Sherwood number along the channel length for $\mathrm{Re}\,Sc\frac{d_e}{L}$ = 10^3 and 10^5 at the wall Peclet number, $\overline{Pe_W}$ =200, is shown in figure 20. The results show the usual trend. The variation of the length averaged Sherwood number with the average wall Peclet number is shown in figure 21. The ratio Q with the extent of suction ($\overline{Pe_W}$) is presented in figure 22. The figures show the expected trend.

4. Conclusion

The Sherwood number relations incorporating the effects of permeation are derived from the first principles for a laminar flow in a tubular module and rectangular channel for three non-Newtonian fluids. Effects of permeation on the mass transfer coefficient have been quantified. Because of permeation, the Sherwood number can increase several times compared to that without permeation depending upon the permeate flux. The derived analytical expressions are useful to the engineers for design of the tubular and spiral wound membrane modules for flow of the non-Newtonian fluids covered in this study.

Nomenclature

A	rhelogical parameter in Eyring fluid
A_1,A_2,A_3	dimensionless parameters in Eqs.(12), (55) and (67)
A_1^0, A_2^0, A_3^0	dimensionless parameters in Eqs.(82), (120) and (132)
$A_{11,22,33}$	dimensionless rheological parameters in Eqs.(14), (56) and (68)
$A_{11,22,33}^0$	dimensionless rheological parameters in Eqs.(83), (121) and (132)
B	rhelogical parameter in Eyring fluid
B_1	constant in Eq.(21)
B_1^0	constant in Eq.(87)
c	solute concentration, kg/m^3
c_0	feed concentration, kg/m^3
c_p	permeate concentration, kg/m^3
c^*	dimensionless concentration
c_m	membrane surface concentration, kg/m^3
D	solute diffusivity, m^2/s
d	tube diameter, m
F	pressure gradient across the channel length (*-dP/dx*), Pa/m
f	friction factor
$I_{1,2,3}$	definite integrals in Eqs. (27), (59) and (71)
$I_{1,2,3}^0$	definite integrals in Eqs. (93), (124) and (136)

K	parameter in Eq.(64)
$K_{1,2}$	integration constants in Eq.(24)
$K_{1,2}^{0}$	integration constants in Eq.(96)
k	mass transfer coefficient, m/s
L	channel length, m
P	pressure, Pa
Pe_w	dimensionless permeate flux (wall Peclet number)
$\overline{Pe_w}$	length averaged non-dimensional permeate flux
R	tube Radius, m
Re	Reynolds number
R_r	real retention of the membrane
r	radial direction, m
Sh	Sherwood number
$\overline{Sh_L}$	length averaged Sherwood number
Sc	Schmidt number
u_0	average velocity across the cross section, m/s
v_x	x-component velocity, m/s
v_y	y-component velocity, m/s
v_w	permeate flux, m^3/m^2s
x	axial dimension, m
x^*	dimensionless axial dimension
y	dimension normal to the flow direction, m
y^*	dimensionless normal dimension

Greek letters:

α	Ellis fluid rheological parameter
δ	concentration boundary layer thickness, m
δ^*	dimensionless concentration boundary layer thickness
φ_0, φ_1	Ellis fluid rheological parameters
τ_{yx}	Shear stress, Pa
μ_0, μ_∞	rheological parameters in Eq.(50), Pa.s
μ_{eff}	effective viscosity, Pa.s
$\eta, \xi, \phi, \eta_0, \xi_0, \phi_0$	similarity parameters
ρ	density, kg/m^3
τ_s	rheological parameters in Eq.(50), Pa

References

[1] Bouchard, C. R.; Carreau, P. J.; Matsuuara, T.; Sourirajan, S. (1994). Modeling of ultrafiltration: prediction of concentration polarization effects. *J. Membrane Sci., 97,* 215-229.

[2] Kleinstreuer, C ; Paller, M. S. (1983). Laminar dilute suspension flows in plate and frame ultrafiltration units. *AIChE J., 29*, 533-539.

[3] van den Berg, G. B; Racz, I. G.; Smolders, C. A. (1989). Mass transfer coefficients in cross flow ultrafiltration, *J. Membrane Sci., 47*, 25-50.

[4] Gekas, V; Hallstrom, B. (1987). Mass transfer in the membrane concentration polarization layer under turbulent cross flow. I. Critical literature review and adaptation of existing Sherwood correlations to membrane operations. *J. Membrane Sci., 80,* 153-169.

[5] De, S.; Bhattacharjee, S.; Bhattacharya, P. K. (1995). Development of correlations for mass transfer coefficient in ultrafiltration systems. *Develop. Chemical Engg. Mineral Proc., 3,* 187-206.

[6] Girard, B.; Fukumoto, L. R. (2000). Membrane processing of fruit juices and beverages: a review. *Crit. Rev. Food Sci. Nutrition, 40 (2)*, 91-157.

[7] Cheryan, M. *Ultrafiltration Handbook*, Technomic Publishing Co. Ltd.: Lancaster, PA, 1986, pp. 349-369.

[8] Pepper, D.; Orchard, A.C. J.; Merry, A. J. (1985). Concentration of tomato juice and other fruit juices by reverse osmosis. *Desalination, 53,* 157-166.

[9] Thomas, R. L.; Gaddis, J. L.; Westtfall, P. H.; Titus, T. C.; Ellis, N. D. (1987) Optimization of apple juice production by single pass metallic membrane ultrafiltration. *J. Food Sci., 52,* 1263-1266.

[10] Aptel, P., and Clifton, M. (1983). Ultrafiltration. In P. M. Bungay, H. K. Lonsdale and M. N. de Pinho (Eds.), *Synthetic Membranes: Science, Engineering and Applications* (pp. 249-305). Dordrecht : D. Reidel Publishing Co.

[11] Porter, M. C. (2005). Ultrafiltration. In *Handbook of Industrial Membrane Technology* (pp. 136-256). New Delhi: Crest Publishing House.

[12] Chhabra, R. P.; Richardson, J. F.; Non-Newtonian flow in the Process Industries: Fundamentals and Engineering Applications; Butterworth Heinemann: Oxford, 1999, pp. 77.

[13] Charcosset, C; Choplin, C. (1996). Ultrafiltration of non-Newtonian fluids. *J. Membrane Sci., 115*, 147-160.

[14] Howell, J. A; Field, R.; Wu, D. (1996). Ultrafiltration of high viscosity solutions: theoretical developments and experimental findings. *Chem. Engg. Sci., 51*, 1405-1415.

[15] Pritchard, M.; Howell, J. A.; Field, R.; Wu, D. (1995). The ultrafiltration of viscous fluids. *J. Membrane Sci., 102*, 223-235.

[16] De, S.; Bhattacharya, P. K. (1997). Prediction of mass transfer coefficient with suction in the applications of reverse osmosis and ultrafiltration. *J. Membrane Sci., 128,* 119-131.

[17] Minnikanti, V. S.; DasGupta, S.; De, S. (1999). Prediction of mass transfer coefficient with suction for turbulent flow in cross flow ultrafiltration. *J. Membrane Sci., 137,* 227-239.

[18] Ranjan, R.; DasGupta, S.; De, S. (2004). Mass transfer coefficient with suction for laminar non-Newtonian flow in application to membrane separations. *J. Food Engg., 64*, 53-61.

[19] Ranjan, R; DasGupta, S.; De, S. (2004). Mass transfer coefficient with suction for turbulent non-Newtonian flow in application to membrane separations. *J. Food Engg., 65*, 533-541.

[20] Bird, R. B.; Stewart, W. E.; Lightfoot, E. N. *Transport Phenomena;* Wiley: N.Y.,1960; pp 13-14.

[21] De, S.; Bhattacharjee, S.; Sharma, A.; Bhattacharya, P. K. (1997). Generalized integral and similarity solutions of the concentration profiles for osmotic pressure controlled ultrafiltration. *J. Membrane Sci., 130*, 99-121.

[22] Opong, W. S.; Zydney, A. L. (1991). Diffusive and convective protein transport through asymmetric membranes. *AIChE J., 37,* 1497-1510.

[23] Yurusoy, M.; (2003). A study of pressure distribution of a slider bearing lubricated with Powell-Eyring fliuid, *Turkish J. Eng. Env. Sci., 27*, 299-304.

[24] White, F. M. *Viscous Fluid Flow;* McGraw Hill Inc.: Singapore, 1991; pp. 123.

Appendix

A.1. Effective Viscosity (μ_{eff})

From the definition of friction factor, *f* [12],

$$f = \frac{\tau_w}{\frac{1}{2}\rho u_0^2} \tag{A1}$$

From the definition of the wall shear stress [12],

$$\tau_w = \left(-\frac{dP}{dx}\right)\frac{d}{4} = F\frac{d}{4} \tag{A2}$$

From Eqs. (A1) and (A2), the expression of friction factor becomes,

$$f = \frac{Fd^2}{2\rho u_0^2} \tag{A3}$$

For laminar flow, $f = \dfrac{16}{\mathrm{Re}}$ (A4)

Hence, from Eqs.(A3) and (A4), $$\mu_{eff} = \frac{Fd^2}{32u_0} \tag{A5}$$

A.2. Similarity Parameter

Evaluating Eq.(12) at the edge of the concentration boundary layer,

$$A_1\delta^* \frac{\Delta c^*}{x^*} \approx \frac{\Delta c^*}{\delta^{*2}} \tag{A6}$$

From the above equation, $\delta^* = \left(\frac{x^*}{A_1}\right)^{\frac{1}{3}}$

Similarity parameter is defined as, $$\eta = \frac{y^*}{\delta^*} = A_1^{1/3}\frac{y^*}{x^{*1/3}} \tag{A7}$$

A.3. Effective Viscosity for Power Law Fluid

Flow Through a Tube

In this case, $\varphi_0 = 0$. From Eqs.(46) and (47), the explicit expression of F becomes,

$$F = 2^{\frac{\alpha+1}{\alpha}} \frac{(\alpha+3)^{\frac{1}{\alpha}} u_0^{\frac{1}{\alpha}}}{\varphi_1^{\frac{1}{\alpha}} d^{\frac{\alpha+1}{\alpha}}} \tag{A8}$$

From Eqs. (A5) and (A8), the expression of effective viscosity is obtained in this case,

$$\mu_{eff} = \frac{1}{16}\left(\frac{u_0}{d}\right)^{\frac{1-\alpha}{\alpha}}\left(\frac{2(\alpha+3)}{\varphi_1}\right)^{\frac{1}{\alpha}} \tag{A9}$$

Flow through a Rectangular Thin Channel

In this case, $\varphi_0 = 0$. From Eqs.(111) and (112), the explicit expression of F becomes,

$$F = 4^{\frac{\alpha+1}{\alpha}} \frac{(\alpha+2)^{\frac{1}{\alpha}} u_0^{\frac{1}{\alpha}}}{\varphi_1^{\frac{1}{\alpha}} d_e^{\frac{\alpha+1}{\alpha}}} \tag{A10}$$

From Eqs. (A5) and (A10), the expression of effective viscosity is obtained in this case,

$$\mu_{eff} = \frac{1}{8}\left(\frac{u_0}{d_e}\right)^{\frac{1-\alpha}{\alpha}} \left(\frac{4(\alpha+2)}{\varphi_1}\right)^{\frac{1}{\alpha}} \tag{A11}$$

In: Fruit Juices: Properties, Consumption and Nutrition
Editor: Pauline G. Scardina
ISBN: 978-1-60741-505-3

Chapter 9

Membrane Based Clarification/Concentration of Fruit Juice*

Sirshendu De, Sunando DasGupta and S. Ranjith Kumar
Department of Chemical Engineering, Indian Institute of Technology, Kharagpur, India

Abstract

This chapter discusses the effect of externally applied d.c electric field during cross-flow ultrafiltration of synthetic juice (mixture of sucrose and pectin) and mosambi (Citrus Sinensis (L.) Osbeck) fruit juice using 50000 (MWCO) polyerthersulfon membrane. Pectin, completely rejected by the membrane, forms a gel type layer over the membrane surface. Under the application of an external d.c. electric field across the membrane, gel layer formation is restricted leading to an enhancement of permeate flux. During ultrafiltration of synthetic juice, application of d.c. electric field (800 V/m) increases the permeate flux to almost threefold compared to that with zero electric field. A theoretical model based on integral method assuming suitable concentration profile in the boundary layer is developed. The proposed model is used to predict the steady state permeate flux in gel-layer governed electric field assisted ultrafiltration. A gel polarization model is also proposed incorporating continuous as well as pulsed electric field and numerically solved to quantify the flux decline and growth of the gel layer thickness. The gel layer thickness is also measured with high-resolution video microscopy and successfully compared with results from the numerical solution of the model under various operating conditions. Predictions of the model are

* A version of this chapter was also published in *Electric Field Enhanced Membrane Separation System: Principles and Typical Applications*, by Sirshendu De, Ranjith Kumar and Sunando DasGupta published by Nova Science Publishers, Inc. It was submitted for appropriate modifications in an effort to encourage wider dissemination of research.

successfully compared with the experimental results under a wide range of operating conditions.

Application of d.c. electric field during ultrafiltration of mosambi juice has resulted in significant improvement of permeate flux. A steady state gel polarization model has been applied to evaluate the gel layer concentration, effective diffusivity and effective viscosity of the juice within the concentration boundary layer, by optimizing the experimental flux data. Application of pulsed electric field is found to be more beneficial in terms of energy consumption, and equally effective in terms of flux augmentation as compared to constant field.

Nomenclature

A	Constant defined by Eq.(2.25)
A’	Membrane surface area, m^2
$a_{1,2,3}$	Coefficients in Eq.(2.29)
c	Concentration of pectin, kg/m^3
c_o	Pectin concentration at bulk, kg/m^3
c_g	Pectin concentration in gel, kg/m^3
c^*	Dimensionless concentration (c / c_o)
c_g^*	Dimensionless gel concentration (c_g / c_0)
d_p	Equivalent spherical diameter of pectin, m
d_e	Equivalent diameter, m
D	Diffusivity of pectin, m^2/s
D_i	Dielectric constant, dimensionless
E	Electric field, V/m
E_{total}	total energy consumption, kWh/m^3
E_{pump}	pump energy consumption, kWh/m^3
$E_{electrical}$	energy consumption due to external electric field, kWh/m^3
I	current, amp
h	Half of channel height, m
K	Boltzmann constant (1.38×10^{-23}), J/K
k	Mass transfer coefficient, m/s
L	Channel length, m
M_w	Molecular weight, kg/k.mol
N	fraction of on time, dimensionless
P	power consumption per unit volume of permeate, watt hr/m^3
Q	permeation rate, m^3/s

$\overline{Pe_w}$	Average peclet number (dimensionless flux)
Pe_e	Peclet number due to electric field (dimensionless flux)
Re	Reynolds number at the bulk condition
Sc	Schmidt number at the bulk condition
T	Absolute temperature, ^oC
t	time, s
t_1	on-time, s
t_2	off-time,s
t_{total}	total operational time, s
u_e	Electrophoretic mobility, ms^{-1}/Vm^{-1}
v_e	Electrophoretic velocity, m/s
v_w	Permeate flux, m^3/m^2 s
$v_{w, pure}$	pure water flux, m^3/m^2 s
v_w^{exp}	experimental permeate flux, m^3/m^2 s
v_w^{cal}	calculated permeate flux, m^3/m^2 s
u	Axial velocity, m/s
u_0	Average bulk velocity, m/s
v	Velocity component in normal direction, m/s
x	Coordinate from the membrane, m
y	Normal distance, m
y*	Dimensionless normal distance (y/h)
x*	Dimensionless axial distance (x/L)
z	Parameter in Eq. (2.12), kg/kmol.m^3

Greek Letters

μ	Viscosity, Pa s
δ_g	Gel layer thickness, m
δ_c	Thickness of concentration boundary layer, m
δ_c^*	Dimensionless concentration boundary layer thickness (δ_c / h)
ζ	Zeta potential of particle, V
ε_o	Permittivity of vacuum (8.854×10^{-12}), $CV^{-1}m^{-1}$
ρ	Bulk density, kg/m^3
ρ_g	gel density, kg/m^3
ΔP	transmembrane pressure drop, kPa
ΔP_{pump}	pump pressure drop, kPa

ρ_g gel density, kg/m^3

η_{pump} efficiency of pump

$\eta_{d.c.\ power\ supply}$ efficiency of d.c. power supply

2.1. Importance and Techniques of Clarification of Fruit Juice

India is the second largest producer of fruits in the world, but only 2% of the produced fruits are processed. In India, the production per capita availability is very low (120-130 g/day against 300g recommended) due to wastage caused by inadequate post-harvest facilities. Hence to minimize the post harvest losses due to spoilage and to meet the increasing market demand, there is a need to process the fruit juice with increased shelf-life and to retain the properties of fresh fruit, as well as color, aroma, nutritional value and structural properties. The composition of fruit juice depends on the variety, origin, weather, processing procedure and storage. The major components of fruit juice are sugar (in the form of sucrose, glucose, fructose, etc.), salts, acids, proteins, pectin, starch, minerals, vitamins, flavor and aroma compounds. The organic flavor and aroma compounds contain alcohols, esters, aldehydes etc., which are highly volatile in nature. The raw fruit juice obtained after extraction is very viscous, turbid, rich in color and contains significant amount of colloidal materials (100-1000 ppm) which are stabilized in suspension by pectin, starch etc.,[1]. Hence, raw juice needs to be clarified prior to its commercial use. Clarification of juice involves the removal of haze–forming components such as suspended solids, colloidal particles, pectins, proteins etc. For clarification of fruit juice, traditional methods involve several labor-intensive and time consuming batch operations, e.g., use of enzyme (pectinase), fining agent (gelatine, bentonite etc.), filter aids (diatomaceous earth, kieselguhr etc.) etc. However, the use of these additives (fining agent, filter aids) give bitter taste in the juice. Moreover, the solids obtained after filtration contains enzyme, fining agent and filter aids. This can not be reused and causes pollution problems due to their disposal [2]. For concentrating clarified juice, evaporation is the most common technique but it causes the loss of aroma and flavor compounds and requires high energy consumption [3].

In this regard, membrane based separation processes have gradually become a cost effective alternative to conventional fining and clarification technique. These processes are athermal and involve no phase change or addition of chemicals. Apart from it, other advantages of these processes are low energy consumption, less processing time, production of additive free high quality juice with natural fresh taste.

The major problem associated with membrane based clarification of fruit juice is the flux decline due to concentration polarization and membrane fouling during the operation. The objective of ultrafiltration of fruit juice is to retain high molecular weight pectin and its derivative (which have a tendency to form gel on the membrane surface) and to allow low molecular weight solute like sucrose, acid, salt etc., to permeate through the membrane. In fruit juice, typical concentration of pectic substances is up to 1.0 % [4]. Pectins are acidic polysaccharides that originate in the cell membrane structure in plants which is composed of a rahmno-galacturonan backbone in which 1-4 linked α-D-galacturonan chain are interrupted and bent at the intervals by the insertion of 1-2 linked α-L-rahmnopyranosyl residue. One of the important properties of pectin is that it forms gel in presence of sugar and acid. Pectin gel is nothing but network of cross-linked polymer molecules in a liquid medium [5]. The strength and characteristics of pectin gel depend on degree of methoxylation, presence of sugar, average molecular weight, ionic strength, pH, temperature and charge density etc. Based on degree of esterification, pectins are classified into high methoxyl-pectin (> 50% esterified) and low methoxyl-pectin (<50% esterified). High methoxyl-pectins form gel in presence of sugar and acid (pH<3.6) by the formation of hydrogen-bonding and hydrophobic interactions. Gelation of low methoxyl-pectin occurs in presence of divalent cations, such as calcium ion, which binds the pectin molecules and acts as a bridge between two carboxyl groups of pectin [5]. Apart from gel forming characteristics, other important properties of pectin is that it carries a negative charge and its charge density depends on pH and degree of methoxylation. The variation of zeta potential with pectin concentration at different solution pH and glucose contents is discussed by Sulaiman et al. [6]. Gelation of pectin is largely affected by the charge distribution in rahmno-galacturonan backbone.

Gel forming pectin molecules are found to behave as significant organic foulants of membranes [7]. Therefore, depectinization of juice is a common pretreatment method before membrane clarification. In order to reduce the pectin content, an enzymatic treatment of the raw juice is usually carried out with enzyme such as pectinase. Pectinase hydrolyses pectin resulting in a flocculation of pectin-protein complex. This enzyme treatment reduces the amount of pectin in the juice and makes the filtration process easier by lowering its viscosity. During ultrafiltration of fruit juice, the left over pectin even after enzyme treatment is sufficient to cause a formation of gel type layer over the membrane surface which offers extra resistance to the permeate flow in series with the hydraulic resistance of the membrane [8,9] and thereby drastically reduces the permeate flux. Hence improvement of permeate flux during fruit juice clarification is an interesting challenge.

2.2. Application of External Field

Application of various external fields such as acoustic, magnetic, and d.c. electric field for the reduction of concentration polarization and membrane fouling have been discussed in Chapter 1. Among the various external fields, use of d.c. electric field is explored here to improve the membrane performance. Several studies have been focused to reduce concentration polarization and membrane fouling but very few reports are available in literature regarding the use of external electric field to the enhancement of permeate flux. In electro-ultrafiltration, the concentration polarization is reduced by applying an external d.c. electric field across the membrane. A number of excellent publications on electro-ultra filtration are available in literature (see section 1.4.4). The major problems associated with the use of continuous electric field during ultrafiltration include changes in feed properties due to electrode reaction [10-13], requirement of high energy, rise of temperature, etc. The method can not be effectively used for feeds of high electrical conductivity and heat sensitivity. These problems can be circumvented by the use of pulsed electric field instead of a continuous one. A few references of the use of pulsed electric fields are available in literature (see section 1.4.4). During electro-ultrafiltration, electrolysis may take place at the electrode. When electric field is applied, the passage of current causes the reaction at the two electrodes and may lead to change in pH near the electrode. Rabie et al. [14] and Vijh [15] have discussed the possible electrode reactions in detail. Most possible electrode reactions are as follows:

Reduction at the cathode:

$$2H_2O + 2e^- \rightarrow H_2 + 2OH^- \quad (2.1)$$

$$M_c^{n+} + ne^- \rightarrow M_c \quad (2.2)$$

Oxidation at the anode:

$$M_a \rightarrow M_a^{n+} + ne^- \quad (2.3)$$

$$6H_2O \rightarrow O_2 + 4H_3O^+ + 4e^- \quad (2.4)$$

where, M_c and M_a represent the cathode and anode material, respectively. Reaction (2.1) leads to the evolution of hydrogen gas and OH^- ions near the cathode. Reaction (2.2) takes place if the cathode metal is positioned below hydrogen in the electrochemical series. Since the porous cathode plate is placed below the membrane, the produced OH^- ions are washed out with the permeate stream resulting an increase in pH of the permeate. Reaction (2.3) can be avoided by using inert material such as platinum, silver, gold, etc. and reaction (2.4) causes the evolution of oxygen gas and H_3O^+ that leads to decrease of pH near the anode.

2.2.1. Application of Electric Field during Fruit Juice Clarification

Pectin being negatively charged, application of external d.c. electric field during cross-flow ultrafiltration of fruit juice appears to be promising. Application of an appropriate external electric field across the membrane significantly reduces the gel-type layer formation by the charged pectin molecules, thereby increasing the permeate flux (and possible reduction of membrane fouling). This observation has encouraged us to investigate the effect of electric field on the permeate flux in the clarification of fruit juice.

Several models have been attempted to simulate the ultrafiltration performance of fruit juice. The most conventional models are gel-polarization model [16], osmotic pressure model [17], boundary layer model [18], resistance in series model etc. Shen et al. [19] have developed a similarity solution model and Probstein et al. [20] have proposed an integral method to model gel layer controlled ultrafiltration. Permeation of sucrose through a gel forming material (PVA) is studied and modeled by De et al. [16]. In contrast, a suitable mathematical model for electric field enhanced ultrafiltration of gel forming particle is rare in literature.

In this chapter, the potential of an externally applied electric field for the reduction of pectin gel type layer formation over the membrane surface has been explored. A cross-flow ultrafiltration in presence of electric field has been carried out under a wide range of operating conditions for the clarification of synthetic juice (a mixture of pectin and sucrose) and mosambi (*Citrus Sinensis (L.) Osbeck*) juice. Effects of operating conditions, e.g. electric field, feed concentration, pressure and cross flow velocity on the permeate flux are investigated in detail. The integral method of solution under the frame work of boundary layer analysis of Probstein et al. [20] is extended for the prediction of steady state permeate flux in gel controlled ultrafiltration of synthetic juice in presence of an external d.c. electric field. The gel type layer thickness during ultrafiltration of a synthetic juice solution of pectin and sucrose mixture is measured using high-resolution video microscopy. A theoretical model for the growth of the gel-type layer over the membrane surface under various operating conditions is proposed, numerically solved and successfully compared with optically measured values of gel thickness. It is appeared from the earlier discussion that use of a pulsed electric field may be able to address some of the inherent limitations and shortcomings associated with the application of a continuous field. There has been no report in the literature about the use of pulsed electric field for fruit juice clarification. The present work also investigates to study the effects of pulsed electric field, cross flow velocity and feed concentration on the permeate flux during clarification of synthetic and mosambi juice. A theoretical model based on resistance-in-series model for prediction of permeate flux and gel layer thickness over the membrane surface is proposed in presence of pulsed electric field. Mosambi juice is a complex mixture of several components, the viscosity and diffusivity values are difficult to obtain. The gel concentration of the actual juice is also different from that of pure pectin. Moreover, the variation of viscosity and diffusivity within concentration polarization layer near the membrane surface is significant due to sharp variation in the concentration. For the difficulty in estimating the concentration dependence of viscosity and diffusivity of the real juice, an optimization technique has been developed to evaluate the effective values of these parameters. The value of mass transfer coefficient required for the above mentioned optimization has been deduced from the Sherwood number relationship derived in integral solution method for synthetic juice. Knowing these parameters, transient flux decline is quantified by a resistance-in-series model during ultrafiltration of mosambi juice in presence of continuous as well as pulsed electric field.

2.3. Membrane Experiment

2.3.1. Cross-flow Electro-ultrafiltration Cell

The experiments are conducted in continuous mode of operation. From the feed tank, feed solution is pumped and allowed to flow tangentially over the membrane surface through a thin channel of 37 cm in length, 3.6 cm in width and 6.5 mm in height. The anode is platinum coated titanium sheet (length 33.5 cm, width 3.4 cm, thickness 1.0 mm) obtained from Ti Anode Fabricators, Chennai (India), and mounted parallel to the flow position just above the ultrafiltration channel. External electric field from a regulated DC power supply is applied across the membrane surface. The retentate is recycled to the feed tank. The flow rate is measured by a rotameter in the retentate line. Pressure inside the electro ultrafiltration cell is maintained by operating the bypass valve and measured by a pressure gauge. Permeate is collected from bottom of the cell. The effective filtration area is 133.2 cm^2. The details of schematic of the experimental set up are shown in Figure 2.1 and 2.2.

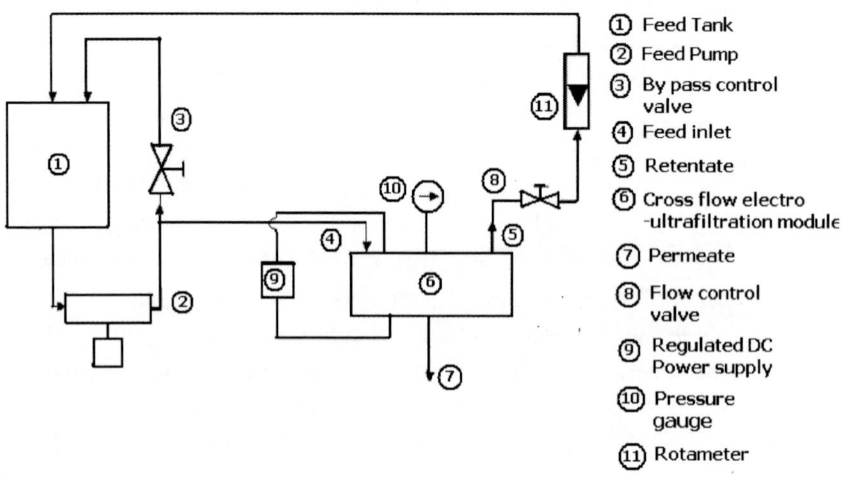

Figure 2.1. Schematic diagram of electro-ultrafiltration system.

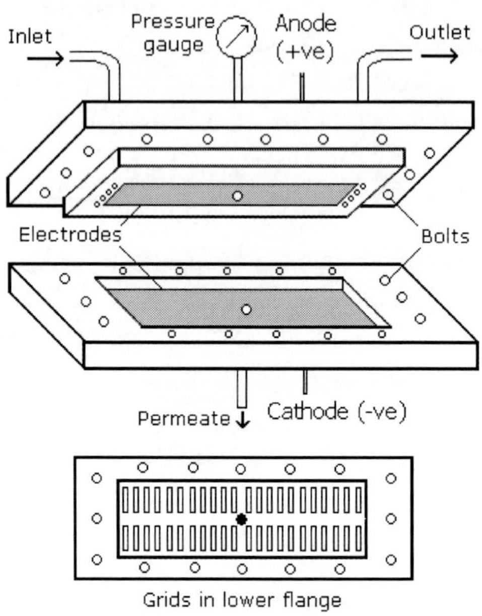

Figure 2.2. Continued on next page.

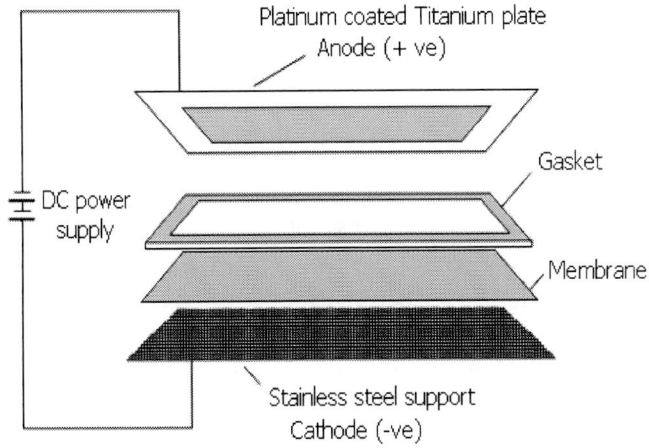

Figure 2.2.Configuration of the electro-ultrafiltration chamber.

2.3.2. Procedure for Conducting Experiments

2.3.2.1. Materials

Mosambi (*Citrus sinensis (L.) Osbeck*) fruits were collected from local market. In industries, membranes having a wide range of pore sizes, with molecular weight cut-off (MWCO) 18 kDa to 0.2 μm are generally used for clarification of fruit juice [21]. Since the average molecular weight of pectin is approximately 65 kDa, flat sheet polyethersulfone membrane of MWCO 50 kDa is chosen for electric field assisted clarification of synthetic juice as well as mosambi juice. Membranes obtained from M/s, Permionics Membranes Pvt. Ltd., Boroda, Gujarat, (India), have been used for the experiments.

2.3.2.2. Operating Conditions

Electro-ultrafiltration experiments are designed to observe the effects of variations in operating conditions (transmembrane pressure, cross-flow velocity, electric field, feed concentration and pulse ratio). The electrical conductivity of mosambi fruit juice (4.0 m S/cm) is significantly higher compared to that of the synthetic juice (0.17 m S/cm). Due to the high electrical conductivity of mosambi juice, use of higher electric field results in significant water hydrolysis at the electrodes leading to evolution of oxygen (O_2) and hydronium ions (H_3O^+) at the anode and hydrogen (H_2) and hydroxyl ions (OH^-) at the cathode. This may change the properties of the feed as well as the permeate and may result in rise of temperature. To avoid electrolytic reactions, maximum operating electric field has been restricted to 500 V/m.

2.3.2.3. Preparation of Feed

Three different mixtures of pectin and sucrose are prepared in double distilled water (Pectin: 1 kg/m^3, Sucrose: 14 Brix; Pectin: 3 kg/m^3, Sucrose: 12 Brix; Pectin: 5 kg/m^3, Sucrose: 10 Brix) and used for the experiments. Mosambi juice was extracted by a manually operated 'screw type juice extractor'. Pectinase from *Aspergillus nigar* with activity 3.5-7.0 units/mg protein (Lowry) (SIGMA-ALDRICH (USA) was used to treat the mosambi juice at an enzyme concentration of 0.01% v/v at 44°C (in a bath at constant temperature) for 120 minutes. After the treatment, the suspension was heated to 90°C for 5 minutes in a water bath to inactivate the remaining enzyme in the sample. The decanted, depectinized juice was used for electro-ultrafiltration.

2.3.2.4. Conduction of Experiments

The membrane is compacted at a pressure of 690 kPa (higher than the highest operating pressure used in this study) for 3 hours using distilled water. Pure water fluxes at different operating pressures are measured next and plotted against pressure difference. The membrane permeability is obtained from the slope of this curve as $1x10^{-10}$ m/Pa s for 50 kDa. During ultrafiltration experiment, permeate samples are collected at different time. The duration of each experiment is 30-40 minutes. All experiments are conducted at 30±2°C. After each experiment, the membranes are cleaned using the following procedure:

Table 2.1. Operating conditions used in experiment

Juice	Variable	Operating conditions
Synthetic juice	Feed	Pectin: 1 kg/m^3; Sucrose: 14 Brix Pectin: 3 kg/m^3; Sucrose: 12 Brix Pectin: 5 kg/m^3; Sucrose: 10 Brix
	Transmembrane pressure (kPa)	220, 360, 500, 635
	Cross flow velocity (m/s)	0.09, 0.12, 0.15, 0.18
	Electric field (V/m)	0, 300, 600, 800,1000, 1200,1600, 2000
	Pulse ratio (off time always set to 1 sec).	1:1, 2:1, 3:1, 4:1, constant electric field
Real juice	Mosambi juice	
	Transmembrane pressure (kPa)	220, 360, 500, 635
	Cross flow velocity (m/s)	0.09, 0.12, 0.15, 0.18
	Electric field (V/m)	0, 200, 300,400, 500
	Pulse ratio (off time always set to 1 sec).	1:1, 2:1, 3:1, 4:1, constant electric field

After completion of an experiment membrane was washed thoroughly for 45minutes by recirculating distilled water at room temperature 30±2°C, followed by 45 minutes of static acid (pH 3.0) washing using HCl, 30 min of washing using distilled water, 30 minutes of alkaline (pH 10) washing and finally membrane was washed with distilled water. After such thorough washing, water flux was measured with distilled water. This procedure is allowed for recovery of the pure initial water flux within 95%. All the steps are carried out at room temperature i.e., 30±2°C. The membranes are also cleaned in situ in some of the experiments in the same way as mentioned before. In both the cases results are almost same. It has been found that the original permeability of the membrane is completely recovered in most cases.

Application of external d.c. electric field has a significant effect on membrane fouling. In presence of electric field the deposition over the membrane surface is less and therefore less time is needed for its cleaning compared to without electric field.

2.3.2.5. Analysis of the Feed and Permeate

The concentrations of pectin and sucrose in the synthetic juice as well as in the permeate and retentate are determined using a Genesys2 Spectrophotometer. For pectin concentration, a wavelength of 230 nm is used and distilled water is taken as a blank. For pectin-sucrose mixture, the pectin free solution containing same amount of sucrose is used as blank. The sucrose contents in the sample are assessed with a refractometer (Thermospectronic). The raw mosambi juice and clarified juice samples were analyzed for color, clarity, total soluble solid, titrable acidity, pH, viscosity, pectin content, and conductivity. Color was measured by absorbance at 420 nm and clarity by transmittance at 660 nm using Genesys2 Spectrophotometer (Thermospectronic, USA). The total soluble solid was measured by refractometer, (Thermospectronic, USA). The acidity of the sample was determined by titration against 0.1 M NaOH and expressed as % of anhydrous citric acid. The viscosity was measured by using an Ostwald viscometer. Zeta potential is obtained by measuring electrophoretic mobility and then by using Henry equation. The electrophoretic mobility of the particle is measured by Laser Doppler Velocimetry. The conductivity is measured by an autoranging conductivity meter, Toshniwal Instrument (India). Alcohol insoluble solid (AIS) was used as a measure for pectin content in the juice. AIS values were measured by mixing 20 g juice with 300 ml 80% alcohol solution and simmering the mixture for 30 minutes. The filtered residue was washed with 80% alcohol solution. The residue was dried at 100°C for 2 hour and is expressed in weight percentage [22]. Pectin content of the juice was about 0.38 times of AIS value as obtained from a calibration curve. The zeta potential of mosambi juice at its natural pH was measured by a zeta meter (Zetasizer, Nano-ZS, Malvern Instruments, UK). Physico-chemical properties of synthetic juice and mosambi juice are presented in Table 2.2 and 2.3.

Table 2.2. Physico-chemical properties of synthetic juice

Pectin + Sucrose mixture	pH	Conducti -vity (mS/cm)	Viscosity x 10^3 (Pa s)	Density x 10^{-3} (kg/m^3)	Zeta potential (mV)	Diffusivity x 10^{11}(m^2/s)
(1 kg/m^3 + 14 Brix)	3.5	57.0	1.83	1.06	-19.4	5.11
(3 kg/m^3 + 12 Brix)	3.2	127.0	2.72	1.05	-20.5	3.44
(5 kg/m^3 + 10 Brix)	3.16	170.0	3.10	1.04	-20.1	3.02

The particle size of the mosambi juice are determined by Malvern Zetasizer (Nano ZS, ZEN3600, Malvern, England). It measures the particle size using the technique of dynamic light scattering (DLS). The suspended particles are in brownian motion. DLS measures the brownian motion of the particle to calculate the size of the particle. In this system Helium-Neon red laser is used to provide the source of light at a wavelength of 638.2 nm and a detector is used to measure the intensity of scattered light at an angle of 173°, called backscattered detection. The rate of intensity fluctuation is used to calculate the size of the particle. Thus DLS gives a measure of intensity particle size distribution shown in Figure 2.3. The average particle size are found to be 1.676 μm, 1.495 μm and 0.145 μm for actual mosambi juice, enzyme treated juice and permeate respectively.

Table 2.3.1. Physico-chemical properties of mosambi juice

Juice	Pectin (kg/m^3)	TSS (^{0}Brix)	pH	Density $\times 10^{-3}$ (kg/m^3)	Viscosity $\times 10^3$ (Pa s)	Conductivity (mS/cm)
Mosambi juice	2.5	8.5	4.10	1.04	2.45	4.0
Mosambi juice (enzyme treated)	1.6	8.5	4.15	1.03	1.05	4.0

Table 2.3.2. Physico-chemical properties of mosambi juice

Juice	Color	Clarity	Acidity as Citric acid (kg/m^3)	Zeta potential (mV)
Mosambi juice	1.33	38.50	7.1	-21.0
Mosambi juice (enzyme treated)	0.96	40.50	5.4	-21.8

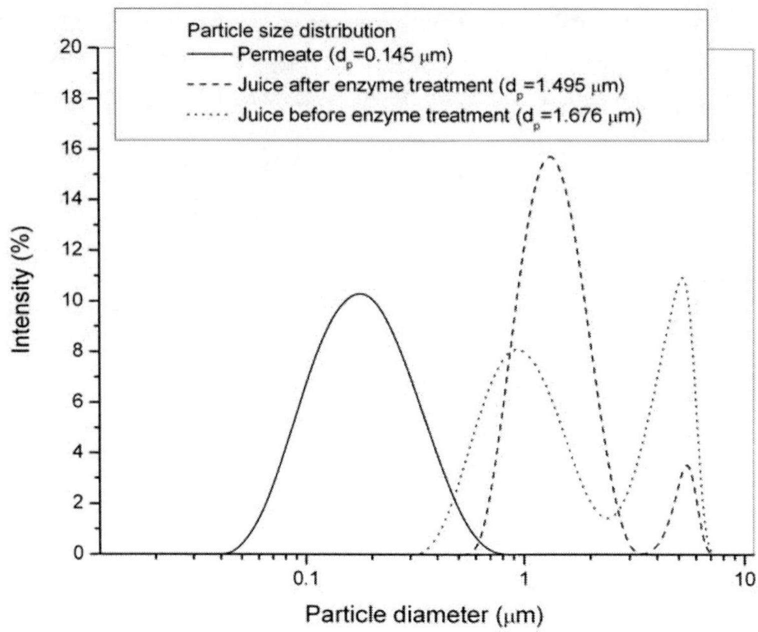

Figure 2.3. Particle size distribution of mosambi juice.

Variation of Zeta Potential of Synthetic Juice (A Mixture of Pectin and Sucrose) with pH

Table 2.4 illustrates the variations of zeta potential with different pH values of pectin sucrose solution, indicating the significant increase of the zeta potential with increasing suspension pH. From the table it is clear that with increasing pH, pectin becomes more negative. Similarly, for a fixed value of solution pH, the pectin becomes more positive with increasing sucrose contents. For an example, at a pectin concentration of 1 kg/m^3, the measured zeta potential decreases from -35 mV to -54 mV with an increase of pH from 3.5 to 9.0; whereas, at pH 5.0, zeta potential increases from -56.2 mV to -39.0 mV with the addition of 14 Brix sucrose to the pectin suspension. The presence of sucrose in pectin suspension causes the electrostatic repulsion between the pectin molecules to decrease and also promotes hydrophobic interaction between the ester methyl groups of pectin and hence facilitates the formation of stable gel [6].

Table 2.4. Values of zeta potential of synthetic juice for various solution pH

Pectin: 1 kg/m^3, Sucrose: 14Brix		Pectin: 3 kg/m^3, Sucrose: 12Brix		Pectin: 5 kg/m^3, Sucrose: 10 Brix	
pH	Zeta potential (mV)	pH	Zeta potential (mV)	pH	Zeta potential (mV)
3.5	-35.0	3.5	-26.6	3.5	-19.5
4.0	-51.0	3.8	-40.6	3.8	-32.8
6.0	-56.2	4.0	-45.0	4.0	-36.1
7.0	-53.7	5.0	-46.5	5.0	-40.0
7.9	-53.5	7.0	-42.8	7.0	-36.5
9.0	-54.0	9.0	-41.6	9.0	-34.0

2.3.2.6. Optical Studies

Immediately after each experimental run, the filtration chamber is opened, carefully removing the top but leaving the lower gasket undisturbed that essentially hold the gel formed along with a layer of the solution. The soft gel over the membrane is partially dried by illuminating the surface with high power lamps to prevent any unwanted motion and loss during transportation for final drying in vacuum desiccators. After two hours of vacuum drying, the deposited membranes are then cut carefully to avoid any beveling or physical depression in the cutting edge. A large number of pieces are then cut from relevant locations. The sample pieces are cut in 4mm x 3mm size pieces. Each sample piece is fixed vertically with its edge held up at the edge of a glass slide. The glass slide with the membrane piece projecting out is then placed under a high-resolution optical microscope (ε POL 400 of Nikon, Japan). Multiple images are obtained of the top of the projected part of the membrane (which essentially is the cross section of the original deposited membrane) and further analyzed to quantify deposition. For each such mounted membrane piece, images are captured at large number of locations and averaged to eliminate local fluctuations. The sampling of the membrane after each experiment is done carefully to encompass the whole area of the membrane by analyzing at many points on the two diagonals of the rectangular membrane piece.

The optical measurements are done in reflection mode of incident light. The membrane sample pieces are viewed under the microscope as well as in a LCD display interfaced with the microscope and a high-resolution digital camera. The captured images are digitized and then analyzed to evaluate the thickness of different layers of the membrane, voids in the substrate material, deposition over the membrane surfaces. A standard grating element having 2000 lines per inch is used to calibrate the magnification of the microscope (500 X) coupled with the camera.

2.4. Prediction of the Permeate Flux and Deposition Thickness

2.4.1. Analysis of Transient Flux

2.4.1.1. Theoretical Aspects

The schematic of a cross flow electro-ultrafiltration system along with development of gel-layer and external concentration boundary layer with and without external d.c. electric field are shown in Figure 2.4 (a and b) respectively. During ultrafiltration, solutes are convected by the transmembrane pressure gradient towards the membrane surface. The lower molecular weight solutes permeate through the membrane whereas; higher molecular weight solutes are retained, forming a gel-layer over the membrane surface. Since the bulk concentration of higher molecular weight solute is much less than that of the gel layer concentration, a concentration boundary layer forms from the bulk of the solution up to the gel layer. This prompts diffusion of gel forming solutes from the gel layer towards the bulk of the solution due to concentration gradient. The formation of external concentration boundary layer and gel layer over the membrane surface without electric field is shown in Figure 2.4a. In presence of external d.c. electric field (with the top surface maintains opposite polarity as that of the charged particles), the particles move away from the gel layer due to electrophoresis. At steady state, the rate of convective movement of solute particles towards the membrane surface is equal to the rate of migration of solute particles away from the membrane surface due to both back diffusion and electrophoresis (Figure 2.4b).

As has been pointed out before, high-methoxylated pectin, as is used herein for experiments, can form gel even in the absence of divalent cations such as Ca^{+2}, if the conditions are acidic and in presence of sugar. Visual observations of the membrane after the experiments confirm the presence of a gel-type layer on the surface. Furthermore, the osmotic pressure contribution of the feed solution is estimated, based on Vant Hoff's equation, and is found to be significantly small compared to the applied transmembrane pressure (less than 1%). Experimentally the permeate flux exhibits almost a pressure independence further indicating that the filtration is carried out under gel-controlled regime. Based on the above considerations, the model equations are developed. In Figure 2.4a, δ_g is the gel layer thickness and δ_c is the thickness of the concentration boundary layer over the gel layer. c_g

and c_0 are the gel concentration and bulk concentration of solute respectively. Solute concentration in permeate (c_p) can be neglected by considering very high rejection of solute (by selecting a membrane with low molecular weight cutoff).

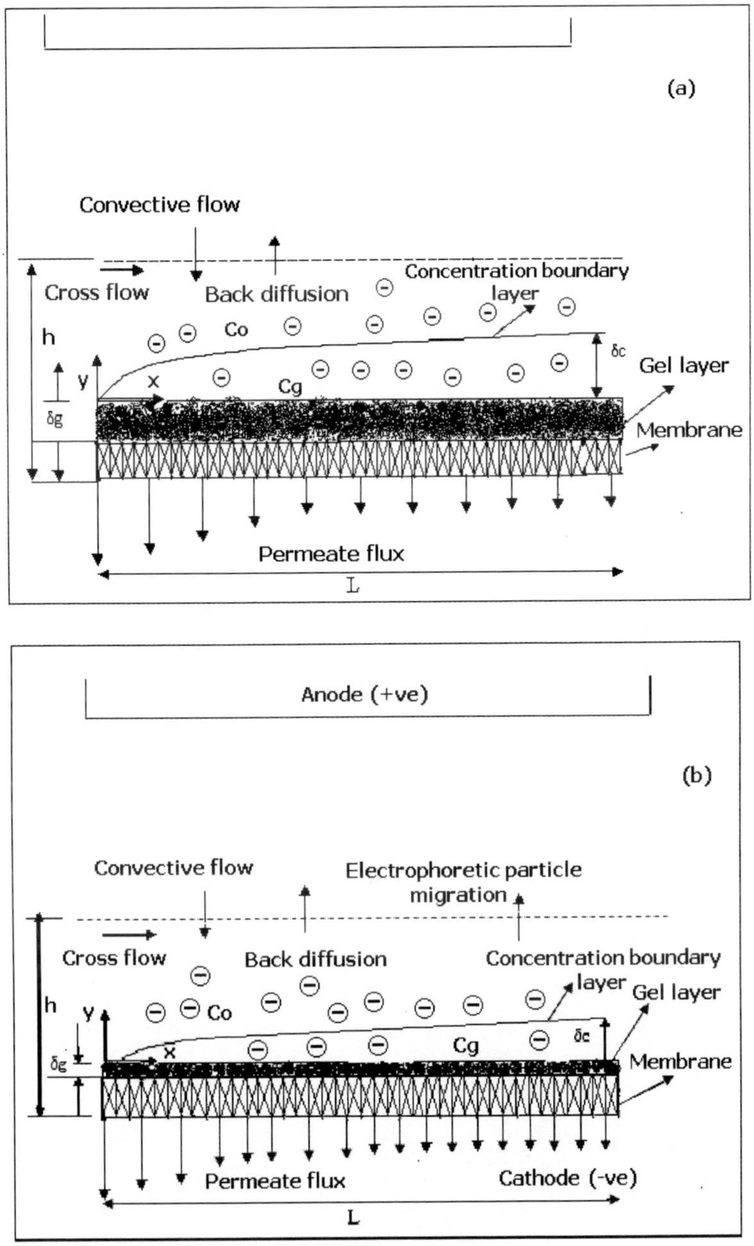

Figure 2.4. Schematic of formation of external concentration boundary layer and gel layer over the membrane surface (a) with out electric field (b) with electric field.

The rate of gel layer formation on the membrane surface is given by a solute mass balance as,

$$\rho_g \frac{dL}{dt} = \left(v_w - v_e\right)c + D\,\frac{dc}{dy} \tag{2.5}$$

The concentration of gel layer is considered to be constant. Therefore, the relevant boundary conditions are

$$c = c_0 \text{ at } y = \delta_g + \delta_c \tag{2.6}$$

$$c = c_g \text{ at } y = \delta_g \tag{2.7}$$

The electrophoretic velocity (v_e) is related with the electrophoretic mobility by the following equation,

$$v_e = E\, u_e \tag{2.8}$$

where, E is the applied electric field. The electrophoretic mobility, u_e can be expressed by Helmholtz-Smoulochowski's equation [23] as

$$u_e = \frac{\varepsilon_0 D_i \xi}{\mu} \tag{2.9}$$

where, ε_o is permittivity of vacuum, D_i is the dielectric constant and μ is the viscosity. Eq. (2.5) can be solved using the boundary conditions, to obtain the growth of the gel layer thickness as

$$\rho_g \frac{dL}{dt} = \left[\frac{c_g - c_0 \exp\left(\frac{v_w - v_e}{k}\right)}{1 - \exp\left(\frac{v_w - v_e}{k}\right)}\right]\left(v_w - v_e\right) \tag{2.10}$$

where, k is the mass transfer coefficient, defined as $\frac{D}{\delta_c}$ and D is diffusion coefficient. The diffusion coefficient is given by Einstein equation as,

$$D = \frac{KT}{3\pi\mu d_p} \tag{2.11}$$

where, K, T, μ, d_p are the Boltzmann constant, absolute temperature, viscosity of the solution and equivalent spherical diameter of the particle respectively. The average diameter of the gel forming pectin molecule is estimated assuming spherical molecule and using the following relationship [24]

$$M_w = z\, d_p^3 \qquad (2.12)$$

where, M_w is the average molecular weight of gel forming material, the value of z taken as $6\text{x}10^{29}$ gm/gm-mole.m^3 [24]. For synthetic juice, the pectin used has a molecular weight range from 30-100 kDa and hence 65 kDa is taken as an average molecular weight. The corresponding value of equivalent spherical diameter of pectin is found to be $4.77\text{x}10^{-9}$ m. The gel concentration of pectin used is 38 kg /m^3 [25]. Hence, permeate flux can also be expressed by a resistance in series formulation including the flow resistance due to the membrane itself and the deposited gel layer. For pure water, the flux can be expressed as

$$v_{w,\,pure} = \frac{\Delta P}{\mu R_m} \qquad (2.13)$$

In case of a gel forming macromolecular solution,

$$v_w(t) = \frac{\Delta P}{\left[\mu\left(R_m + R_g(t)\right)\right]} \qquad (2.14)$$

where, R_m and R_g are membrane hydraulic resistance and gel layer resistance respectively.

Gel layer formation is similar to that of gel formation in classical filtration. Thus the gel layer resistance (R_g) can be expressed in term of gel layer thickness as,

$$R_g(t) = \alpha\left(1 - \varepsilon_g\right)\rho_g L(t) \qquad (2.15)$$

Where α is specific gel resistance which is obtained from Kozeny-Carman equation as,

$$\alpha = 180\,\frac{\left(1 - \varepsilon_g\right)}{\varepsilon_g^3 d_p^2 \rho_g} \qquad (2.16)$$

where, ε_g, ρ_g and d_p are the porosity, density, and diameter of the gel forming particles respectively.

The specific gel layer resistance (α) and the permeate flux are obtained by solving the model equations in an iterative manner following the sequence of steps as outlined below.

1. For known input parameters of operating conditions, membrane parameter and physical properties such as ΔP, c_o, E, R_m, c_g, Di, μ, ρ_g, ξ, ε_o, d_p, a value of specific gel layer resistance (α) is guessed.
2. In case of constant electric field ultrafiltration, applied electric field remains constant throughout the operation. In case of pulsed electric field ultrafiltration, at a particular operational time, t, the applied electric field (either E or 0) is determined and used for subsequent calculations.
3. v_e is calculated using Eqs.(2.8) and Eq.(2.9).
4. V_w^{cal} is calculated by solving the coupled differential and algebraic equations, Eqs. (2.10), (2.14), (2.15) and (2.16) including the effect of pulsed electric field (i.e. constant electric field during on-time and zero electric field during off-time) with the initial condition, L = 0 at t = 0.
5. The time, t, is increased to t +Δt next.
6. Steps 2 to 4 are repeated till t = t_{total}.
7. If $\sum_{i=1}^{N_{total}} \left(\frac{V_w^{exp} - V_w^{cal}}{V_w^{exp}} \right)^2 \leq 0.001$ the program is terminated and transient profiles of permeate flux are obtained. The corresponding value of α is recorded. If not another value of α is guessed in step1 and the process is continued till the given convergence is achieved. It needs to be pointed out that the values of the specific gel resistance,α, cannot be calculated a-priori, and the porosity ε_g, can be a function of the operating conditions (e.g. pressure).

2.4.1.2. Analysis of Transient Flux Decline of Synthetic Juice

Effect of Constant Electric Field

As discussed in earlier, the value of specific gel layer resistance, α is estimated by minimizing the root mean square error associated measured and calculated flux values. The profile of permeate flux is calculated. It may be observed that the value of α increases with operating pressure but at higher pressure it becomes invariant (Table 2.5). The probable cause for this observation is that the gel layer behaves like a compressible one up to 360 kPa and its compressibility becomes almost invariant for higher pressure. For a constant gel concentration, the specific gel layer resistance, α, varies with operating pressure which is observed in the present study as well as other studies; e.g., Bhattacharjee et al. [26]. The specific gel layer resistance, α is related with gel porosity by Kozeny-Carman equation. Since α typically increases with pressure (resulting in gel compaction), porosity shows a decreasing trend with increase in pressure.

Figure 2.5 (a, b and c) to 2.6 (a, b and c) represent the transient profile of permeate flux and gel layer thickness at different operating pressure differences for fixed values of feed concentration, electric field and cross flow velocity. The symbols are the experimental data and solid lines are the model predictions. The flux values are higher for higher operating pressure, increased as expected, due to increased convection. The initial rapid decline in flux is due to the building up of concentration polarization and subsequent formation of gel layer over the membrane. It is clear that steady state values in terms of flux are reached within 3 to 4 minutes. From the figures it is clear that gel layer thickness decreases with increase in applied electric field. Applied electric field reduces the gel layer formation by electrophoresis of the pectin molecules in the reverse direction i.e., opposite to the convective flow of filtrate resulting in decrease of gel layer thickness. It is evident from the figure that the thickness (steady state) becomes about half at 800 V/m compare to that of the no electric field case.

Table 2.5. Variation of specific gel layer resistance (α) with operating pressure for synthetic juice

Transmembrane pressure, ΔP (kPa)	Specific gel layer resistance, α (m/kg)
220	22.3 x 10^{15}
360	28.1 x 10^{15}
500	28.1 x 10^{15}

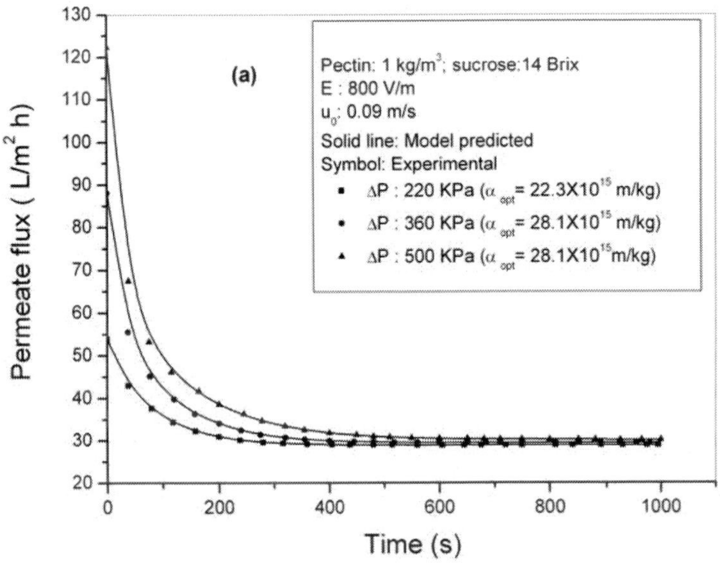

Figure 2.5. Continued on next page.

Figures 2.7 and 2.8 represent the effect of applied electric field on permeate flux and gel layer thickness. The symbols are experimental data and solid lines are predictions from the model. The sharp decrease observed at the beginning can be attributed to the rapid adsorption of pectin molecules on the membrane and buildup of concentration polarization at the beginning of the experiment. As the time of operation progresses, there is more accumulation of solutes over the membrane surface leading to severe concentration polarization. The smoother and slower flux decline at later stages can be attributed to gel layer formation on the membrane surface. With applying electric field, the pectin molecules tend to move away from the membrane surface due to electrophoresis and gel layer formation is reduced leading to substantial increase of permeate flux. For example, the steady state flux at an electric field of 800 V/m is 18.0 L / m^2 h, showing about 200 % increase over the zero electric field flux of 5.9 L / m^2 h (Figure 2.7). With the same increment of electric field gel layer thickness decreases from 8.88 μm to 2.315 μm (Figure 2.8)

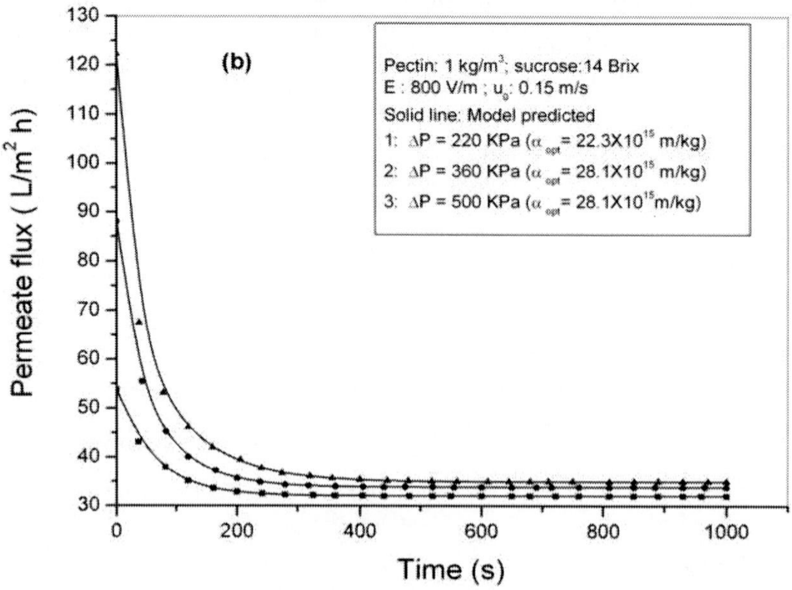

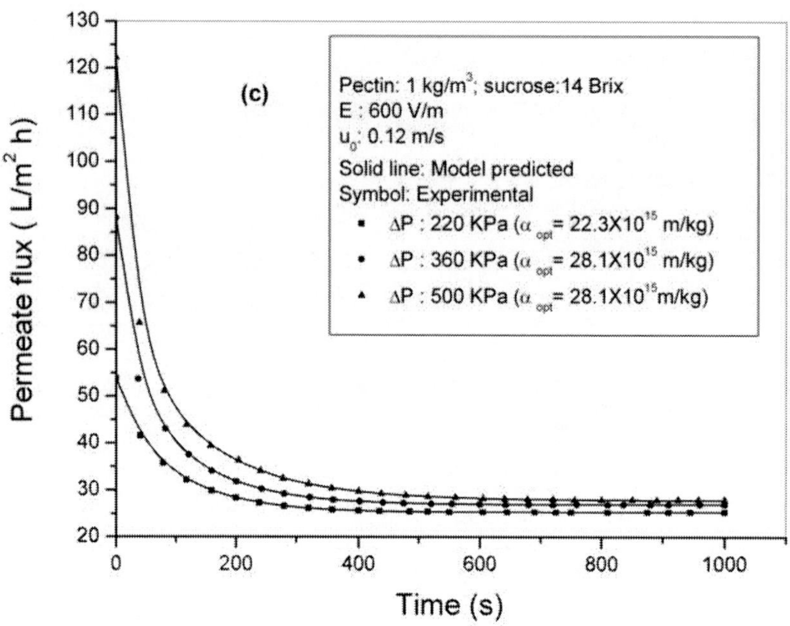

Figure 2.5. Variation of permeate flux with time for synthetic juice (Pectin: 1 kg/m^3 + Sucrose: 14 Brix) (a) E = 800 V/m, u_0 = 0.09 m/s; (b) E = 800 V/m, u_0 = 0.15 m/s; (c) E = 600 V/m, u_0 = 0.12 m/s.

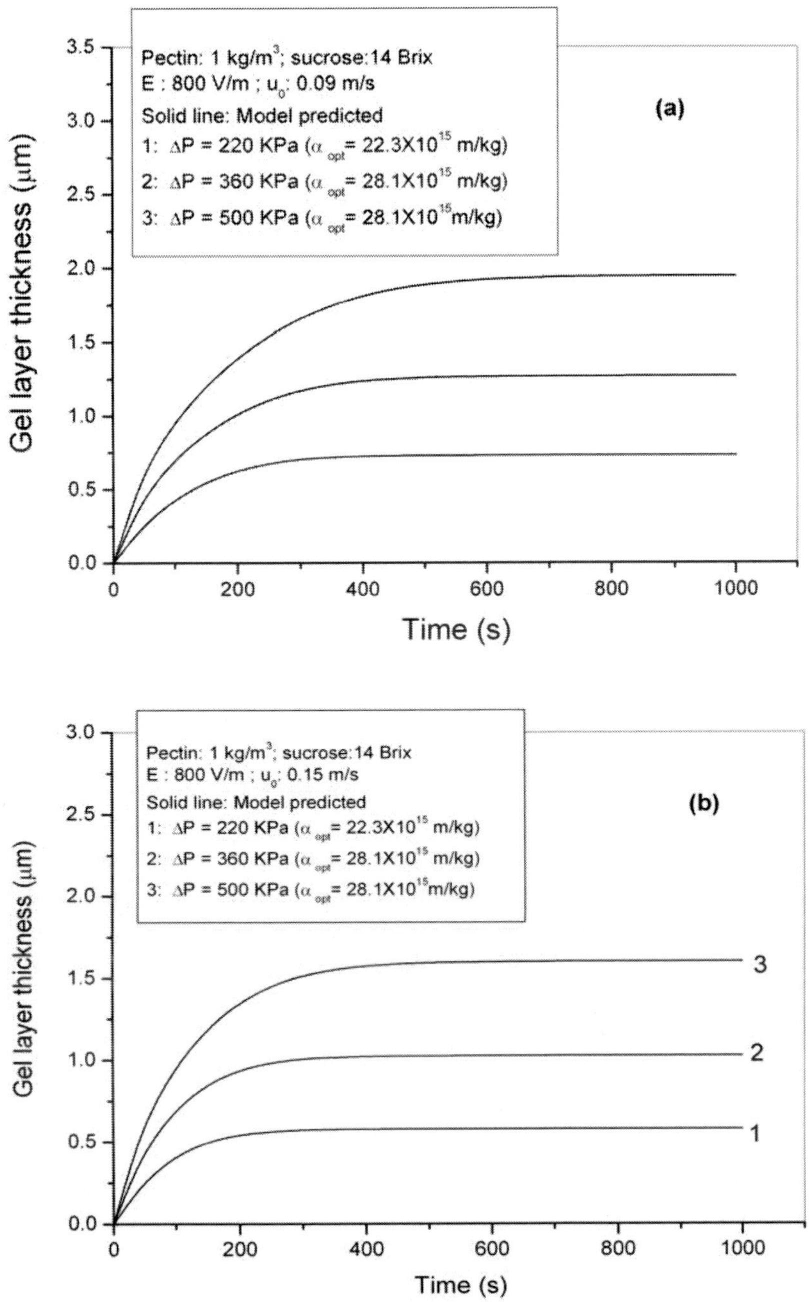

Figure 2.6. Continued on next page.

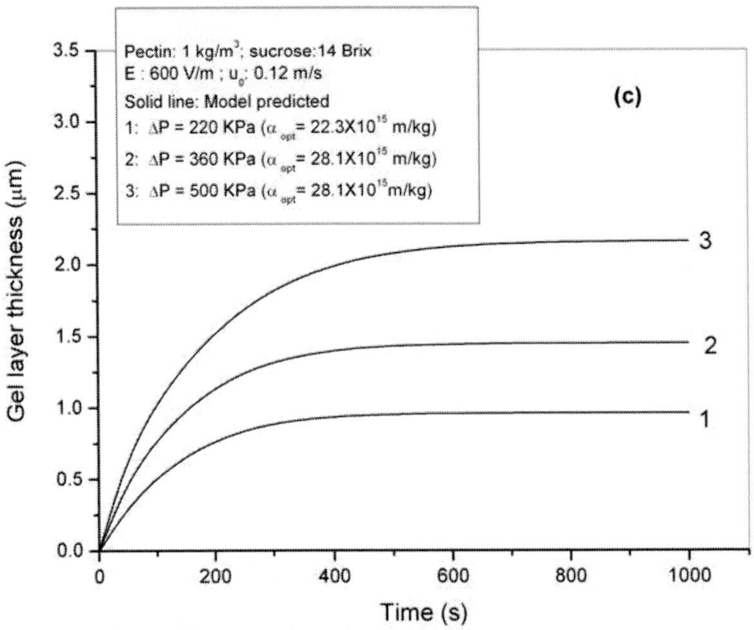

Figure 2.6. Variation of gel layer thickness with time for synthetic juice (Pectin: 1 kg/m^3 + Sucrose: 14 Brix) (a) E = 800 V/m, u_0 = 0.09 m/s; (b) E = 800 V/m, u_0 = 0.15 m/s; (c) E = 600 V/m, u_0 = 0.12 m/s.

Optical Quantification of Gel Layer Thickness

The images of the deposited membrane after electro-ultrafiltration are analyzed using software, Radical Microcam of Radical Instruments (India) to obtain the thickness of the deposit. The measurements are taken at several positions and then averaged to eliminate local fluctuations. The microscopic observation confirms the decrease in deposition thickness with increase in applied electric field while other parameters remain constant. For example, the deposition decreases from 8.63 microns to 5.52 microns (Figure 2.9) with increase in electric field from 0 V/m to 800 V/m. for a fixed feed concentration (3 kg/m^3+12 Brix), pressure (360 kPa) and cross-flow velocity (0.09 m/s). The gel layer thicknesses for all the ten operating conditions reported in this study are measured optically. However a calibration is required before comparison of optically measure gel layer thickness and those predicted from the numerical solution of the model [27,28]. The comparison between the predicted values of the gel thickness and the experimental measurement is depicted in Table 2.6 which clearly shows the excellent match between these two sets. Table 2.6 also summarizes the effect of different operating parameters. For example the highest gel layer thickness is observed in the case with zero electric field. As expected, it can be seen from the table that gel layer thickness decreases with increasing electric field, increasing cross-flow velocity and decreasing feed concentration. For example, the gel layer thickness (steady state) at an electric field of 800 V/m is 2.069 μm compared to 5.3 μm for no electric field case keeping other operating conditions (pressure, flow rate and feed concentration) unchanged. Gel layer thickness increases with feed concentration. For example, gel layer thickness increases from 1.68 μm to 3.238 μm with increases in feed concentration from 1 kg/m^3 pectin to 5 kg/m^3 pectin while other operating conditions remain unaltered. Again for a fixed value of electric field and pressure, with increases in cross flow velocity from 0.09 m/s to 0.15 m/s, gel layer thickness (steady state) decreases from 2.582 μm to 2.062 μm.

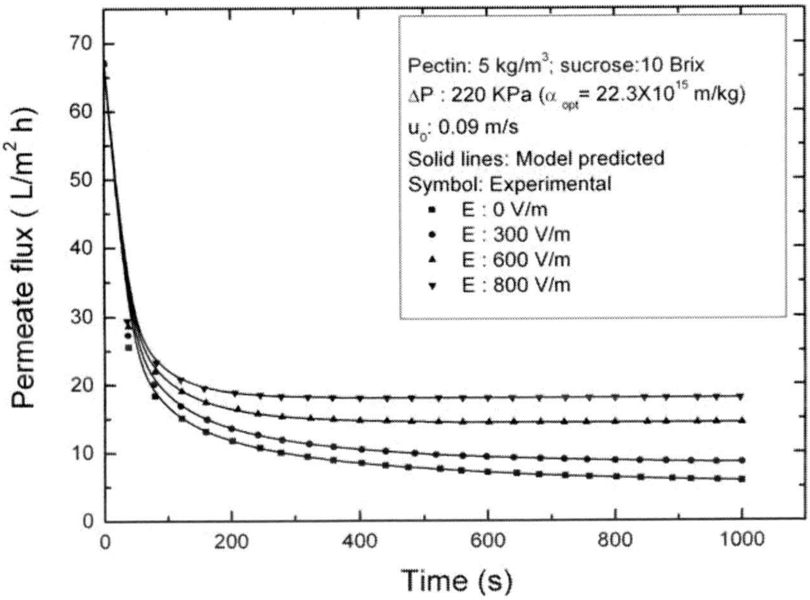

Figure 2.7. Variation of permeate flux with time for different electric fields during clarification of synthetic juice.

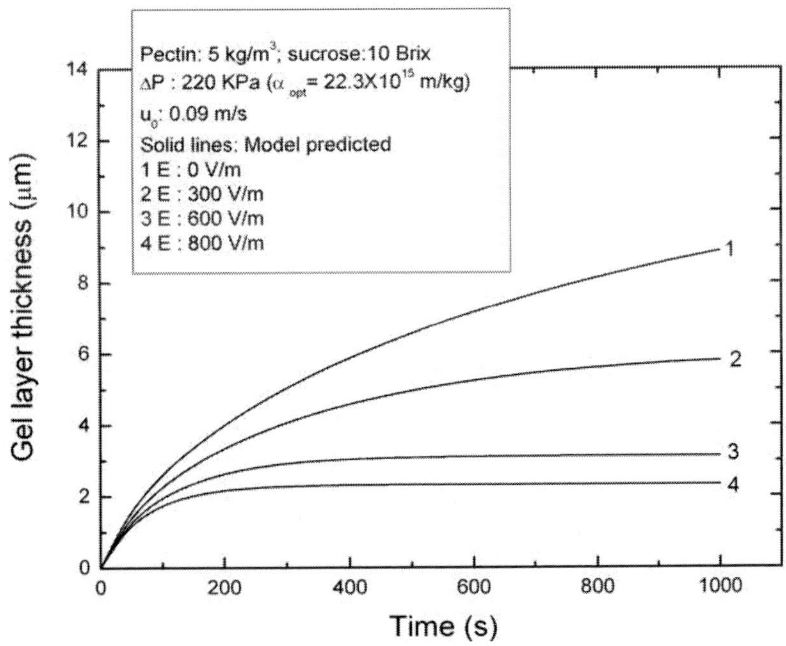

Figure 2.8. Variation of gel layer thickness with time for different electric fields during clarification of synthetic juice.

Table 2.6. Comparison of predicted and experimental gel thickness values

Different parametric conditions	Gel porosity, ε_g	Theoretically obtained gel thickness from flux values (A) (micron)	Modified values of optically measured gel height D = B-C (micron)
(3kg/m^3 +12 Brix) ΔP : 360 kPa u_0: 0.09 m/s E: 300 V/m	0.4775	3.619	*
(3kg/m^3 +12 Brix) ΔP : 360 kPa, u_0: 0.09 m/s E: 600 V/m	0.4775	2.582	*
(.3kg/m^3 +12 Brix) ΔP : 220 kPa, u_0: 0.09 m/s E: 600 V/m	0.5062	2.042	*
(3kg/m^3 +12 Brix) ΔP : 500 kPa, u_0: 0.09 m/s E: 600 V/m	0.4775	3.42	*
(3kg/m^3 +12 Brix) ΔP : 360 kPa, u_0: 0.12 m/s E: 600 V/m	0.4775	2.173	*
(3kg/m^3 +12 Brix) ΔP : 360 kPa, u_0: 0.15 m/s E: 600 V/m	0.4775	2.062	2.073
(5kg/m^3 +10 Brix) ΔP : 360 kPa u_0: 0.09 m/s E: 600 V/m	0.4775	3.238	3.363
(1kg/m^3 +14 Brix) ΔP : 360 kPa, u_0: 0.09 m/s E: 600 V/m	0.4775	1.68	1.573
(3kg/m^3 +12 Brix) ΔP : 360 kPa, u_0: 0.09 m/s E: 0 V/m	0.4775	5.3	5.193
(3kg/m^3 +12 Brix) ΔP : 360 k Kpa, u_0: 0.09 m/s E: 800 V/m	0.4775	2.069	2.083

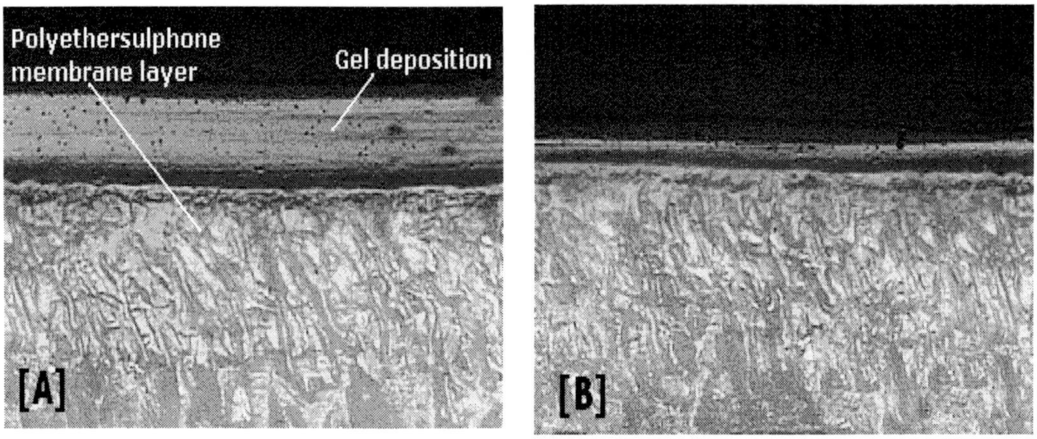

Figure 2.9. Reduction of gel layer thickness with applied d.c. electric field for a synthetic juice (Pectin: 3 kg/m^3, Sucrose: 12 Brix), pressure (360 kPa) and cross flow velocity (0.09 m/s); (A) E = 0 V/m, (B) E = 800 V/m.

Effect of Pulsed Electric Field

The variation of permeate flux with time for different pulse (on-time/off-time ratio) ratio at a transmembrane pressure of 360 kPa and cross flow velocity of 0.12 m/s during clarification of synthetic juice (a mixture of pectin: 3 kg/m^3 and sucrose: 12 Brix) is shown in Figure 2.10 The symbols are experimental data and solid lines are model predictions. For a given set of operating conditions, the value of specific gel resistances (α) is obtained by minimizing the root mean square error between the measured and calculated flux values. For a feed (Pectin: 3 kg/m^3, Sucrose: 12 Brix), at a transmembrane pressure of 360 kPa, cross flow velocity of 0.12 m/s, and electric field of 1000 V/m, the optimum value of α is found to be 21.3 x 10^{15} m/kg which is consistent with the results reported in literature [25]. It is evident from the figure that permeate flux declines rapidly as the gel layer grows and reaches a steady value. The same trend can be observed for all operating conditions. It may be observed from the figure, that for the pulse ratio of 3:1 the end of operation flux declines from 82.4 L/m^2 h to 22.0 L/m^2 h whereas, for zero electric field it declines to 8.12 L/m^2 h, denoting a sharp rise in steady state permeate flux with electric field application.

2.4.1.3. Mosambi (Citrus Sinensis (L.) Osbeck) Juice

Effect of Constant Electric Field

The variation of permeate flux and gel layer thickness with time for different electric field at a transmembrane pressure of 360 kPa and cross flow velocity of 0.12 m/s during clarification of mosambi juice is shown in Figures 2.11 and 2.12 respectively. The symbols are experimental data and solid lines are model predictions. For a given set of operating conditions, the value of specific gel resistances (α) is obtained by minimizing the root mean square error between the measured and calculated flux values. For mosambi juice, at a transmembrane pressure of 360 kPa, cross flow velocity of 0.12 m/s, and electric field of 400 V/m, the optimum value of α is found to be 2.34 x10^{16} m/kg. It is also observed that value of α is invariant with electric field. It is evident from the figure that permeate flux declines rapidly as the gel layer grows and reaches a steady value. The same trend can be observed for all operating conditions. It may be observed from the figure, that at an electric field of 400 V/m, at the end of operation flux declines from 130 L/m^2 h to 11.95 L/m^2 h and gel layer thickness grows up to 3.8 μm whereas, for zero electric field flux declines to 8.67 L/m^2 h and gel layer grows up to 5.4 μm, denoting a sharp rise in steady state permeate flux with electric field application.

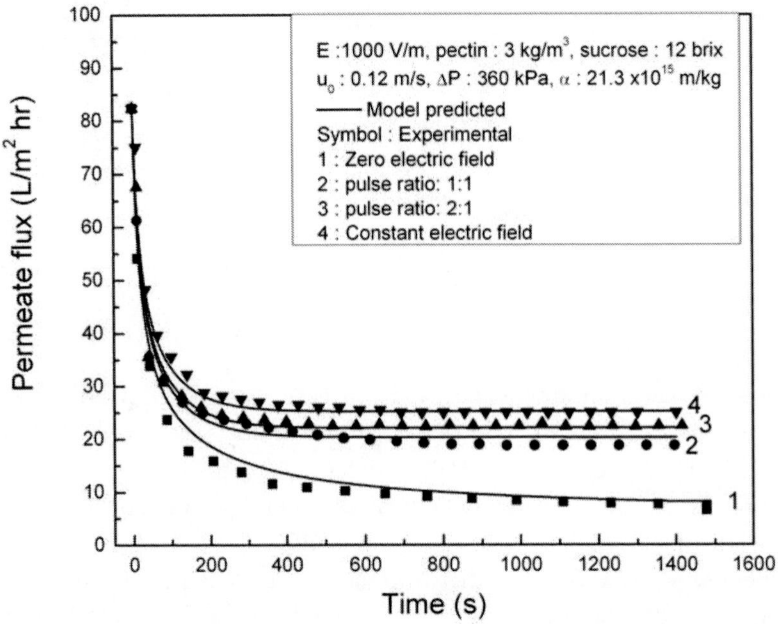

Figure 2.10. Variation of permeate flux with time for different on pulse ratio during clarification of synthetic juice.

The values of specific gel resistances (α), at an operating condition is selected based on the best-fit value i.e. by minimizing the root mean square error associated measured and calculated flux values. The corresponding values of ε_g are calculated from Eq. 2.16. The variation of specific gel resistances (α) and gel porosity (ε_g) with operating pressure are shown in Table 2.7. It may be observed that the value of α increases sharply for lower pressure and gradually for higher pressure values. For example, with increase in pressure from 220 kPa to 635 kPa, the value of ε_g increase by a factor of 2.24. This observation indicates the compressible nature of the gel layer over the range of operating pressure considered here. At higher pressure, the compressibility of gel layer becomes less compared to lower pressure. Since α typically increases with pressure (resulting in gel compaction), gel porosity shows a decreasing trend with increase in pressure. The evaluated optimum values of α are correlated with operating pressure by a simple relation,

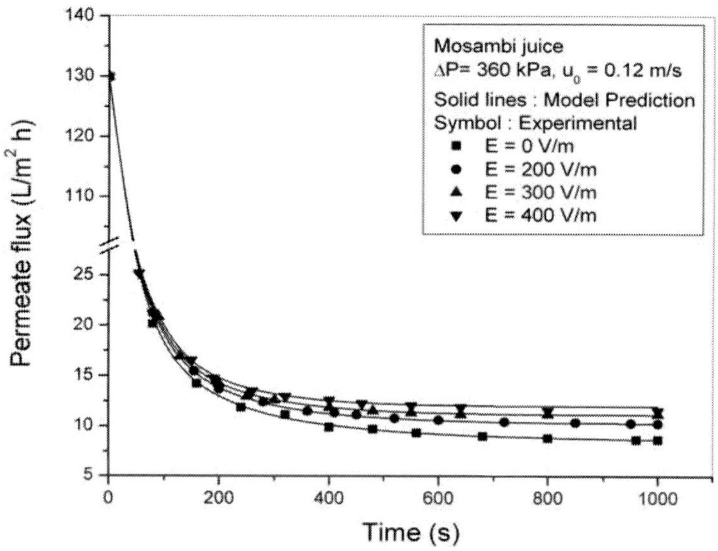

Figure 2.11. Variation of permeate flux with time for different electric field during clarification of mosambi juice.

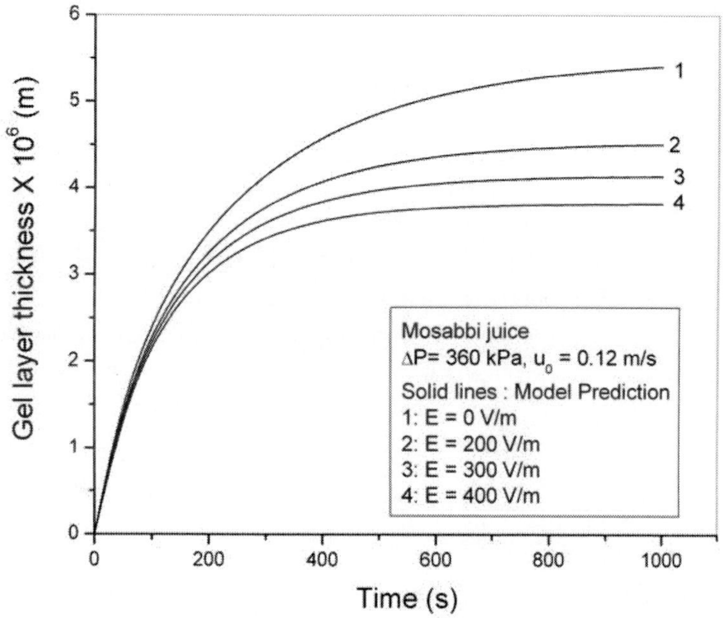

Figure 2.12. Variation of gel layer thickness with time for different electric field during clarification of mosambi juice.

$$\alpha = \alpha_0 \left(\Delta P\right)^{0.784} \qquad (2.17)$$

where, $\alpha_0 = 1.313 \times 10^{15}$ m/kg and ΔP is in Pa.

Table 2.7. Variation of specific gel layer resistance (α) with operating pressure for mosambi juice

Transmembrane pressure, ΔP (kPa)	Specific gel layer resistance, α (m/kg)
220	15.6×10^{15}
360	23.4×10^{15}
500	31.1×10^{15}
635	35.0×10^{15}

Effect of Pulsed Electric Field

The variation of permeate flux and gel layer thickness with time for different pulse (on-time/off-time ratio) ratio at a transmembrane pressure of 360 kPa and cross flow velocity of 0.12 m/s during clarification of mosambi juice are shown in Figures 2.13 and 2.14 respectively. The symbols are for the experimental permeate flux, whereas, the solid lines are model predicted permeate flux and the dashed lines are estimated gel layer thickness. For a given set of operating conditions, the value of specific gel resistances (α) is obtained by minimizing the root mean square error between the measured and calculated flux values. For example, at a transmembrane pressure of 360 kPa, cross flow velocity of 0.12 m/s, and electric field of 400 V/m, the optimum value of α is found to be 2.34×10^{16} m/kg. It is also observed that the value of α is independent of pulse ratio. It is evident from the figure that permeate flux declines rapidly as the gel layer grows and reaches a steady value. The same trend can be observed for all pulse ratios. In this study, the off-time is always fixed at 1s. It can clearly be seen that an increase in pulse ratio (i.e., increase in on-time) results in a decrease in the estimated gel layer thickness (less resistance to flow) and associated with increase in flux. For a fixed electric field, with increase in pulse ratio i.e., on-time, charged pectin molecules move at a faster rate from the membrane surface. This restricts the formation of gel-type layer over the membrane surface and leads to an enhancement of permeate flux. For example, at 400 V/m, a transmembrane pressure of 360 kPa, a cross flow velocity of 0.12 m/s, and at a pulse ratio of 1:1 (i.e., 1 s on followed by 1 s off time), permeate flux declines from 130 L/m^2 h to 10.4 L/m^2 h and gel layer thickness grows up to 4.45 μm at the end of operation whereas, at a pulse ration of 3:1(i.e., 3 s on followed by 1 s off time), the permeate flux declines to 11.35 L/m^2 h with a gel layer thickness of 4.04 μm keeping other operating conditions unaltered.

2.4.2. Analysis of Steady State Flux

2.4.2.1. Theoretical Aspect

The steady state solute mass balance in the rectangular channel within the concentration boundary layer is given by

$$u\frac{\partial c}{\partial x} + (v + v_e)\frac{\partial c}{\partial y} = D\frac{\partial^2 c}{\partial y^2} \tag{2.18}$$

where, V_e is the electrophoretic velocity which can be obtained from Eq. (2.8). The electrophoretic mobility (u_e) can be obtained from Eq. (2.9). The diffusion coefficient (D) is given by Einstein equation (Eq. (2.11)). Assuming hydrodynamic velocity profile to be fully developed, the x-component velocity becomes [29]

$$u = \frac{3}{2} u_0 \left[1 - \left(\frac{y-h}{h} \right)^2 \right] \tag{2.19}$$

The above equation of velocity is obtained assuming the permeation velocity of solvent through the membrane is small enough so that the x-component velocity profile is not distorted [30]. Within the thin concentration boundary layer, the term $\frac{y^2}{h^2}$ can be neglected and the x-component velocity profile can be simplified as,

$$u = \frac{3u_0 y}{h} \tag{2.20}$$

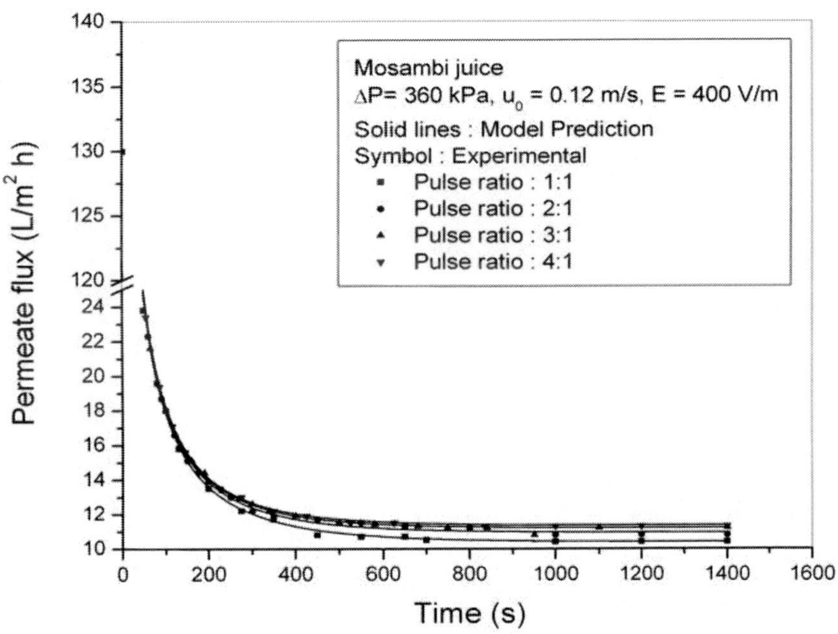

Figure 2.13. Variation of permeate flux with time for different pulse ratio during clarification of mosambi juice.

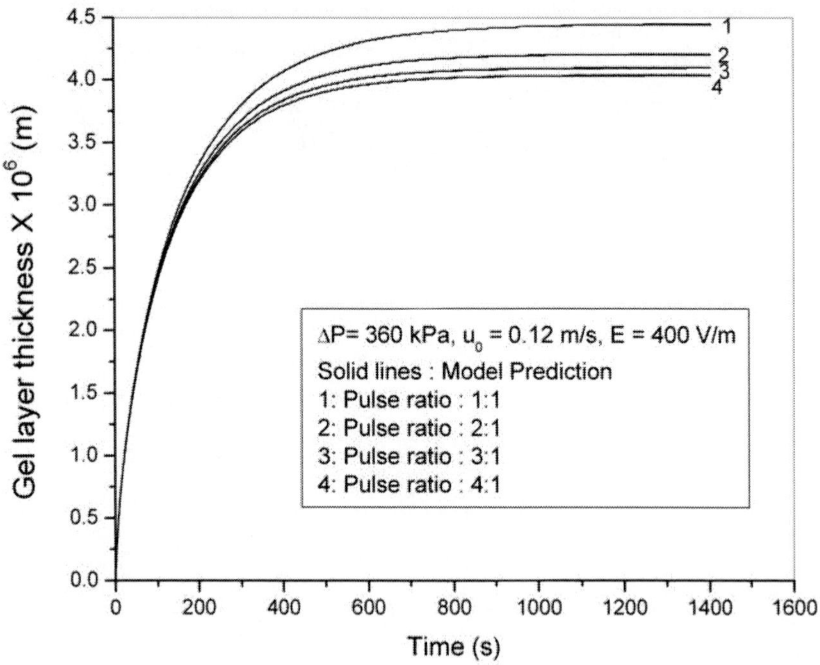

Figure 2.14. Variation of gel layer thickness with time for different pulse ratio during clarification of mosambi juice.

Since the thickness of concentration boundary layer is extremely small as $\delta_c \propto \frac{1}{Sc^{\frac{1}{3}}}$ and Schmidt number is quite large due to lower diffusivity of pectin molecule, the y-component velocity within concentration boundary layer is approximated as,

$$v = -v_w \tag{2.21}$$

The boundary conditions of Eq. (2.18) are,

$$\text{at } x = 0\text{, } c = c_0 \text{ at } y = \delta_c\text{, } c = c_0 \tag{2.23}$$

where, δ_c is the thickness of the concentration boundary layer.

The boundary condition at the gel-solution interface can be written as (equality of convective movement of the solutes towards the membrane to the diffusive and electrophoretic movement away from the membrane),

$$\text{at } y=0, \quad D\frac{\partial c}{\partial y} + (v_w - v_e)c_g = 0 \tag{2.24}$$

Inserting the velocity profiles i.e., Eqs. (2.20) and (2.21), the governing mass balance equation (Eq.(2.18)) can be non-dimensionalized as,

$$Ay^* \frac{\partial c^*}{\partial x^*} + \left(\frac{Pe_e - Pe_w}{4}\right)\frac{\partial c^*}{\partial y^*} = \frac{\partial^2 c^*}{\partial y^{*2}} \tag{2.25}$$

where $x^* = \dfrac{x}{L}$; $c^* = \dfrac{c}{c_0}$; $A = \dfrac{3}{16}\left(ReSc\dfrac{d_e}{L}\right)$

$$Pe_e = \frac{v_e d_e}{D}, \quad Pe_w = \frac{v_w d_e}{D}, \quad y^* = \frac{y}{h}$$

The initial and boundary conditions are non-dimemsionalized as,

$$\text{at } x^* = 0, \quad c^* = 1 \tag{2.26}$$

$$\text{at } y^* = \delta_c^*, \quad c^* = 1 \tag{2.27}$$

$$\text{and at } y^* = 0, \quad \frac{\partial c^*}{\partial y^*} + \left(\frac{Pe_w - Pe_e}{4}\right)c_g^* = 0 \tag{2.28}$$

Using the integral approach, the following concentration profile is assumed:

$$c^* = \frac{c}{c_0} = a_1 + a_2\left(\frac{y^*}{\delta_c^*}\right) + a_3\left(\frac{y^*}{\delta_c^*}\right)^2 \tag{2.29}$$

where, $\delta_c^* = \dfrac{\delta_c}{h}$

Eq. (2.29) satisfies the following boundary conditions:

$$\text{at } y^* = \delta_c^*, \quad c^* = 1 \tag{2.30}$$

$$\text{at } y^* = \delta_c^*, \quad \frac{\partial c^*}{\partial y^*} = 0 \tag{2.31}$$

$$\text{at } y^* = 0, \quad c^* = \frac{c_g}{c_0} = c_g^* \tag{2.32}$$

where, c_g is the gel concentration.

With the help of the above boundary conditions Eq. (2.29) can be written as,

$$c^* = c_g^* - 2(c_g^* - 1)(\frac{y^*}{\delta_c^*}) + (c_g^* - 1)(\frac{y^*}{\delta_c^*})^2 \tag{2.33}$$

Substituting the partial derivative of c^* with respect to x^* and y^* from Eq. (2.33) into the non-dimentionalized governing equation (Eq.(2.25)), the following equation is obtained;

$$A\left(\frac{y^*}{\delta_c^*}\right)^2\left(1-\frac{y^*}{\delta_c^*}\right)\frac{d\delta_c^*}{dx^*}+\left(\frac{Pe_w - Pe_e}{4\delta_c^*}\right)\left(1-\frac{y^*}{\delta_c^*}\right)=\frac{1}{\delta_c^{*2}} \tag{2.34}$$

Multiplying both sides of Eq. (2.34) by dy^* (taking zeroth moment) and then integrating across the boundary layer thickness, i.e. from 0 to δ_c^* the following expression is obtained:

$$A\frac{d\delta_c^*}{dx^*}\int_0^{\delta_c^*}\left(\frac{y^{*2}}{\delta_c^{*2}}-\frac{y^{*3}}{\delta_c^{*3}}\right)dy^* + \left(\frac{Pe_w - Pe_e}{4}\right)\int_0^{\delta_c^*}\left(\frac{1}{\delta_c^*}-\frac{y^*}{\delta_c^{*2}}\right)dy^* = \frac{1}{\delta_c^{*2}}\int_0^{\delta_c^*}dy^* \tag{2.35}$$

After integration of Eq. (2.35), the following expression is obtained:

$$\frac{A\,\delta_c^{*2}}{12}\frac{d\delta_c^*}{dx^*}+\frac{(Pe_w - Pe_e)\,\delta_c^*}{8}=1 \tag{2.36}$$

Following equation is obtained by substituting the partial derivative of c^* with respect to y^* from Eq. (2.33) into the Eq. (2.28).

$$(Pe_w - Pe_e)\,\delta_c^* = \frac{8(c_g^*-1)}{c_g^*} \tag{2.37}$$

Substituting Eq. (2.37) into Eq. (2.36) and after simplification the following expression is obtained:

$$\frac{A\delta_c^{*2}}{12}\frac{d\delta_c^*}{dx^*} = \frac{1}{c_g^*} \tag{2.38}$$

$$\text{at } x^* = 0, \ \delta_c^* = 0 \tag{2.39}$$

The solution of the above expression can finally be written as,

$$\delta_c^* = \left(\frac{36x^*}{Ac_g^*}\right)^{\frac{1}{3}} \tag{2.40}$$

Substituting the Eq. (2.40) into Eq. (2.37) the following expression is finally obtained:

$$Pe_w = Pe_e + \frac{8(c_g^*-1)}{c_g^{*\frac{2}{3}}}\left(\frac{A}{36x^*}\right)^{\frac{1}{3}} \tag{2.41}$$

The above solution provides the variation of permeate flux along the length of the channel for different electric field, feed concentration and cross flow velocity.

Finally, length averaged permeate flux is obtained by integrating the Eq. (2.41) as,

$$\overline{Pe_w} = \int_0^1 Pe_w(x^*)\, dx^* \tag{2.42}$$

$$\overline{Pe_w} = Pe_e + 2.1\left(ReSc\frac{d_e}{L}\right)^{\frac{1}{3}}\frac{(c_g^*-1)}{c_g^{*\frac{2}{3}}} \tag{2.43}$$

Eq. (2.43) can be simplified as,

$$\overline{Pe_w} = Pe_e + 2.1\left(ReSc\frac{d_e}{L}\right)^{\frac{1}{3}} \ln c_g^* \ \text{ when, } c_g^* < e^3 \tag{2.44}$$

2.4.2.2 Analysis of Steady State Flux of Synthetic Juice

Effect of Constant Electric Field

Figure 2.15 and 2.16 represent the variations of permeate flux with applied external d.c. electric field for different values of feed concentration and transmembrane pressure. The symbols are experimental data and the solid lines are model predictions. It may be observed from the figure that permeate flux increases almost linearly with applied electric field. When external d.c. electric field is applied with appropriate polarity, the electrophoretic movement of pectin towards the positive electrode causes reduction of deposition on the membrane surface and gel layer formation is restricted. As a result, permeate flux increases. From the Figure 2.6 it is observed that the permeate flux increases by a factor 2.78 with an increase in electric field from 0 to 800 V/m for a fixed feed concentration (1 kg/m^3 +14 Brix), pressure (220 kPa) and cross-flow velocity (0.12 m/s). Similar trends are observed in case of other cross flow velocity i.e., at 0.09 m/s, the permeate flux increases by a factor 2.87 with the same increment of electric field (Figure 2.16). Moreover, from the results shown in this figure, lower feed concentration results in higher permeate flux due to less concentration polarization on the membrane surface with other operating conditions held constant.

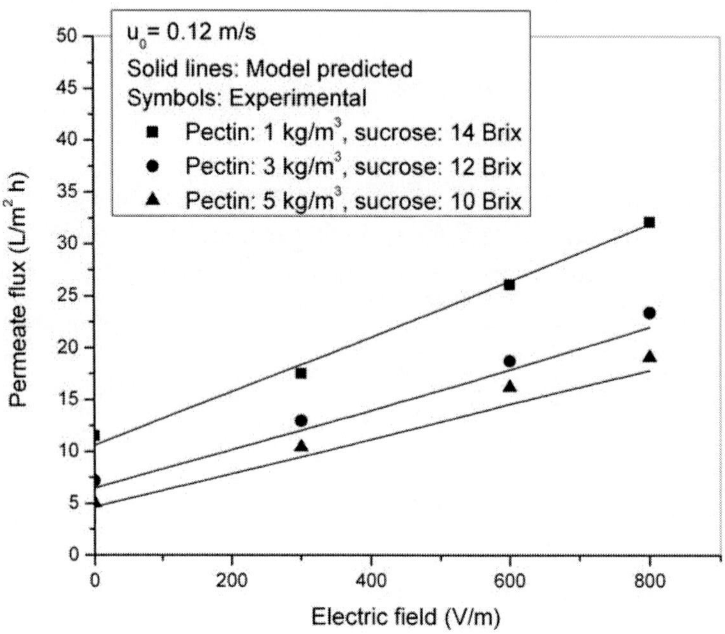

Figure 2.15. Variations of permeate flux with electric field for different feed concentration at a pressure of 220 kPa and cross velocity of 0.12 m/s.

Effect of Transmembrane Pressure

During gel-layer governed ultrafiltration, for a fixed values of feed concentration, cross flow velocity and electric field, the permeate flux is, by definition, independent of pressure. The enhanced driving force for solvent flux due to increase in pressure is fully compensated by the resistance offered by the growing gel layer on the membrane surface and/or due to compaction of the gel layer in an ideal situation. However, weak pressure dependence is observed in our experimental results, especially at higher values of operating pressure (360 kPa). Nevertheless, the average deviation is of the order of 10% only. This may be due to departure from the ideal gel layer controlled operation (as described above). This trend is more clear if the permeate fluxes are plotted as a function of electric field at different operating pressures (Figures 2.17 and 2.18). The departure from pressure independence of permeate flux are more pronounced for higher transmembrane pressure (as is evident from the slight positive slopes of the four solid lines connecting the experimental data points).

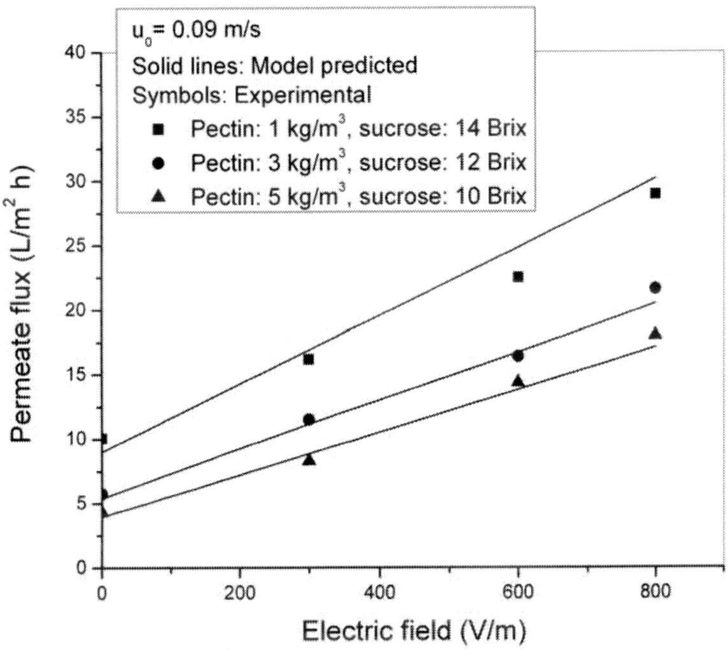

Figure 2.16. Variations of permeate flux with electric field for different feed concentration at a pressure of 220 kPa and cross velocity of 0.09 m/s.

Effect of Cross Flow Velocity

The variations of permeate flux with cross flow velocity for different electric fields are presented in Figure 2.20. From the results shown in this figure, it is clear that for a fixed electric field permeate flux increases with increase in cross flow velocity. At higher cross flow velocity, gel layer thickness on the membrane surface is lower due to forced convection. Therefore, the back diffusion from membrane surface to the bulk increases as the concentration gradient from the membrane surface to the bulk increases. This leads to an increase of permeate flux at higher cross flow velocity. For example, for feed concentration (1 kg/m^3 +14 Brix), at 600 V/m, permeate flux increases from 22.5 L /m^2 h to 27.0 L /m^2 h with an increase of cross flow velocity from 0.09 m/s to 0.18 m/s. The calculated values of permeate flux using the developed model are also presented by the solid lines in Figure 2.19. It is clear from this figure that the model predictions are within 10% of the experimental data.

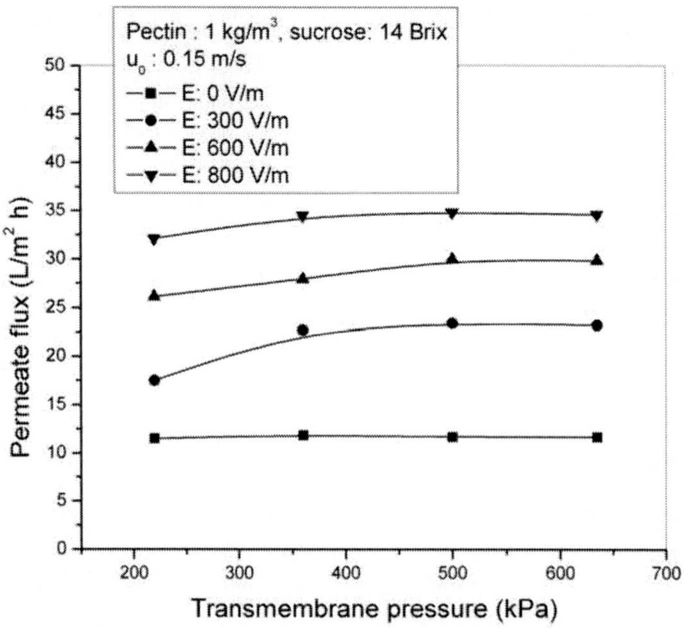

Figure 2.17. Variations of experimental permeate flux with transmembrane pressure difference for different electric field. The solid lines are only guides for the reader.

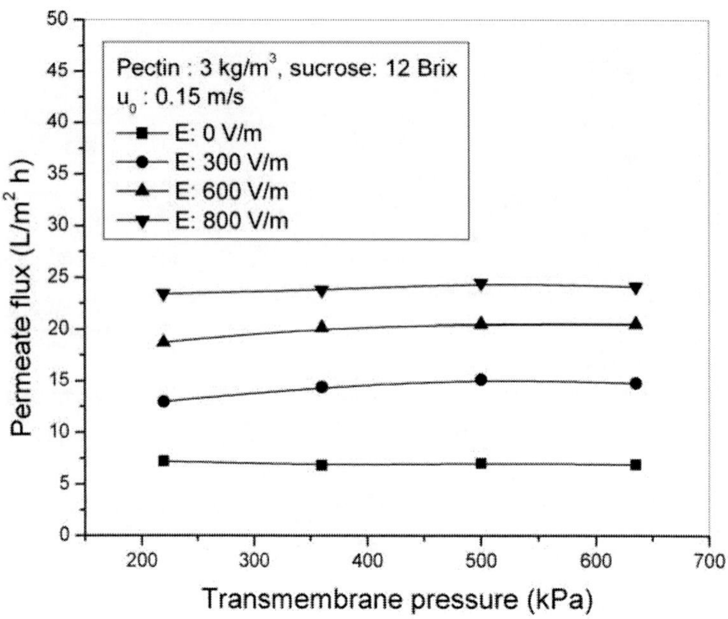

Figure 2.18. Variations of experimental permeate flux with transmembrane pressure difference for different electric field. The solid lines are only guides for the reader.

Variation of Permeate Flux with Axial Position

Figures 2.20 to 2.24 show the variation of permeate flux along the dimensionless length of the ultrafiltration channel for various feed concentration and cross flow velocity. It is observed from the figures that during the initial part of the channel, flux decline is very rapid and then gradual for the later part of the channel. This may be due to the sluggish development of concentration boundary layer in the downstream of the channel because of the forced convection imposed by the cross flow. For example, for feed concentration (1 kg/m^3+14 Brix), at 800 V/m and a cross flow velocity of 0.15 m/s, permeate flux decreases from 77.4 L /m^2 h to 33.6 L /m^2 h along the length of the channel. At any position of the channel an increase in flux is increased with increase in cross flow velocity and decrease in feed concentration. For example, at a cross flow velocity of 0.12 m/s permeate flux is about 22.0 L /m^2 h for feed concentration (3 kg/m^3+12 Brix) and that is for feed concentration (5 kg/m^3+10 Brix) is about 18.07 L /m^2 h at the end of the channel; whereas, at a cross flow velocity of 0.15 m/s, permeate flux is about 22.55 L /m^2 h for feed concentration (3 kg/m^3+12 Brix).

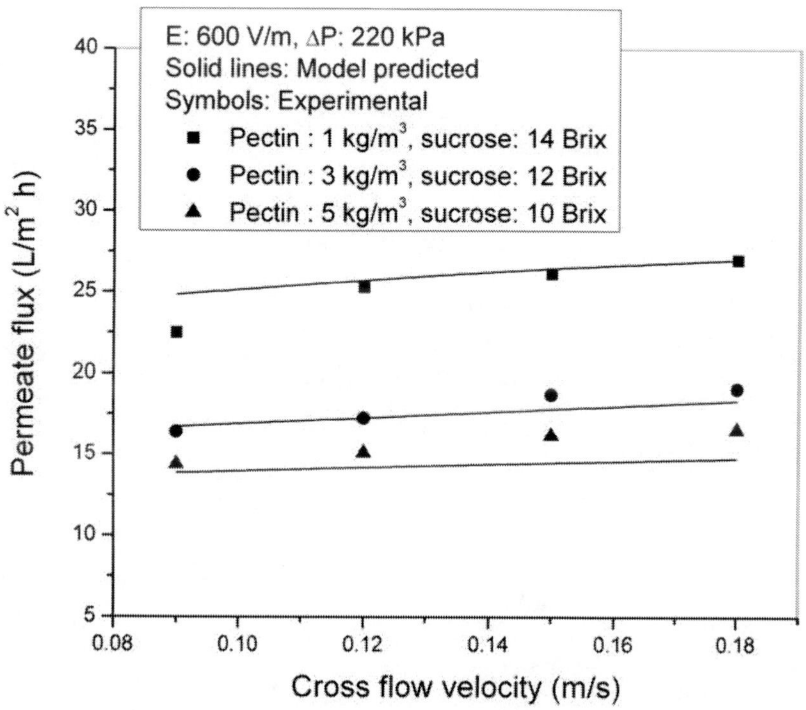

Figure 2.19. Variations of permeate flux with cross flow velocity for different electric field at a fixed pressure of 220 kPa and an electric field of 600 V/m.

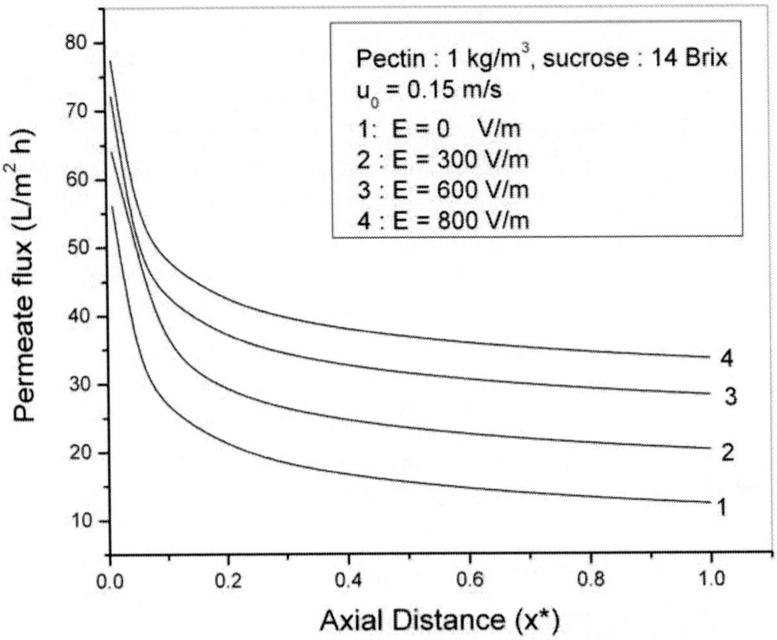

Figure 2.20. Variations of permeate flux along the channel length for different values of feed concentration of pectin: 1 kg/m^3, sucrose: 14 Brix and cross flow velocity of 0.15 m/s.

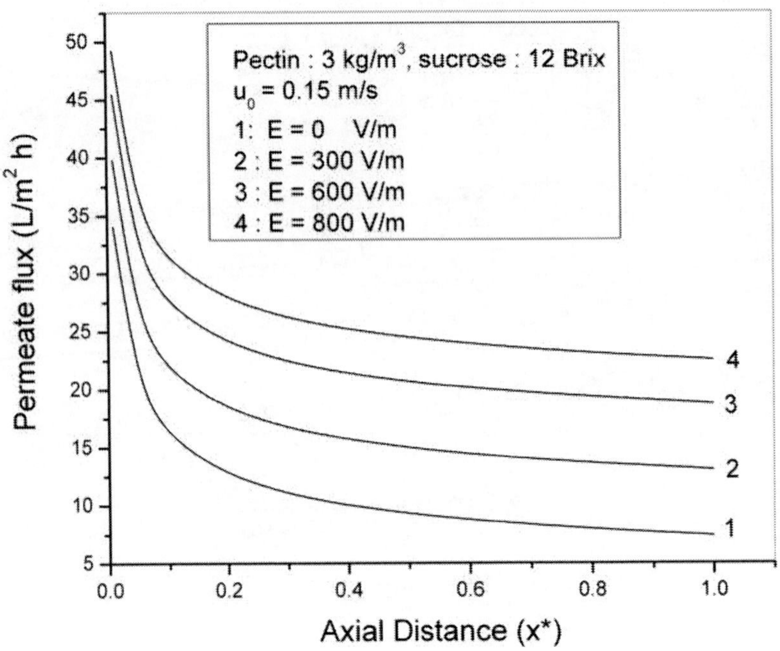

Figure 2.21. Variations of permeate flux along the channel length for different values of feed concentration of pectin: 3 kg/m^3, sucrose: 12 Brix and cross flow velocity of 0.15 m/s.

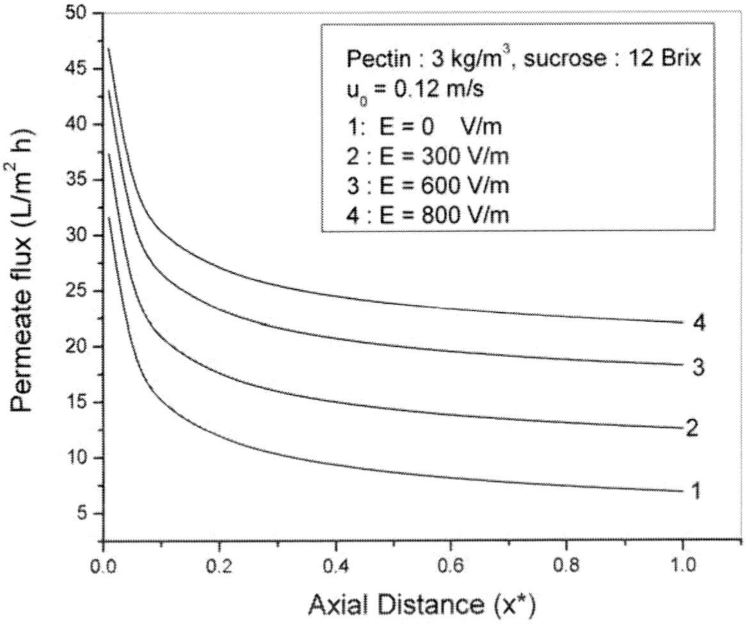

Figure 2.22. Variations of permeate flux along the channel length for different values of feed concentration of pectin: 3 kg/m^3, sucrose: 12 Brix and cross flow velocity of 0.12 m/s.

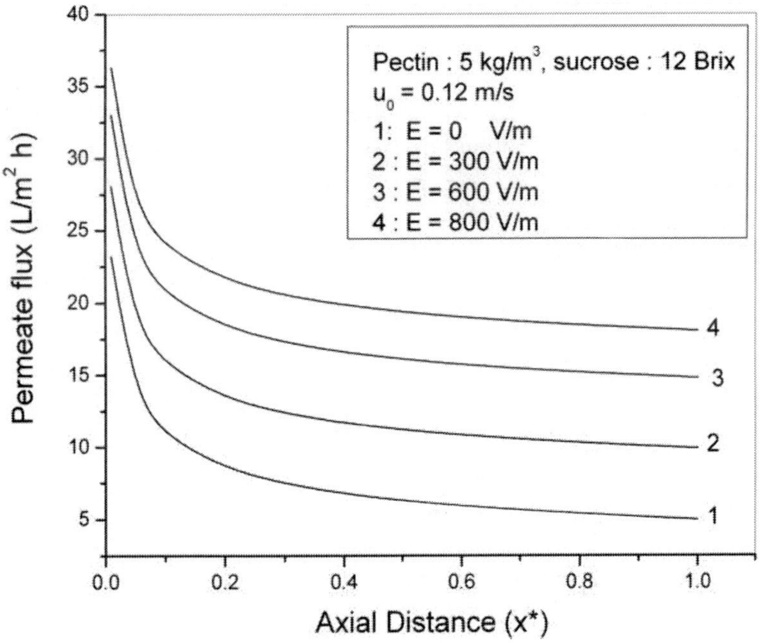

Figure 2.23. Variations of permeate flux along the channel length for different values of feed concentration of pectin: 5 kg/m^3, sucrose: 10 Brix and cross flow velocity of 0.12 m/s.

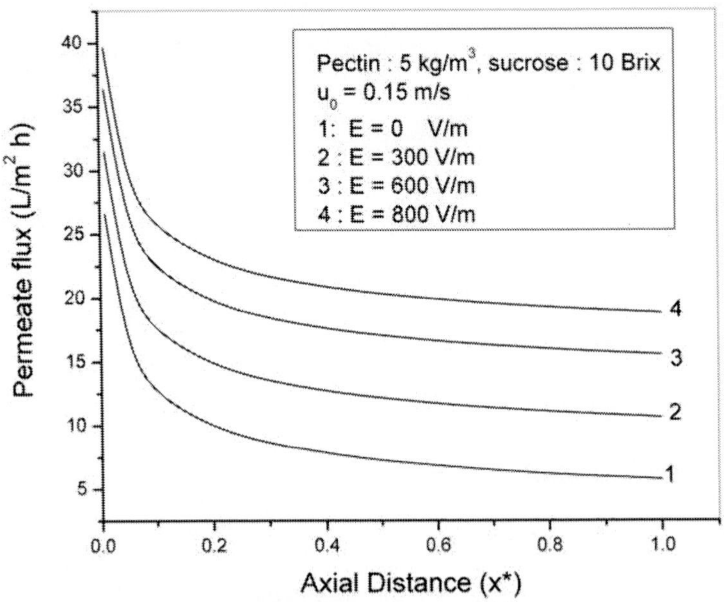

Figure 2.24. Variations of permeate flux along the channel length for different values of feed concentration of pectin: 5 kg/m^3, sucrose: 10 Brix and cross flow velocity of 0.15 m/s.

Effect of Pulsed Electric Field

Effect of Pulse Ratio

Figures 2.25 and 2.26 show the variation in steady state average permeate flux and gel layer thickness with pulse (on time/off time) ratio for various electric field at a transmembrane pressure of 360 kPa and a cross flow velocity of 0.12 m/s during clarification of synthetic juice respectively. In Figure 2.15, the symbols are for the experimental permeate flux, whereas, the solid lines are model predicted permeate flux. As can be seen from the figure, the predictions are very close to the experimental values of permeate flux. In fact it can be seen that the model predictions are within ±5% of the experimental results. The off-time is always fixed at 1s. It can clearly be seen that an increase in electric field results in a decrease in the estimated gel layer thickness (less resistance to flow) and associated increase in flux. With increase in electric field, movement of charged pectin molecules away from the membrane surface increases. This restricts the formation of gel-type layer over the membrane surface and leads to an enhancement of permeate flux. For example, for a feed consisting of 3 kg/m^3 Pectin and 12 Brix of Sucrose, at a transmembrane pressure of 360 kPa, cross flow velocity of 0.12 m/s, pulse ratio of 3:1 and electric field of 2000 V/m, the permeate flux is augmented by a factor of 6.0 compared to zero electric field and corresponding values of gel layer thickness decreases from 10.68 μm to 1.3 μm (Figure 2.26). Experimental results confirm that for a given set of operating conditions, 94.5-97.8% of the maximum permeate flux (electric field always on) is obtained at a pulse ratio of 3:1(i.e., 3 s on followed by 1 s off time). Further increase in pulse ratio does not improve the permeate flux significantly and similar trends are observed for all electric fields.

Figures 2.27 and 2.28 illustrate the variation in steady state average permeate flux and gel layer thickness with pulse ratio for various feed concentrations (mixture of pectin and sucrose) at a transmembrane pressure of 360 kPa and a cross flow velocity of 0.12 m/s during clarification of synthetic juice respectively. In Figure 2.17, the symbols are for the experimental permeate flux, whereas, the solid lines are model predicted permeate flux. It may be observed that the predicted flux values are within ±5% to the experimental results. From the figure it is clear that almost same level of the maximum achievable permeate flux (electric field always on) can be obtained at the pulse ratio of 3:1. As can be seen from the figure, permeate flux decreases with increase in feed concentration while other operating conditions are kept unchanged. At higher feed concentration, concentration polarization becomes more severe and results in higher value of gel layer thickness. This increases the resistance to solvent flow through the membrane and hence permeate flux decreases at higher feed concentration. For example, at a transmembrane pressure of 360 kPa, cross flow velocity of 0.12 m/s, pulse ratio of 3:1 and electric field of 800 V/m, with increase in feed concentration from a mixture consisting of 1 kg/m^3 Pectin and of 14 Brix Sucrose to a mixture consisting of 5 kg/m^3 Pectin and of 10 Brix Sucrose, the permeate flux declines from 31.1 L/m^2 h to 15.9 L/m^2 h and corresponding values of gel layer thickness over the membrane surface increases from 1.56 μm to 5.1 μm (Figure 2.28). It may also be observed that application of electric field is more effective at higher feed concentrations. This result is found to be consistent with that reported in the literature [31]. The thickness of gel type layer is quite thin at lower feed concentration. Hence the beneficial effect of electric field is less prominent as compared to the higher concentration cases. For example, at 800 V/m, with increase in feed concentration (from Pectin: 1 kg/m^3, Sucrose: 14 Brix to Pectin: 5 kg/m^3, Sucrose: 10 Brix), flux enhancement factor increases from 2.8 to 3.3.

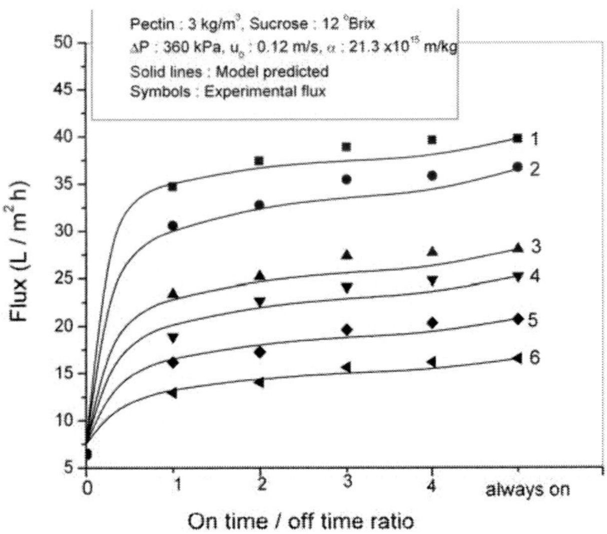

Figure 2.25. Variation in steady state average permeate flux with pulse ratio for various electric fields during clarification of synthetic juice. ■, Curve 1 for E = 2000 V/m; ●, Curve 2 for E = 1600 V/m; ▲, Curve 3 for E = 1200 V/m; ▼, Curve 4 for E = 1000 V/m; ♦, Curve 5 for E = 800 V/m; ◄, Curve 6 for E = 600 V/m.

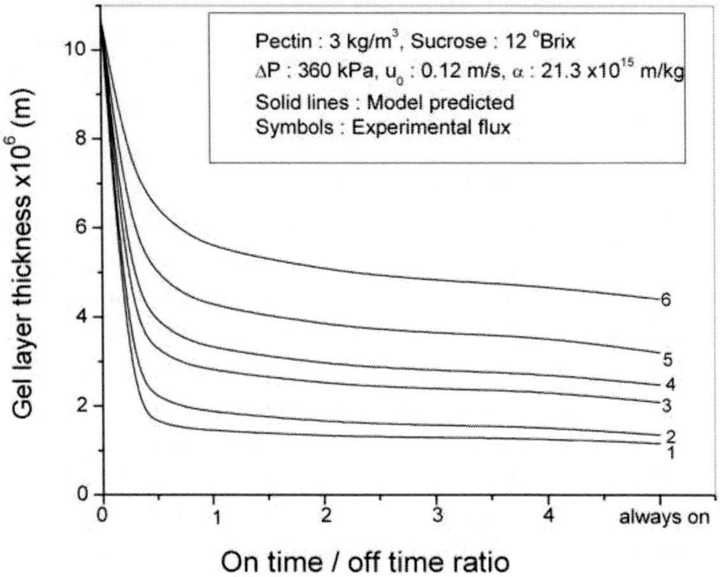

Figure 2.26. Variation in steady gel layer thickness with pulse ratio for various electric fields during clarification of synthetic juice. Curve 1 for E = 2000 V/m; Curve 2 for E = 1600 V/m; Curve 3 for E = 1200 V/m; Curve 4 for E = 1000 V/m; Curve 5 for E = 800 V/m; Curve 6 for E = 600 V/m.

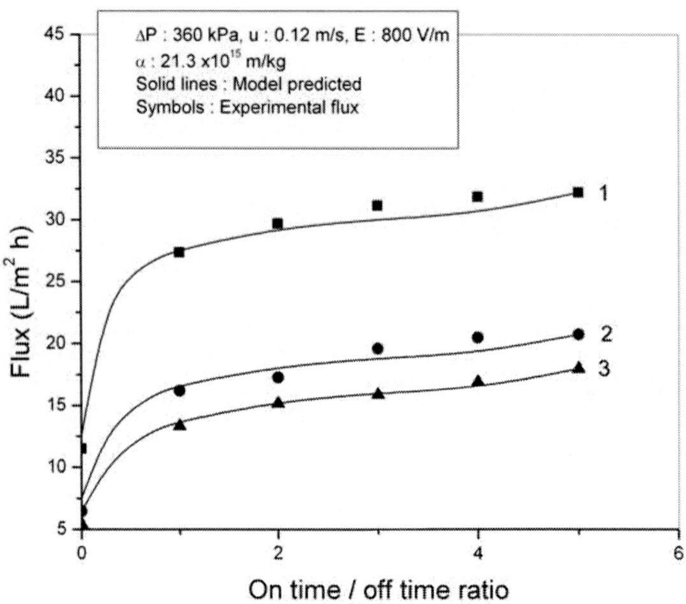

Figure 2.27. Variation in steady state average permeate flux with pulse ratio for various feed concentration during clarification of synthetic juice. ■, Curve 1 for $c_o = 1$ kg/m^3, 14 Brix; ♦, Curve 2 for $c_o = 3$ kg/m^3, 12 Brix; ▲, Curve 3 for $c_o = 5$ kg/m^3, 10 Brix.

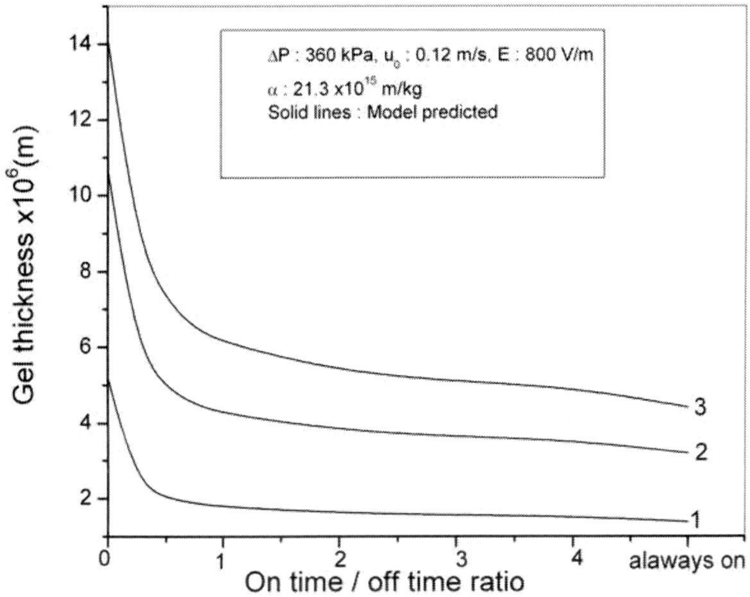

Figure 2.28. Variation in steady state gel layer thickness with pulse ratio for various feed concentration during clarification of synthetic juice. Curve 1 for $c_o = 1$ kg/m^3, 14 Brix; Curve 2 for $c_o = 3$ kg/m^3, 12 Brix; Curve 3 for $c_o = 5$ kg/m^3, 10 Brix.

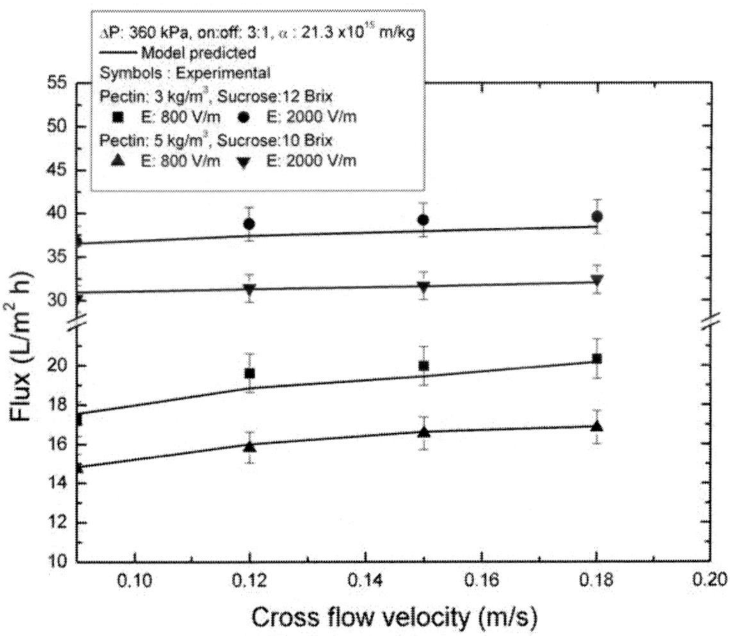

Figure 2.29. Variation in steady state average permeate flux with cross flow velocity for different electric field and a fixed pulse ratio of 3:1 during clarification of synthetic juice.

Effect of Cross Flow Velocity

Variations in steady state average permeate flux with cross flow velocity at a transmembrane pressure of 360 kPa and pulse ratio of 3:1 during clarification of synthetic juice are reported in Figure 2.29. The symbols are the experimental data and solid lines are model predictions and they are within ±5% of each other. It may be observed from the figure that with increase in cross flow velocity, permeate flux increases as the gel thickness over the membrane surface is reduced by enhanced forced convection. For example, for a specific feed concentration (Pectin: 3 kg/m^3, Sucrose: 12 Brix), transmembrane pressure of 360 kPa, pulse ratio of 3:1 and at an electric field of 800 V/m, an increase in cross flow velocity from 0.09 m/s to 0.18 m/s leads to an enhancement of permeate flux by about 17.7 % whereas, at 2000 V/m, this enhancement is about 7.8 %. This also indicates that the effect of cross flow velocity is more pronounced at 800 V/m compared to 2000 V/m. At a higher electric field the thickness of gel-type layer is already thin and an increase in cross flow velocity may not have an appreciable effect.

Estimation of Electric Power Consumption per Unit Volume of Permeate

Total energy consumption is the summation of energy required to run the pump and energy to supply the external d.c. electric field. Pump-dissipated power is directly proportional to the pressure drop and can be expressed as the product of pressure drop and feed flow rate. Electric power is related to the applied voltage. Hence, the total specific energy consumption i.e., energy consumption per unit volume of permeate can be written as,

$$E_{total} = E_{pump} + E_{electical} \tag{2.45}$$

$$E_{total} = \frac{Q\,\Delta P_{pump}}{v_w A'\,\eta_{pump}} + \frac{V\,I\,N}{v_w A'\,\eta_{d.c\ power\ supply}} \tag{2.46}$$

where, Q, ΔP_{module}, V, I, N, v_w, A, η_{pump}, $\eta_{d.c.\ power\ supply}$ are the feed flow rate, pressure drop, applied voltage, current, fraction of on time, permeate flux, membrane area, efficiency of pump and d.c. power supply respectively.

The variation of pH and electric power consumption of the permeate at various electric fields and pulse ratios during clarification of synthetic juice (Pectin: 3 kg/m^3, Sucrose: 12 Brix) and mosambi juice at a transmembrane pressure of 360 kPa and cross flow velocity of 0.12 m/s are shown in Figures 2.30 and 2.31 respectively. It is generally observed that power consumption and pH of the permeate increases with increase in electric field as well as with pulse ratio. As observed in Figure 2.27, for a given electric field, nearly the maximum flux value is achieved at a pulse ratio of 3:1 which corresponds to (27-33) % less energy consumption compared to the constant electric field. From experimental results, it can be seen that pH of the permeate is maximum at constant electric field compared to pulsed electric field. At constant field, electrode reactions resulting in evolution of oxygen (O_2) and hydronium ions (H_3O^+) at the anode and hydrogen (H_2) and hydroxyl ions (OH^-) at the cathode are more pronounced compared to that with the pulsed electric field, these hydroxyl ions (OH^-) are carried with the permeate stream and may result an increase in pH of permeate. Electrolytic gases are released near the membrane resulting in a reduction of permeate flux. For example, pH of the permeate is increased from 6.0 to 9.3 with increase in constant electric field from 0 V/m to 800 V/m, whereas, with a pulse ratio of 3:1, the pH of the permeate increases up 9.0.

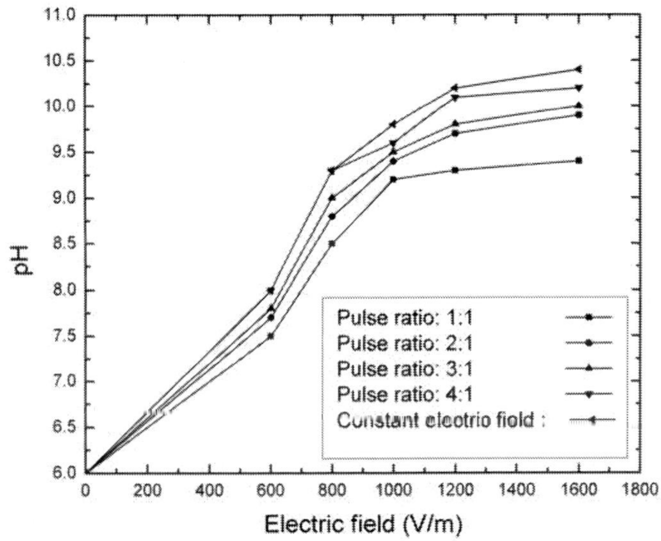

Figure 2.30. Variation of pH of the permeate with d.c. electric field at various pulse ratios at a pressure of 360 kPa and cross flow velocity of 0.12 m/s during clarification of synthetic juice (pectin: 3 kg/m^3, sucrose: 12 Brix).

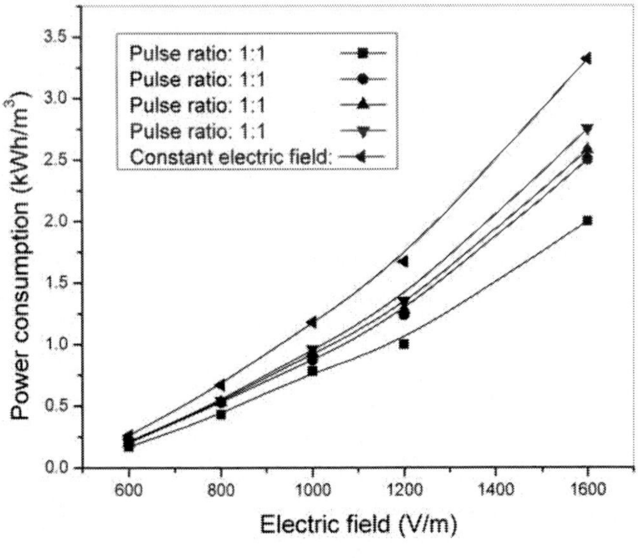

Figure 2.31. Variation of electric power consumption per unit volume of the permeate with d.c. electric field at various pulse ratios at a pressure of 360 kPa and cross flow velocity of 0.12 m/s during clarification of synthetic juice (pectin: 3 kg/m^3, sucrose: 12 Brix).

Table 2.8. Variation of energy ratio of pulse to constant electric field with pulse ratio for different electric fields

ΔP: 360 kPa, u_0 : 0.12 m/s	E = 200 V/m	E = 300 V/m	E = 400 V/m
Pulse	$E_{pulse}/E_{constant}$	$E_{pulse}/E_{constant}$	$E_{pulse}/E_{constant}$
0	0	0	0
1	0.25	0.34	0.41
2	0.38	0.49	0.56
3	0.56	0.58	0.67
4	0.67	0.71	0.76
Constant electric field	1.0	1.0	1.0

Table 2.8 illustrates the variation of energy ratio of pulse to constant electric field with pulse ratio for different electric field. It is evident from the figure that with increase in pulse ratio, the dimensionless energy, $E_{pulse}/E_{constant}$, increases for a fixed value of transmembrane pressure and cross flow velocity. It can be observed from experimental results that at an electric field of 400 V/m, at a pressure of 360 kPa, a cross flow velocity of 0.12 m/s and at the pulse ratio of 3:1, the dimensionless energy, $E_{pulse}/E_{constant}$ is about 0.67. This indicates that during pulsed electro-ultrafiltration, about 97.5% of the maximum attainable permeate flux (electric field always on) is achieved (Figure 2.27) with saving of 33% electrical energy.

Table 2.9 represents the variations of energy consumption per unit volume of permeate with external applied constant d.c. electric field for a fixed pressure of 360 kPa and a cross flow velocity of 0.12 m/s. It is observed from the figure that with increase in electric field, energy consumption due to applied d.c. electric field increases but the energy consumed by the pump decreases. However, total energy consumption per unit volume of permeate decreases. This can be explained by the fact that for a fixed pressure and cross flow velocity, with increase in electric field, energy consumption due to d.c electric field is increases. Though at the same time, with increase in electric field, permeate flux increases due to decrease of gel layer thickness (migration of gel forming materials away from the membrane surface), the overall increase of energy consumption per unit of permeate volume due to d.c electric field ($E_{electrical}$) is observed. For example, at 400 V/m, the value of $E_{electrical}$ is about 1.72 kWh/m^3 of permeate. For the calculation of pump energy consumption, there is no contribution of d.c. electric field. Hence, consumption of pump energy per unit volume of permeate (E_{pump}) decreases with increase of electric field as permeate flux increases with increase in electric field. For example, E_{pump} decreases from 123.8 to 92.85 kWh/m^3 of permeate with increase in electric field from 0 to 400 V/m. Moreover, since the contribution of $E_{electrical}$ to the calculation of E_{total} is less than 2%, with increase in electric field, total energy consumption per unit volume of permeate (E_{total}) decreases. Therefore, the energy consumption due to application of external electric field insignificant compared to that for running the pump.

Table 2.9. Variation of energy consumption with electric field.

E (V/m)	E_{pump} (kWh/m^3)	$E_{electrica}$ (kWh/m^3)	E_{total}(kWh/m^3)
0	123.8	0	123.8
200	104.4	0.15	104.55
300	96.5	0.63	96.65
400	92.85	1.73	94.58

Table 2.10 illustrates the variations of energy consumed by pump per unit volume of permeate for different transmembrane pressures and cross flow velocities at an electric field of 400 V/m and pulse ratio of 3:1. It is evident from the figure that energy consumed by the pump per unit volume of permeate increases with increase in both transmembrane pressure as well as cross flow velocity. This is because, increase in cross flow velocity and transmembrane pressure lead to enhancement of power consumption of pump as it is directly proportional to both cross flow velocity and pressure drop. For example, at a cross flow velocity of 0.12 m/s, with increase in transmembrane pressure from 220 kPa to 635 kPa, pump energy consumption increases from 63.7 kWh /m^3 to 158.8 kWh /m^3 whereas, at a transmembrane pressure of 360 kPa, with increase in cross flow velocity from 0.09 m/s to 0.18 m/s, pump energy consumption increases from 76.83 kWh /m^3 to 127.32 kWh /m^3.

Table 2.10. Variation of pump energy and electrical energy for different transmembrane pressure and cross flow velocity at an electric field of 400 V/m and pulse ratio of 3:1

	E_{punp} (kWh/m^3)				$E_{electrical}$ (kWh/m^3)			
u_0 (m/s) →	0.09	0.12	0.15	0.18	0.09	0.12	0.15	0.18
ΔP (kPa)	↓							
220	50.43	63.70	75.64	83.80	1.34	1.27	1.20	1.11
360	76.83	95.20	112.5	127.32	1.25	1.16	1.10	1.03
500	103.15	128.90	149.5	171.92	1.20	1.13	1.05	1.0
635	126.78	158.80	181.95	212.44	1.16	1.01	1.0	0.98

Table 2.10 also shows the variations of energy consumed by d.c. electric field per unit volume of permeate for different transmembrane pressures and cross flow velocities at an electric field of 400 V/m and a pulse ratio of 3:1 are presented in Figure 2.24. It can be observed from the figure that the energy consumption per unit volume of permeate due to applied d.c. electric field decreases with increase in both cross flow velocity and transmembrane pressure. This can be explained by the fact that increase in both cross flow

velocity and transmembrane pressure lead to an increase in permeate flux. Therefore, for a fixed electric field and pulse ratio, energy consumption per unit volume of permeate decreases with increase in both cross flow velocity and transmembrane pressure. For example, at a cross flow velocity of 0.12 m/s, with increase in transmembrane pressure from 220 kPa to 635 kPa, energy consumption due to d.c. electric field decreases from 1.27 kWh /m^3 to 1.01 kWh /m^3 whereas, at a transmembrane pressure of 360 kPa, with increase in cross flow velocity from 0.09 m/s to 0.18 m/s, it decreases from 1.25 kWh /m^3 to 1.03 kWh /m^3 of permeate.

2.4.2.3. Analysis of Steady State Flux of Mosambi (Citrus Sinensis (L.) Osbeck) Juice

Theoretical Aspect

The expression for steady state permeate flux in case of gel layer controlled electric field assisted ultrafiltration is obtained using film theory as,

$$v_w = v_e + k \ln \frac{c_g}{c_0} \tag{2.47}$$

where, k is the mass transfer coefficient, defined as $\frac{D}{\delta_c}$; D is diffusion coefficient of the gel forming solute; and v_e is the electrophoretic velocity which can be calculated from Eqs. (2.8) and (2.9). The mass transfer coefficient under laminar flow condition can be expressed as:

$$Sh = \frac{k\, d_e}{D} = 2.1\left(ReSc\frac{d_e}{L}\right)^{\frac{1}{3}} \tag{2.48}$$

where, d_e is the equivalent diameter of the flow channel. For a thin channel, the value of d_e is 4h, where h is the half height of the channel. In mosambi juice, apart from major constituents like pectin and sugar, other components are also present such as proteins, microorganisms, acids, salts, aroma and flavor compounds. Since the diffusivity and gel concentration of actual mosambi juice differ from that of pure pectin, the estimation of permeate flux based on the values of diffusivity and gel concentration of pure pectin will be inaccurate. Moreover, the variation of viscosity with concentration has to be incorporated for better prediction. Therefore, instead of using bulk viscosity in Eq. 2.9, an effective viscosity has been suggested. An optimization method has been employed to determine which uses an initial guess for the values of these three parameters in order to minimize the following error function and obtain the correct values of the three parameters:

$$S = \sum_{i=1}^{N}\left(\frac{V_w^{exp} - V_w^{cal}}{V_w^{exp}}\right)^2 \tag{2.49}$$

BCPOL of IMSL Math library using direct complex search algorithm has been used for optimization. As a first guess, the values of diffusivity, gel concentration and effective viscosity are assumed to be the same as those for pure pectin solution. Knowing these parameters, values of steady state permeate flux are predicted. The results obtained are discussed in the subsequent sections.

The values of effective diffusivity, gel concentration and effective viscosity are estimated by optimizing the experimental values of average permeate flux using the optimizer BCPOL of IMSL Math library and the permeate flux is calculated using Eq. (2.47). The values of effective diffusivity, gel concentration and effective viscosity estimated thus are 6.05 x 10^{-11} m^2/s, 48.5 kg/m^3 and 7.03 x 10^{-3} Pa s respectively. The diffusivity is of the same order of magnitude as that obtained for pure pectin from the well known Stokes-Einstein relation (Table 2.1). The value of gel concentration is slightly higher than that reported for pure pectin (38 kg/m^3) by Pritchard et al. [25]. This indicates the presence of other gel forming material apart from pectin in mosambi juice.

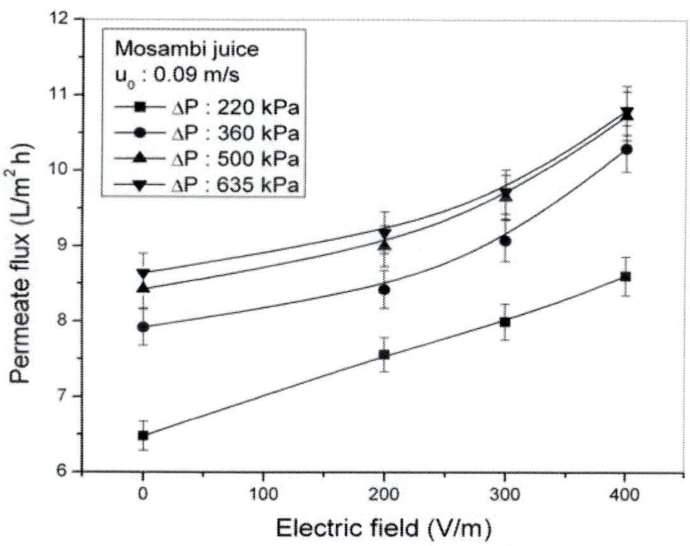

Figure 2.32. Variation of steady state average permeate flux with electric field for various transmembrane pressure during clarification of mosambi juice using 50 kDa membrane.

Effect of Constant Electric Field on Permeate Flux

Figure 2.32 shows the variation of the average steady state average permeate flux with electric field for various transmembrane pressures at a cross flow velocity of 0.12 m/s during clarification of mosambi juice. It is evident from the figure that permeate flux increases with the electric field. This is due to electrophoretic movement of negatively charged pectin molecules away from the membrane surface (i.e. towards the positive electrode).This reduces the deposition of pectin molecules on the membrane surface and prevents the formation of a gel type layer formation over the membrane surface which leads to an enhancement of the permeate flux. For example, at a transmembrane pressure of 360 kPa and cross flow velocity of 0.12 m/s, the application of 400 V/m results in an increase in permeate flux from 8.65 L/m^2 h (in the absence of electric field) to 11.75 L/m^2 h. Furthermore, this figure also indicates that for a fixed electric field, an increase in transmembrane pressure leads to an increase in permeate flux due to enhanced driving force.

Effect of Cross Flow Velocity on Permeate Flux

It has been observed from Figure 2.32 that at the pressure of 360 kPa, with increase in electric field to 400 V/m the permeate flux increases by about 36% (which is an upper limit under the operating conditions employed). At other operating pressures such as 220 kPa, 500 kPa and 635 kPa, with the same increase in electric field, the flux enhancements are 32.5%, 30% and 32%, respectively. Hence the pressure 360 kPa has been selected to discuss the effect of cross flow velocity on permeate flux at different electric field strengths as shown in Figure 2.33. With increase in cross flow velocity, the sweeping effect on the gel layer over the membrane surface increases. This restricts solute particles from being deposited on the membrane surface; further it facilitates backward diffusion of the solutes from the surface to the bulk. Hence, with increase in cross flow velocity, the deposit thickness, and consequently resistance to solvent flow, decreases thereby augmenting the permeate flux. The effect of cross flow velocity on the enhancement in permeate flux is slightly more in the absence of electric field than at 400 V/m. At higher electric field, the layer deposited on the membrane surface is very thin due to electrophoresis. For example, at 400 V/m, with increase in cross flow velocity from 0.09 m/s to 0.18 m/s, the permeate flux increase by about 25% whereas, this augmentation is about 27% in the absence of electric field under otherwise identical operating condition.

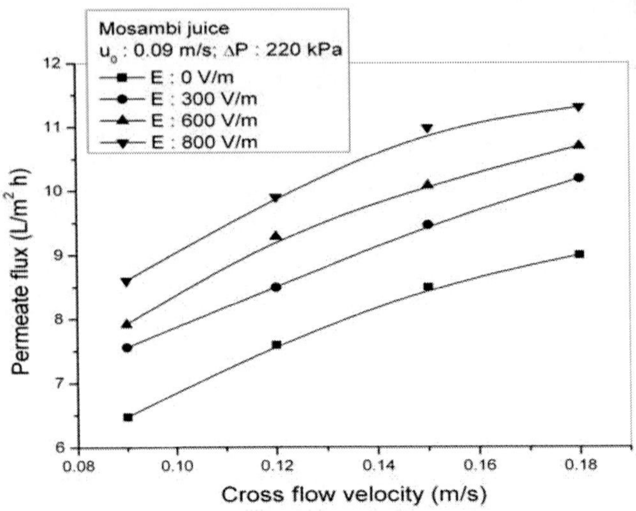

Figure 2.33. Variation of steady state average permeate flux with cross flow velocity during clarification of mosambi juice using 50 kDa membrane.

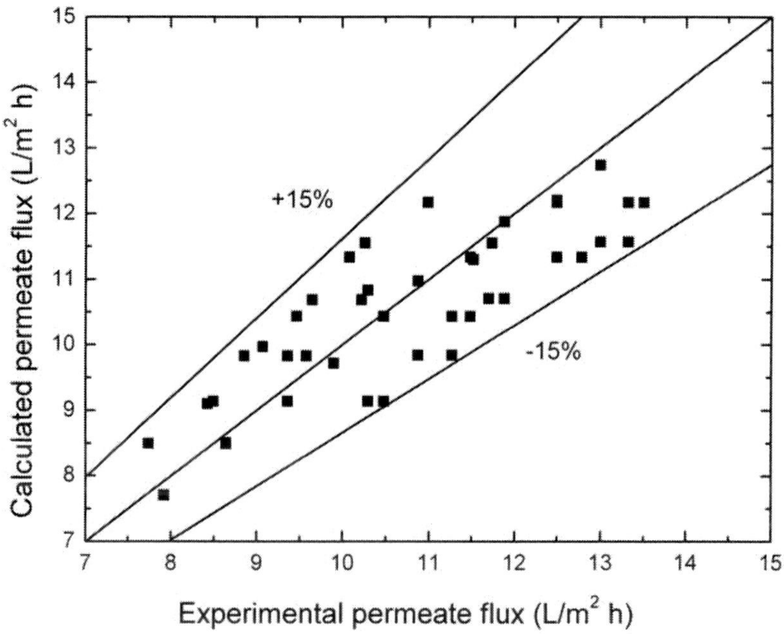

Figure 2.34. Calculated steady state permeate flux using optimized values of effective diffusivity, gel concentration and effective viscosity obtained from the optimization of cross flow electro-ultrafiltration experimental data of mosambi juice.

Figure 2.34 shows the comparison between the experimental and estimated values of average permeate flux under various conditions of cross-flow velocity, electric field and transmembrane pressure. From the figure it is clear that the estimated permeate flux values are within ±15% to the experimental values.

Effect of Pulsed Electric Field

Effect of Pulse Ratio

Figure 2.35 and 2.36 show the variation in steady state average permeate flux with pulse (on time/off time) ratio for various electric field at a transmembrane pressure of 360 kPa and a cross flow velocity of 0.12 m/s during clarification of mosambi juice respectively. The symbols are for the experimental permeate flux, whereas, the solid lines are model predicted permeate flux and the dashed lines are estimated gel layer thickness. As can be seen from the figure, the predictions are very close to the experimental values of permeate flux. In fact it can be seen that the model predictions are within ±5% of the experimental results. The off-time is always fixed at 1s. It can clearly be seen that an increase in electric field results in a decrease in the estimated gel layer thickness (less resistance to flow) and associated increase in flux as observed in case of synthetic juice. As discussed earlier with increase in electric field, movement of charged pectin molecules away from the membrane surface increases leading to restriction of the formation of gel-type layer over the membrane surface. Hence permeate flux increases. For example, at a transmembrane pressure of 360 kPa, cross flow velocity of 0.12 m/s, pulse ratio of 3:1 and electric field of 400 V/m, the permeate flux increases from 8.65 L/m^2 h to 11.2 L/m^2 h compared to zero electric field and corresponding values of gel layer thickness decreases from 5.4 μm to 4.1 μm (Figure 2.36). Experimental results confirm that for a given set of operating conditions, 94-97.5% of the maximum permeate flux (electric field always on) is obtained at a pulse ratio of 3:1(i.e., 3 s on followed by 1 s off time). Further increase in pulse ratio does not improve the permeate flux significantly and similar trends are observed for all electric fields. These results are consistent with the results of synthetic juice.

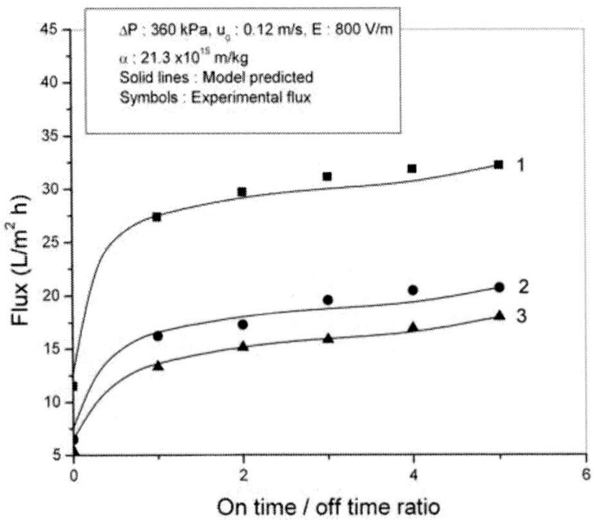

Figure 2.35. Variation in steady state average permeate flux with pulse ratio for various electric field during clarification of mosambi juice. ■, Curve 1 for E = 400 V/m; ●, Curve 2 for E = 300 V/m; ▲, Curve 3 for E = 200 V/m.

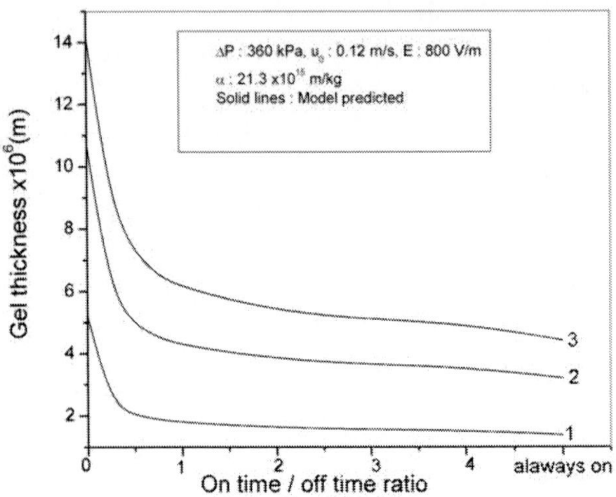

Figure 2.36. Variation in steady state gel layer thickness with pulse ratio for various electric field during clarification of mosambi juice. Curve 1 for E = 200 V/m; Curve 2 for E = 300 V/m; Curve 3 for E = 400 V/m.

Effect of Cross Flow Velocity

The variations of permeate flux and gel layer thickness with cross flow velocity for different electric fields at a pulse ratio of 3:1 are presented in Figures 2.37 and 2.38 respectively. The symbols are for the experimental permeate flux, whereas, the solid lines are model predicted permeate flux and the dashed lines are estimated gel layer thickness. As can be seen from the figure that the model predictions are within ± 3% of the experimental results. From the results shown in this figure, it is clear that for a fixed electric field, with increase in cross flow velocity permeate flux increases and gel layer thickness decreases as observed in case of synthetic juice. At higher cross flow velocity, gel layer thickness on the membrane surface is lower due to forced convection. This is a direct consequence of enhancement of turbulence in the flow channel. Furthermore, the back diffusion from membrane surface to the bulk increases as the concentration gradient from the membrane surface to the bulk increases. This leads to an increase of permeate flux at higher cross flow velocity. For example, at 400 V/m, with an increase of cross flow velocity from 0.09 m/s to 0.18 m/s permeate flux increases from 10.45 L /m^2 h to 12.5 L /m^2 h (Figure 2.38) with decrease in gel layer thickness from 4.4 μm to 3.65 μm (Figure 2.38).

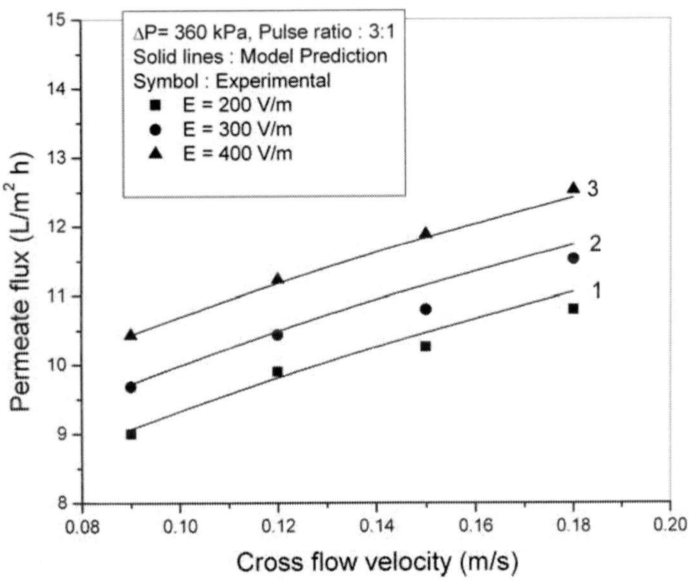

Figure 2.37. Variation in steady state average permeate flux with cross flow velocity at a pulse ratio of 3:1 for various electric field during clarification of mosambi juice. Solid lines and dashed lines are for flux and gel thickness respectively. ■, Curve 1 for E = 200 V/m; ●, Curve 2 for E = 300 V/m; ▲, Curve 3 for E = 400 V/m.

The variations in steady state average permeate flux with pulse ratio for various electric fields at a transmembrane pressure of 360 kPa and cross flow velocity of 0.12 m/s during clarification of mosambi juice are shown in Figure 2.39. It may be observed from the figure that permeate flux very close to the maximum value (always on) is obtained at a pulse ratio of 3:1 as observed in case of synthetic juice (Figure 2.27). As indicated earlier, permeate flux increases with increase in electric field due to enhanced electrophoretic movement of pectin molecules away from the membrane surface (i.e., towards the positive electrode) which reduces the gel type layer formation over the membrane surface. For example, at a transmembrane pressure of 360 kPa, cross flow velocity of 0.12 m/s and pulse ratio of 3:1, by applying an electric field of 500 V/m, permeate flux is improved about 39% compared to zero electric field (0 V/m).

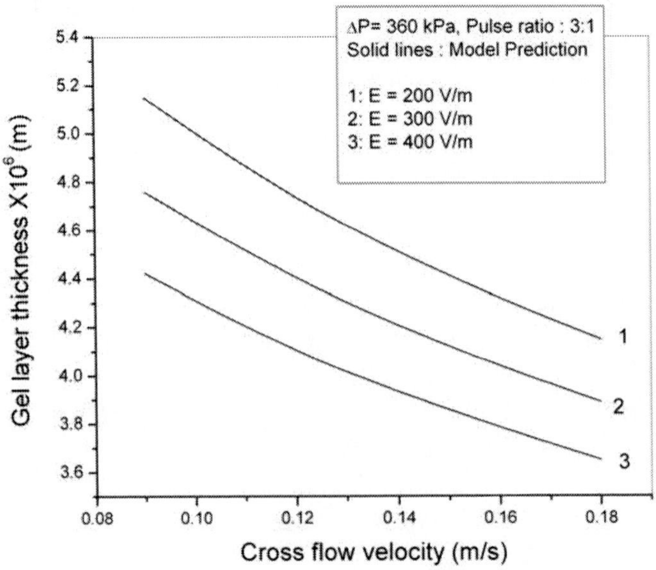

Figure 2.38. Variation in steady state gel layer thickness with cross flow velocity at a pulse ratio of 3:1 for various electric field during clarification of mosambi juice. Curve 1 for E = 400 V/m; Curve 2 E = 300 V/m; Curve 3 for E = 200 V/m.

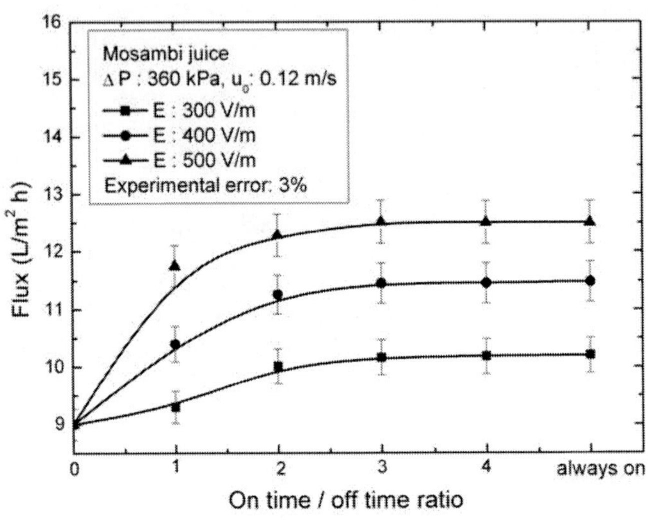

Figure 2.39.Variation in steady state average permeate flux with pulse ratio for various electric field during clarification of mosambi juice using 30 kDa membrane. The solid lines are only guides for the reader.

Characterization of Clarified Mosambi Juice

The physico-chemical properties of permeate after clarification of mosambi juice at a transmembrane pressure of 360 kPa and a pulse ratio of 3:1 are tabulated in Table 2.11. From the results it is clear that density, conductivity, sugar content of both the feed and permeate are practically the same while viscosity is reduced from 2.45×10^{-3} Pa s to 0.87×10^{-3} Pa s due to enzyme treatment and pulsed electro-ultrafiltration. After enzyme treatment color (A_{420}), clarity (T_{660}) and acidity (i.e., as citric acid) of mosambi juice are improved from 1.25 to 1.1, 29.8% to 34% and 0.7 to 0.5 weight % respectively. There is a significant improvement of color (A_{420}) and clarity (T_{660}) after pulsed electro-ultrafiltration and no pectin is found in clarified juice. Color (A_{420}) is decreased from 1.1 to 0.22 and clarity (T_{660}) is improved from 34% to about 98% after pulsed electro-ultrafiltration. A decrease in acidity and consequently an increase in pH of permeate is observed after electro-ultrafiltration. It is further noticed that for a given electric field, with increase in cross flow velocity, pH of the permeate decreases. At higher cross flow velocity, produced OH^- ions by electrode reaction are sheared off from the electrode-membrane interface leading to a decrease in pH of the permeate. For example, with increase in cross flow velocity from 0.09 m/s to 0.18 m/s, pH of the permeate decreases from 4.6 to 4.25.

Table 2.11. Physico-chemical properties of permeate after clarification of mosambi juice at a transmembrane pressure of 360 kPa and a pulse ratio of 3:1

Electric field (V/m)	Cross-flow velocity (m/s)	pH	Color (A_{420})	Clarity % (T_{660})	Sucrose (°Brix)	Conductivity x10^4 (S/m)	Viscosity $\times 10^3$ (Pa s)	Pectin (kg/m^3)	Acidity as Citric acid (kg/m^3)
0	0.09	3.97	0.22	98.4	8.4	4.0	0.87	Nil	4.0
	0.12	3.97	0.21	98.5	8.4	4.0	0.87	Nil	4.0
	0.15	3.98	0.21	98.4	8.4	4.0	0.87	Nil	4.0
	0.18	3.98	0.21	98.6	8.4	4.0	0.87	Nil	4.0
300	0.09	4.30	0.22	96.9	8.4	3.82	0.87	Nil	3.7
	0.12	4.15	0.22	97.8	8.3	3.84	0.87	Nil	3.9
	0.15	4.05	0.21	98.0	8.4	3.90	0.87	Nil	4.0
	0.18	4.00	0.21	97.8	8.3	3.95	0.87	Nil	4.0
500	0.09	4.60	0.22	97.3	8.4	3.86	0.87	Nil	3.5
	0.12	4.40	0.22	98.0	8.4	3.90	0.87	Nil	3.6
	0.15	4.36	0.21	98.5	8.4	3.90	0.87	Nil	3.6
	0.18	4.25	0.22	98.0	8.4	3.95	0.87	Nil	3.7

Power Consumption and pH Variation

The variation of electric power consumption and pH values of the permeate at various electric field and pulse ratio during clarification of mosambi juice at a transmembrane pressure of 360 kPa and cross flow velocity of 0.12 m/s are shown in Figures 2.40 and 2.41 respectively. Experimental result shows that for a fixed electric field of 400 V/m, pH of the permeate increases from 3.97 to 4.6 compared to without electric field, whereas, with the same increment of electric field but with a pulse ratio of 3:1, pH value increases to 4.4. This implies the advantages of a pulsed electric field.

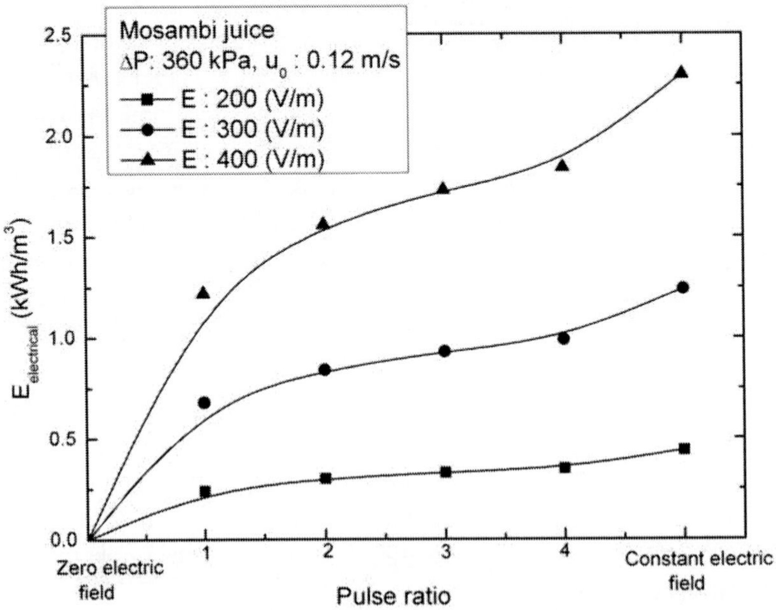

Figure 2.40. Variation of electric power consumption per unit volume of permeate with d.c. electric field at various pulse ratios at a transmembrane pressure of 360 kPa and cross flow velocity of 0.12 m/s during clarification of mosambi juice.

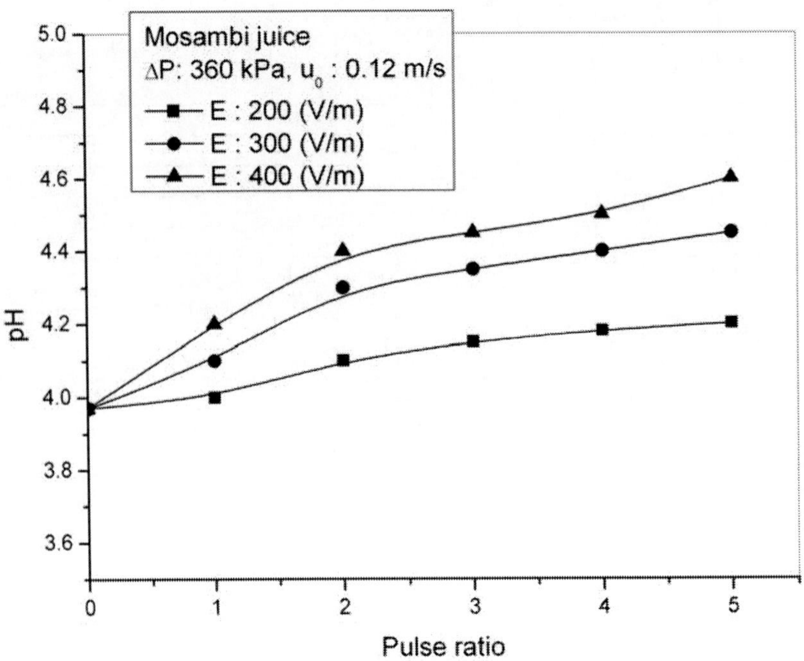

Figure 2.41. Variation of pH of the permeate with d.c. electric field at various pulse ratios at a transmembrane pressure of 360 kPa and cross flow velocity of 0.12 m/s during clarification of mosambi juice.

2.5. Conclusion

The effects of varying electric field during gel controlled ultrafiltration of pectin-sucrose solution are explored in this Chapter. The introduction of an electric field of appropriate polarity substantially improves the permeate flux. The trends are found to be in agreement with the physical understanding of the system. For example, the flux increases with electric field, pressure, cross-flow velocity but decreases with and concentration of pectin in solution. A theoretical approach for the prediction of permeate flux of an electric field enhanced gel controlled cross flow ultrafiltration is proposed in this work. An integral method with appropriate concentration profile in the boundary layer is used for the development of the model. The solutions are obtained for rectangular channel under laminar flow condition. It can also be observed that local permeate flux decreases sharply near the entrance region and then gradually for rest of the channel. The predictions from the proposed model are successfully compared with the experimental results under a wide range of operating conditions. The growth of the gel-type layer has been modeled taking into account the electrophoretic mobility of the charged pectin molecules in an electric field. A resistance-in-series model is proposed considering the hydrodynamic resistance and a resistance due to the growing gel layer. The model equations are solved numerically and the specific gel layer resistances are evaluated at different operating conditions. The thicknesses of the deposited gel-layer have been accurately measured by capturing the images of the deposition over the membrane surfaces using high-resolution video-microscopy and subsequent image analysis. The measured thicknesses under different operating conditions are successfully compared with the model predictions.

The drawbacks of constant electric field ultrafiltration such as high energy consumption, electrode reaction, increase in temperature, limitation to the use of feeds of high conductivity and heat sensitivity etc. can be significantly addressed using pulsed electric field. It can be seen that release of electrolytic gases with the permeate stream is more pronounced at constant electric field associated with higher pH values of the permeate. Apart from flux enhancement, use of pulsed electric field requires less energy and may lead to increase in the membrane service life due to less fouling, less frequent replacement of membrane during operation. For example, for a feed (Pectin: 3 kg/m^3, Sucrose: 12 Brix) mixture, at a transmembrane pressure of 360 kPa and a cross flow velocity of 0.12 m/s, by applying constant electric field of 1000 V/m, permeate flux increases from 6.5 L/m^2 h to 25.2 L/m^2 h compared to zero electric field and associated extra electric power consumption is 0.83 kW h /m^3 of permeate. To yield almost same magnitude of permeate flux, pulsed electro-ultrafiltration with pulse ratio of 3:1 needs 0.65 kW h/m^3 of permeate. For mosambi juice, at a transmembrane pressure of 360 kPa, cross flow velocity of 0.12 m/s and pulse ratio of 3:1, by applying an electric field of 500 V/m, permeate flux is improved about 39% compared to zero electric field. Moreover, significant improvement of color and clarity are observed and no pectin is found in the clarified juice.

This study also highlights the potential utility of using external d.c. electric field to increase the productivity (throughput) during clarification of mosambi juice. For example, at a cross-flow velocity of 0.12 m/s and a transmembrane pressure of 360 kPa the permeate flux increases from 8.65 L/m^2 h to 11.75 L/m^2 h (i.e., 35.8 % flux enhancement) by applying electric field of 400 V/m, and the additional electrical power consumption is 1.16 kW h per m^3 of permeate. A comparison between experimental values of permeate flux and a model developed earlier show that the gel concentration is about 48.5 kg/m^3 and the effective diffusivity of the solute in the juice is about 6×10^{-11} m^2/s. The effective viscosity in the concentration boundary layer adjacent to gel layer is 7.03×10^{-3} Pa s which is about 7 times the bulk viscosity.

According to above findings, the electro-ultrafiltration appears to be a promising alternative for clarification of citrus fruit juice and pectin containing solutions in food processing industries in general. Moreover, the models developed in this study to quantify the effects of electric field on permeate flux should be of immense help for designing electro-ultrafiltration unit.

References

[1] S. Alvarez, F.A. Riera, R. Alvarez, J. Coca, F.P. cuperus, S. Th Bouwer, G. Boswinkel, R.W. van Gemert, J.W. Veldsink, L.Giorno, L. Donato, S. Todisco, E. Drioli, J. Olsson, G. tragardh, S.N. Gaeta, L. Panyor, a new integrated membrane process for producing clarified apple juice and apple juice aroma concentrate, *J. Food Eng.* 46 (2000) 109-125.

[2] Cassano, B. Jiao, E. Drioli, Production of concentrated kiwifruit juice by integrated membrane process, *Food Research International* 37 (2004) 139–148

[3] E. Maccarona, S. Campisi, M.C.C, B. Fallico, C.N. Asmundo, Thermal treatments effect on the red orange juice constituents, *Industria Bevande,* 25 (1996) 335-341.

[4] Girard, L. R. Fukumoto, Membrane processing of fruit juices and beverages: a review. *Critical Reviews in Food Science and Nutrition* 40(2) (2000) 91-157.

[5] R. Thakur, R.K. Singh, A.K. Handa, Chemistry and Uses of Pectin- A Review, *Critical reviews in Food Science and Nutrition* 37 (1) (1997) 47-73.

[6] M.Z. Sulaiman, N.M. Sulaiman, M. Shamel, Ultrafiltration studies on solutions of pectin, glucose and their mixture in a pilot scale cross flow membrane unit, *Chem. Eng. J.* 84 (2001) 557-563.

[7] S. Lee, M. Elimelech, Salt cleaning of organic-fouled reverse osmosis membranes, *Water Res.* 41 (2007) 1134-1142.

[8] P. Rai, G.C. Majumdar, S DasGupta, S. De, Modeling of permeate flux of synthetic fruit juice and mosambi juice (Citrus sinensis (L.) Osbeck) in stirred continuous ultrafiltration, *LWT* 40 (2007) 1765-1773.

[9] P. Rai, C. Rai, G.C. Majumdar, S DasGupta, S. De, Resistance in series model for ultrafiltration of mosambi (Citrus sinensis (L.) Osbeck) juice in a stirred continuous mode, *J. Membr. Sci.* 283 (2006) 116-122.

[10] W.R. Bowen, H.A.M. Subuni, Electrically enhanced membrane filtration at low cross-flow velocities, *Ind. Eng. Res.* 30 (1991) 1573-1579.

[11] W.R. Bowen, H.A.M. Subuni, Pulsed electrokinetic cleaning of cellulose nitrate microfiltration membrane, *Ind. Eng. Res.* 31 (1992) 515-523.

[12] W.R. Bowen, R.S. Kingdon, H.A.M. Subuni, Electrically enhanced separation processes: the basis of in situ intermittent electrolytic membrane cleaning (IIEMC) and in situ electrolytic membrane restoration (IEMR), *J. Membr. Sci.* 40 (1989) 219-229.

[13] C.W. Robinson, M.H. Siegel, A. Condemine, C. Fee, T.Z. Fahidy, B.R. Glick, Pulsed-electric-field cross flow ultrafiltration of bovine serum albumin, *J. Membr. Sci.* 80 (1993) 209-220.

[14] H.R. Rabie, A.S. Majumdar, M.E. Weber, Interrupted electroosmosis dewatering of clay suspensions, *Sep. Technol.* 4(1) (1994) 38-46.

[15] A.K. Vijh, Electrochemical aspects of electroosmotic dewatering of clay suspension, *Drying Technol.* 13 (1-2) (1995) 215-224.

[16] S. De, P.K. Bhattacharya, Modeling of ultrafiltration process for a two-component aqueous solution of low and high (gel forming) molecular weight solutes, *J. Membr. Sci.* 136 (1999) 57-69.

[17] V.S. Minnikanti, S. DasGupta, S.De, Prediction of mass transfer coefficient with suction for turbulent flow in cross flow ultrafiltration, *J. Membr. Sci.* 157 (1999) 227-239.

[18] S. De, S. Bhattarcharya, P.K. Bhattarcharya, A. Sharma, Generalized integral & similarly solution of the concentration profile for osmotic pressure controlled ultrafiltration, *J. Membr. Sci.* 130 (1997) 99-121.

[19] J.S. Shen, R.F. Probstein, On the prediction of limiting flux in laminar ultrafiltration of macromolecular solutes, *Ind. Eng. Chem. Fundam.* 16 (1977) 459-465.

[20] R.F. Probstein, J.S. Shen, W.F. Leung, Ultrafiltration of macromolecular solution at high polarization in laminar channel flow, *Desalination* 24 (1978) 1-16.

[21] M. Cheryan, *Ultrafiltration and Microfiltration Handbook,* Technomic Publishing Company Inc., USA, 1998.

[22] F.L. Hart, H.J. Fisher, *Modern Food Analysis,* Springer, Berlin, 1971.

[23] R.J. Hunter, *Zeta potential in colloid Science: Principles and Applications,* Academic Press, London, 1981.

[24] L. Stryer, *Biochemistry,* Freeman, New York, 1998.

[25] M. Pritchard, J.A. Howell, R.W. Field, The ultrafiltration of viscous fluids, *J. Membr. Sci.* 102 (1995) 223-235.

[26] S. Bhattacharjee, A. Sharma, P.K. Bhattacharya, A unified model for flux prediction during batch cell ultrafiltration, *J. Membr. Sci.* 111 (1996) 243-258.

[27] S. Pal, A. Ghosh, T.B. Ghosh, S. De, S. DasGupta, Optical quantification of fouling during nanofiltration of dyes, *Sep. Purif. Tech.* 52 (2006) 372-379.

[28] B. Sarkar, S. Pal, T.B. Ghosh, S. De, S. DasGupta, A study of electric field enhanced ultrafiltration of synthetic fruit juice and optical quantification of gel deposition, *J. Membr. Sci.* 311 (2008) 112–120.

[29] R.B. Bird, W.E. Stewart, E.N. Lightfoot, *Transport phenomena,* John Wiley, Singapore, 2002.

[30] S. De, S. Bhattarcharya, P.K. Bhattarcharya, A. Sharma, Generalized integral & similarly solution of the concentration profile for osmotic pressure controlled ultrafiltration, *J. Membr. Sci.* 130 (1997) 99-121.

[31] S.M. Oussedik, D. Belhocine, H. Grib, H. Lounici, D.L. Piron, N. Mameri, Enhanced ultrafiltration of bovine serum albumin with pulsed electric field and fluidized activated alumina, *Desalination* 127 (2000) 59-68.

Index

A

B

C

T

U

V

W